Anticonvulsant Therapy

Anticonvulsant Therapy

Pharmacological Basis and Practice

Mervyn J. Eadie

M.D., Ph.D. (Queensland), F.R.A.C.P.
Professor of Clinical Neurology and Neuropharmacology,
University of Queensland.
Neurologist, Royal Brisbane Hospital.

John H. Tyrer

M.D. (Sydney), F.R.C.P. (London), F.R.C.P. (Edinburgh), F.R.A.C.P.
Professor of Medicine, University of Queensland.
Senior Neurologist, Royal Brisbane Hospital.
Honorary Consulting Physician, Mater Misericordiae Hospital,
Brisbane.
Membre d'Honneur de la Société Française de Neurologie

SECOND EDITION

CHURCHILL LIVINGSTONE
EDINBURGH LONDON AND NEW YORK 1980

CHURCHILL LIVINGSTONE
Medical Division of the Longman Group Limited

Distributed in the United States of America by
Churchill Livingstone Inc., 19 West 44th Street, New
York, N.Y. 10036, and by associated companies,
branches and representatives throughout the world

ISBN 0 443 01917 7

First edition 1974
  Italian translation 1976
  Japanese translation 1978
Second edition 1980

British Library Cataloguing in Publication Data
Eadie, Mervyn J.
  Anticonvulsant therapy—2nd ed.
  1. Epilepsy—Chemotherapy
  2. Anticonvulsants
  I. Title II. Tyrer, John Howard
  616.8'53'061   RC375.C48

Printed in Great Britain at The Pitman Press, Bath

Preface

In the five years since the first edition of this book substantial new knowledge about anticonvulsant pharmacology has accumulated. The practice of monitoring plasma anticonvulsant concentrations has grown, and skill in manipulating anticonvulsant dosages on a basis of plasma level data has increased. Inclusion of this new material has led to considerable rewriting and rearrangement of the book, and some expansion of the text.

The book is still intended primarily for clinicians who treat epileptic patients. It acknowledges the generally increased pharmacokinetic awareness of the medical profession by developing a more rigorous pharmacokinetic interpretation of the available material. The techniques of measuring the individual drugs are no longer considered. There has been such a proliferation of analytical methods for individual drugs that the inclusion of these methods would divert the book from its main purpose. The clinician no longer needs some knowledge of individual methods so that he can try to have the assays instigated in his region of practice. Rather, he needs insight into the specificity, accuracy and appropriateness of the assays which are now fairly readily done at his request.

Anticonvulsant therapy is an area of therapeutics in which modern pharmacological knowledge has been intensively applied to the treatment of human disease. Dividends from this approach have appeared in the shape of more efficient, safer and more successful therapy. It is hoped that this book may help to advance the treatment of epilepsy by attempting to consolidate currently available knowledge in this field. By so doing it may point a way to the future.

In the preparation of the new edition of this book we have been helped by several people whose assistance we would acknowledge with gratitude. Miss Jennifer Cole, Mrs. Helen Le Good and Miss Susan Scott typed large portions of the manuscript patiently and accurately while Mr. Danny Sheehy prepared the new illustrations with care and skill, and Mr. G. Jurott photographed them with customary professionalism. Throughout, our publishers provided guidance and encouragement.

This edition contains a number of new illustrations, some previously unpublished and others taken from our published work. For permission to use the latter, we would most gratefully thank the Editors and Publishers of the following journals:
British Journal of Clinical Pharmacology—Figs. 6.19, 8.3, 8.4, 8.5, 8.7, 8.8, 8.13, 8.14, 8.15, 8.16, 8.19, 8.20.

European Journal of Clinical Pharmacology—Figs. 7.3, 7.5, 7.7, 7.15.
Clinical and Experimental Pharmacology and Physiology—Figs. 6.7, 6.8.
Neurology (Minneapolis)—Figs. 6.20, 8.6.
Clinical Pharmacology and Therapeutics—Fig. 7.4.
Clinical Pharmacokinetics—Figs. 7.4, 7.14, 9.4, 9.5, 9.6, 9.7, 9.8, 11.6.
Clinical and Experimental Neurology—Figs. 7.10, 7.11, 7.17, 7.18, 8.9, 8.11, 8.12, 9.1, 9.3, 11.1.
Proceedings of the Australian Association of Neurologists—Figs. 6.24, 6.25, 6.26, 6.28, 7.1, 7.2, 7.9, 7.12, 7.13, 7.16, 7.19, 8.1, 16.7.
Australian and New Zealand Journal of Medicine—Fig. 6.23.
La Clinica Terapeutica—Fig. 7.8.

Brisbane, 1980
Mervyn J. Eadie
John H. Tyrer

Preface to the First Edition

About one in every two hundred persons in our society suffers from epilepsy. Many require treatment for periods of several years, or longer. Recent research in pharmacology and clinical pharmacology has produced much new information relevant to the treatment of epilepsy. When this knowledge has been applied, particularly in conjunction with the measurement of plasma concentrations of anticonvulsant drugs, it has often led to improved control of epilepsy in individual patients, with fewer drug side-effects. Thus the clinical pharmacological approach to the treatment of epilepsy is rapidly becoming part of the routine management of the disorder in everyday clinical practice, particularly in the United States. It therefore seems that there is a place for a book considering the treatment of epilepsy in relation to modern pharmacological knowledge. Such a book would set out the principles of clinical pharmacology at a degree of complexity sufficient for the practising clinician. It would also collate the currently available data on anticonvulsant chemistry and pharmacology in man, and discuss the treatment of epilepsy in continuous correlation with this pharmacological knowledge and with recent views on the classification of the disorder.

The present work has been written with the above intentions. It aims to be useful for neurologists, physicians, psychiatrists, paediatricians and others who treat epilepsy, as well as for pharmacologists and clinical biochemists.

The book falls into three parts—the *first* considers the principles which underlie the treatment of epilepsy, and the basic concepts of clinical pharmacology; the *second* deals with those aspects of the pharmacology of the principal anticonvulsant drugs that are relevant clinically (though excluding corticotrophin and adrenal steroids, which are not ordinarily used as anticonvulsants except in hypsarrhythmia); the *third* discusses the use of anticonvulsants in man.

In writing this book the authors have been greatly helped by the following persons to whom they would like to express their appreciation: Dr. J. M. Sutherland and Mr. W. D. Hooper, who offered most helpful criticism of the text; Drs. D. Evans, B. Lucas, R. Mulhearn and W. Zylstra, who made available information which otherwise would not have been readily accessible; Miss Marnie Harrington, who patiently deciphered and then typed and retyped the manuscript; Mr. D. Hill, who prepared the illustrations with patience and care and Mr. G. Jurott, who photographed them with his customary skill. To each of these colleagues we would acknowledge our deep indebtedness and gratitude.

We would also thank the Editors and Publishers of the following journals for permission to use illustrations from our previously published work: *Journal of Neurological Sciences:* Fig. 5.16; *Archives of Neurology* (Chicago): Fig. 5.11; *Australian and New Zealand Journal of Medicine:* Figs. 3.1, 5.1, 5.2, 5.3, 5.10, 6.2; *Journal of Neurology, Neurosurgery and Psychiatry*: Fig. 5.7; *Clinical Pharmacology and Therapeutics:* Figs. 5.14, 5.15; *Proceedings of the Australian Association of Neurologists:* Figs. 5.5, 5.9, 5.13, 13.1, 13.2, 13.3, 13.4, 13.5, 13.6.

Lastly we would thank our publishers for their guidance and interest during the preparation of the manuscript.

Brisbane, 1973   Mervyn J. Eadie
                                                                 John H. Tyrer

Contents

A note on concentration units

Although increasing use is being made of S.I. units in clinical laboratories, anticonvulsant concentrations are still commonly expressed in terms of micrograms per millilitre (μg/ml) or milligrams per litre (mg/litre), both of which yield the same numerical values. In the present book drug concentrations will continue to be expressed in terms of the older units.

In order to convert μg/ml (or mg/litre) into μ moles/litre (10^{-6} M) the number of μg/ml is multiplied by 1000 and then divided by the molecular weight of the substance in question. The molecular weights of the anticonvulsants considered in this book, together with the conversion factor for changing older units to S.I. units, are as follows:

	M.W.	conversion factor
carbamazepine	236	×4·24
chlormethiazole	162	×6·17
clonazepam	315	×3·17
diazepam	285	×3·51
ethosuximide	141	×7·09
methylphenobarbitone	246	×4·07
nitrazepam	281	×3·56
phenobarbitone	232	×4·31
phenytoin	252	×3·97
primidone	218	×4·59
sulthiame	290	×3·45
troxidone	143	×6·99
valproate	166	×6·02

For rough purposes, multiplying drug concentrations in μg/ml by a factor of 4 converts them to μ moles/litre for the commonly used major anticonvulsants carbamazepine, methylphenobarbitone, phenobarbitone, phenytoin and primidone. For clonazepam the multiplication factor is 3, for valproate it is 6 and for ethosuximide and troxidone, 7.

PART I

Basic principles

1

The decision to treat epilepsy

The decision to treat a patient's epilepsy should be taken after weighing the disadvantages of the disorder against the likely effectiveness-to-risk ratio of its treatment.

The data from the literature on epilepsy, reviewed in Rodin's (1968) monograph, indicated that the results of the treatment of epilepsy were not very satisfactory at that time. Only about one patient in three receiving medical treatment for epilepsy remained without seizures for as long as one year. More recent data (Hauser, Elveback and Kurland, 1973) showed a somewhat better result. Forty per cent of cases were seizure-free for over 2 years.

Epilepsy does not hold a high risk for life itself. However the detrimental effects of epilepsy on the quality of life increase as society becomes more complex and technological (e.g. in driving motor cars, operating machinery). At the same time *increased experience suggests that the treatment of epilepsy can be made safer and more effective by adjusting anticonvulsant drug doses in relation to plasma drug concentrations* (Lund, 1974; Reynolds, Chadwick and Galbraith, 1976; Rowan, Pippenger, McGregor and French, 1975; Terrence, Wisotzkey and Perper, 1975). Thus at the present time epilepsy is becoming an increasing disadvantage for the sufferer, whilst its treatment can often be made safer and more effective. This evolving alteration in the balance between the disadvantages of the disorder and the effectiveness-to-risk ratio of treatment, suggests that the indications for treatment of epilepsy should be reassessed from time to time.

Treatment of epilepsy should aim to cure the disorder completely and permanently. The data cited by Rodin (1968) and the paper of Hauser, Elveback and Kurland (1973) make it abundantly clear that this desirable state has not been reached in the majority of epileptic patients. Rodin's analysis showed a number of important prognostic points related to the control of epilepsy. The shorter the time epilepsy had been present, and the fewer seizures there had been prior to treatment, the greater were the chances that the epilepsy could be controlled. Among Rodin's own patients it was found that the earlier the patient had been referred for specialist treatment the greater were the chances of controlling the epilepsy. There was a control rate of 50 to 60 per cent for all persons with 'grand mal seizures' only, but of merely 20 to 30 per cent for persons with 'psychomotor seizures'. Hauser, Elveback and Kurland (1973) reached similar conclusions regarding generalized and partial epilepsy from their data. These findings may reflect a different therapeutic responsiveness for the different types of seizure. The findings may also in part be due to doctors making a more vigorous and perhaps earlier therapeutic effort to control objectively spectacular convulsive seizures, while being less active as regards the milder, often subjective, partial seizures. Moreover, patients may be more willing to tolerate the comparatively minor partial seizures than major convulsive seizures. Patients may therefore present later in the course of the former type of disorder. The above data suggest that epilepsy should be treated as early as possible, to reduce facilitation of the epileptic process because of repeated discharging in the sufferer's brain. Further, the more vigorous and skilful the initial attempt to treat epilepsy, the better the chances of cure. Rodin (1963) pointed out, and personal experience confirms, that hypsarrhythmia is a medical emergency. Unless it is successfully treated within a few weeks of its beginning, permanent intellectual retardation and residual epilepsy are highly probable (Friedman and Pampiglione, 1971). The finding of Faero, Kastrup, Lykkegaard Neilsen, Melchior and Thorn (1972) that phenobarbitone must be prescribed in dosage sufficient to produce plasma concentrations of the drug in excess of 15 μg/ml to protect against febrile convulsions in infancy, illustrates the need for skilled and vigorous anticonvulsant therapy.

HOW EARLY CAN EPILEPSY BE TREATED?

Unless there is a strong family history of epilepsy one is unlikely to suspect that an individual is at risk from the disorder until his first seizure has occurred. Diagnosis may be further delayed. Sometimes attacks of partial epilepsy, in particular those originating in the temporal lobe, are regarded as epileptic auras or even some type of pre-epilepsy. They may not be recognized as epileptic seizures in their own right. Consequently treatment may be delayed until the attacks interfere appreciably with the patient's life, or until an attack culminates in a major convulsive seizure.

As treatment of epilepsy becomes safer and more effective an increasingly strong case can be made for anticonvulsant therapy to be used before epilepsy has begun in persons judged to be at a high enough risk of developing the disorder. Such a view is sometimes held in relation to certain types of head injury (e.g. penetrating brain wounds) in which there is known to be a substantial risk of post-traumatic epilepsy (Jennett, 1975). A survey of neurosurgeons in the United States showed that 60 per cent do employ anticonvulsants at times to try to prevent epilepsy developing in patients who have suffered head injuries (Rapport and Penry, 1973). Ounsted, Lindsay and Norman (1966) raised the question of epilepsy prophylaxis in children with family histories of febrile convulsions in infancy. They argued that such convulsions may lead to subsequent temporal lobe epilepsy. Ounsted (1967) suggested that in families known to be predisposed to febrile convulsions, children aged between 6 months and 3½ years should receive anticonvulsants during any febrile illness. Apparently he considered that such therapy should be used irrespective of whether or not the individual child had suffered a previous febrile convulsion. This type of thinking may be extended, e.g. to include persons with many types of brain damage or disease, or with a family history of any form of epilepsy. There may be justification for doing this if anticonvulsant therapy can be made sufficiently effective and safe. At the present time it may be more realistic to suggest that *as a general rule therapy should begin at the time of the first recognized epileptic manifestation, unless there is adequate reason for believing that further epileptic attacks are unlikely.*

Most neurologists would probably agree that therapy should begin once the diagnosis of epilepsy is established. However the point at which this diagnosis is made in the individual can sometimes be a contentious matter. For many the term 'epilepsy' carries the connotation, implicit or explicit, that the attacks already are, or will be, recurrent (Williams, 1958). Yet if one waits to be sure that the attacks in a patient are recurrent before treatment, one may reduce the chances of cure by allowing the epileptic process to become more firmly established in the brain. The decision to treat a patient after the first epileptic manifestation (subject to the qualification mentioned above) should be based on the degree of risk and disadvantage of further epileptic manifestations for that patient relative to the effectiveness-to-risk ratio of currently available anticonvulsant therapy. The contemporary improvement in the latter favours the policy of adequate treatment commenced as early as practicable.

HOW MANY PERSONS WILL NEED TREATMENT?

It is widely accepted that approximately 1 in 200 of the population suffers from epilepsy (Lennox and Lennox, 1960). This figure was derived from the number of males rejected from service in the United States Army in the first world war because of epilepsy (Pratt, 1967) and probably refers to persons with recurrent seizures. Other figures are comparable. Kurland (1958) found a minimal prevalence of epilepsy of 3·65 per 1000 in the population of Rochester, Minnesota, U.S.A. Pond, Bidwell and Stein (1960), in a survey of 14 general practices in Britain, found an epilepsy prevalance rate of 6·2 per 1000. Brewis, Poskanzer, Rolland and Miller (1966) in their survey of neurological disease in Carlisle, found an epilepsy prevalence rate of 5·49 per 1000, taking epilepsy to include only persons who had more than one seizure. Further epidemiological data in general conformity with the above figures are available in the monograph edited by Alter and Hauser (1972). However certain authors have found higher prevalences of epilepsy, particularly when febrile convulsions have been considered epileptic. Thus Eisner, Pauli and Livingstone (1959) obtained evidence that one person in fifty has an epileptic disturbance at some stage in his life. Cooper (1965) found that 2·27 per cent of children under two years of age had experienced one or more convulsions. Rose, Penry, Markush, Radloff and Putnam (1973) found that, by the age of 8–9 years, 1·86 per cent of children in one county in the United States had experienced at least one epileptic seizure while Gomez, Arciniegas and Torres (1978) found 1·95 per cent of 8658 persons surveyed in Colombia had suffered two or more non-febrile seizures. Even higher figures exist for the prevalence of epilepsy. Miller, Court, Walter and Knox (1960) found that 7·2 per cent of 1000 children under the age of 5 years in Newcastle upon Tyne had suffered at least one convulsion. Of these children with convulsions 20 per cent had died, all but one prior to the age of one year. Thus about 6 per cent of the survivors would have had one or more convulsions. Thom's (1942) study in Boston had produced a rather similar figure of 6·75 per cent for the same age group.

It is difficult to find overall figures for the frequency with which a solitary epileptic seizure goes on to subsequent attacks. However data are available for certain types of epilepsy, in particular febrile convulsions. Millichap (1968) quoted a 5 per cent risk for a child with a single febrile convulsion subsequently developing non-febrile seizures. This figure should be compared with Livingstone's (1972) figure of a 58·2 per cent risk for the same situation. However Livingstone could distinguish good and poor prognosis groups (*see* Chapter 16) and Millichap probably considered the good prognosis group only. After excluding instances of simple febrile convulsions (the good prognosis group referred to above), Livingstone (1958) followed 200 children aged 3 to 6 years seen after their first (idiopathic) epileptic seizure. Of 100 treated with phenobarbitone, 19 had further attacks within 4 years; of 100 who were untreated, 91 had further epilepsy over the same period. Other figures are quoted below.

If all persons receive treatment from the time of their first epileptic event, the above prevalence figures suggest that use of anticonvulsant drugs would constitute a major field of therapeutic endeavour.

CONSEQUENCES OF EARLY TREATMENT

Epileptic manifestations appear to have a higher prevalence in children than in the overall population. If all epilepsy (including febrile convulsions) is treated from the time of its first manifestation, many of those treated, at least in childhood, may not have required their treatment, since their disorder tends to recover even without treatment. Thus Hauser and Kurland (1975) found only a 2·5 per cent risk of febrile seizures of infancy going on to non-febrile epilepsy. Nelson and Ellenberg (1976) found a 3 per cent risk, while Wallace (1977) put the risk higher, at 17 per cent for the occurrence of non-febrile fits, and at 12 per cent for the development of recurrent fits. However it could also be argued that if treatment of epilepsy is delayed until it is clearly necessary because seizures recur, those who do need the treatment have a reduced chance of being cured by it. Therefore, if treatment can be made safe enough, and effective enough, the disadvantages of unnecessary but not harmful treatment of some persons may be offset by the greater success and shorter duration of the therapy in those who do require it.

After weighing the above considerations the clinician should determine when to treat epilepsy in a given patient, basing the decision on an evaluation of the patient's risk of, and probably degree of disability from, subsequent epilepsy as well as the likelihood of adverse effects of therapy. It is suggested that, as a general rule, epilepsy should be treated once the first epileptic manifestation has been recognized, unless it appears likely that further attacks will not occur. In consequence of this view the word 'epilepsy' in this book is taken to include the first and any subsequent epileptic manifestation, without requiring it to be known that manifestations are recurrent. Once the decision to treat epilepsy is taken the treatment should be as adequate as possible.

AIMS OF TREATMENT

Ideally, a treatment should cure the disorder for which it is prescribed by removing the cause of the disorder and restoring normal function. In epilepsy the primary cause usually cannot be removed. Often the cause is either a genetic tendency or else is a pathological process which has ceased to progress long before clinical epilepsy began. However this pathological process has induced a tendency to 'occasional, excessive and disorderly discharge' (Jackson, 1870) in the part of the brain affected. Thus hypoxia at birth causing temporal lobe damage may lead to temporal lobe epilepsy years later in adolescence. Here the damage cannot be corrected and the treatment of epilepsy usually must be directed at restoring to normal the excitability of the epileptogenic area of the brain. This aim may be achieved by continuously suppressing with drugs the abnormal electro-chemical activity in the epileptogenic area. If this activity can be suppressed for long enough it may not recur after drugs are withdrawn. Thus the patient's epilepsy may be cured. Apart from the psychological and social management of the affected person, the treatment of epilepsy is largely a matter of such drug therapy.

The remainder of this book is concerned with the possibility of making such anticonvulsant therapy more adequate and more safe.

REFERENCES

Alter, M. & Hauser, W. A. (1972) The epidemiology of epilepsy. A workshop. *Department of Health, Education and Welfare Publication No. (NIH)*, 73–390.

Brewis, M., Poskanzer, D. C., Rolland, C. & Miller, H. (1966) Neurological disease in an English city. *Acta Neurol. Scand.*, **42**, Suppl. 24, 1–89.

Cooper, J. E. (1965) Epilepsy in longitudinal survey of 5000 children. *Brit. Med. J.*, **1**, 1020–1022.

Eisner, V., Pauli, L. L. & Livingstone, S. (1959) Hereditary aspects of epilepsy. *Bull. Johns Hopkins Hosp.*, **105**, 245–271.

Faero, O., Kastrup, K. W., Lykkegaard Neilsen, E., Melchior, J. C. & Thorn, I. (1972) Successful prophylaxis of febrile convulsions with phenobarbital. *Epilepsia* (Amst.), **13**, 279–285.

Friedman, E. & Pampiglione, G. (1971) Prognostic implications of electroencephalographic findings in hypsarrhythmia in first year of life. *Brit. Med. J.*, **4**, 323–325.

Gomez, J. G., Arciniegas, E. & Torres, J. (1978) Prevalence of epilepsy in Bogota, Colombia. *Neurology* (Minneap.), **28**, 90–94.

Hauser, W. A., Elveback, L. R. & Kurland, L. T. (1973) Remission rates in epilepsy: a total population study. *Epilepsia* (Amst.), **14**, 93.

Hauser, W. A. & Kurland, L. T. (1975) The epidemiology of epilepsy in Rochester, Minnesota, 1935 through 1967. *Epilepsia* (Amst.), **16**, 1–66.

Jackson, J. H. (1870) A study of convulsions. *Transactions of the Saint Andrews Medical Graduates Association*, **3**, 162–204; reprinted in *Arch. Neurol. (Chic.)* (1970), **22**, 184–188.

Jennett, B. (1975) *Epilepsy after non-missile head injuries.* 2nd edition, London: Heinemann Medical Books.

Kurland, L. T. (1958) Descriptive epidemiology of selected neurologic and myopathic disorders with particular reference to a survey in Rochester, Minnesota. *J. Chron. Dis.*, **8**, 378–418.

Lennox, W. G. & Lennox, M. A. (1960) *Epilepsy and related disorders*, Vol. I. Boston, Toronto: Little, Brown and Co.

Livingstone, S. (1958) Convulsive disorders in infants and children in *Advances in Pediatrics* Vol. X ed. Levine, S. Z. Chicago: Year Book Publishers.

Livingstone, S. (1972) *Comprehensive management of epilepsy in infancy, childhood and adolescence.* Springfield: Charles C. Thomas.

Lund, L. (1974) Anticonvulsant effect of diphenydantoin relative to plasma levels. A prospective three-year study in ambulant patients with generalized epileptic seizures. *Arch. Neurol.* (Chicago), **31**, 289–294.

Miller, F. J. W., Court, S. D. M., Walton, W. S. & Knox, E. G. (1960) *Growing up in Newcastle on Tyne.* London: Oxford University Press.

Millichap, J. G. (1968) *Febrile convulsions.* New York: Macmillan Co.

Nelson, K. B. & Ellenberg, J. H. (1976) Predictors of epilepsy in children who have experienced febrile seizures. *New Engl. J. Med.*, **295**, 1029–1033.

Ounsted, C. (1967) Temporal lobe epilepsy: the problem of aetiology and prophylaxis. *J. Roy. Coll. Phycns.*, **1**, 273–284.

Ounsted, C., Lindsay, J. & Norman, R. (1966) *Biological factors in temporal lobe epilepsy.* London: W. Heinemann Medical Books.

Pond, D. A., Bidwell, B. H. & Stein, L. (1960) A survey of epilepsy in fourteen general practices. I. Demographic and medical data. *Psychiat. Neurol. Neurochir.*, **63**, 217–236.

Pratt, R. T. C. (1967) *The genetics of neurological disorders.* London: Oxford University Press.

Rapport, R. L. II & Penry, J. K. (1973) A survey of attitudes towards the pharmacological prophylaxis of post-traumatic epilepsy. *J. Neurosurg.*, **38**, 159–166.

Reynolds, E. H., Chadwick, D. & Galbraith, A. W. (1976) One drug in the treatment of epilepsy. *Lancet* i, 923–926.

Rodin, E. A. (1968) *The prognosis of patients with epilepsy.* Springfield: Charles C. Thomas.

Rose, S. W., Penry, J. K., Markush, R. E., Radloff, L. A. & Putnam, P. L. (1973) Prevalence of epilepsy in children. *Epilepsia* (Amst.), **14**, 133–152.

Rowan, A. J., Pippenger, C. E., McGregor, P. A. & French, J. H. (1975) Seizure activity and anticonvulsant drug concentration. *Arch. Neurol.*, (Chicago) **32**, 281–288.

Terrence, C. F. Jr., Wisotzkey, H. M. & Perper, J. A. (1975) Unexpected, unexplained death in epileptic patients. *Neurology* (Minneap.), **25**, 594–598.

Thom, D. A. (1942) Convulsions of early life and their relation to the chronic convulsive disorders and mental defect. *Amer. J. Psychiat.*, **98**, 574–580.

Wallace, S. J. (1977) Spontaneous fits after convulsions with fever. *Arch. Dis. Childh.*, **52**, 192–196.

Williams, D. (1958) Modern views on the classification of epilepsy. *Brit. Med. J.*, **1**, 661–663.

2

Principles of clinical pharmacology

When any drug enters the body, depending on its solubility, it may become distributed through the various body fluids and tissues. It may be altered by metabolic transformation within the body. In time the drug, and its metabolites, may be excreted from the body. While present in the body the drug, and possibly the metabolites, may exert biological activity.

MECHANISMS OF DRUG ACTION

Although there are certain exceptions (Goldstein, Aranow and Kalman, 1975), drugs usually exert their effects within the body as a consequence of forming various types of physico-chemical bond with functionally important tissue molecules. These tissue molecules are regarded as receptors in relation to the drug under consideration. The drug-receptor bonding is nearly always readily reversible under physiological conditions. How drug-receptor interactions lead to the biological effects of drugs often remains obscure. The most generally applicable theory of drug action suggests that the intensity of effect produced by a particular dose of a drug is related to the proportion of receptor sites occupied by drug molecules provided by the drug dose. This theory may be refined to meet certain special situations (Rang, 1971; Goldstein, Aranow and Kalman, 1975). In terms of this theory and its modifications, *the extent of a drug's action is related to the drug's concentration around its sites of action (i.e. to its concentration in the so-called 'biophase')*. The law of mass action governs the reversible combining of drug and receptor. Ideally, one would wish to measure drug concentration around its sites of biological action, to obtain a useful index of drug action when the drug's effect cannot be measured directly. For drugs like anticonvulsants, which exert their desired action within the brain of man, it is clearly impossible to obtain material to measure drug concentration around receptor sites, except in the most unusual circumstances (e.g. at diagnostic brain biopsy). However, knowledge of the way in which a drug is distributed throughout the body shows that it still may be possible to obtain a convenient index of drug concentration around its sites of biological activity.

DRUG DISTRIBUTION

The distribution of a drug within the body can be represented by a series of dynamic equilibria, as follows:

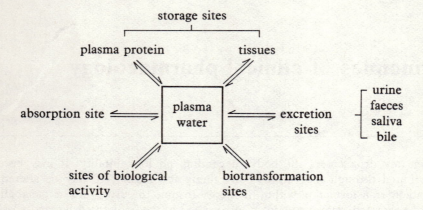

There is an increased interest in describing these equilibria and their time courses mathematically as the science of pharmacokinetics develops (Wagner, 1975; Gibaldi and Perrier, 1975). It seems doubtful whether detailed consideration of pharmacokinetics is yet necessary for the purposes of the practicing clinician, though it may be useful for him to know a little about the more commonly quoted pharmacokinetic parameters.

Much of the total amount of a drug distributed throughout the body may be bound to tissue molecules at sites where this bonding produces no apparent biological activity. This bound drug may be released again from these storage sites, which include plasma protein, to replace drug molecules which are eliminated from the body by biotransformation or excretion.

From the equilibria shown above it can be seen that drug molecules in the biophase around the sites of biological activity are in equilibrium with drug molecules in plasma water. A drug may have several sites of biological activity, and may be at different concentrations at different sites because of local physico-chemical factors. However the drug in the biophase at each receptor site will be in equilibrium with the common concentration of the drug in plasma water. Whole plasma is readily obtained in man, but it is cumbersome to separate plasma water from plasma protein as a routine. Drug in plasma water is also in equilibrium with any drug bound to plasma protein. *Therefore drug concentration in whole plasma (i.e. the pooled concentrations of the drug in plasma water and any drug bound to plasma protein) is usually measured in man as the best available convenient index of drug concentration in the biophase.* Obviously drug concentration in whole plasma is a less proximate measure of drug concentration at receptor sites than is the drug level in plasma water. Further, the whole plasma drug concentration can be altered by changes in the plasma protein binding of the drug, even though neither drug concentration at receptor sites nor drug concentration in plasma water is altered. The whole plasma concentration of a drug can be looked on as a convenient but occasionally distorting mirror reflecting drug concentration around its sites of biological activity.

The concept of the therapeutic range of plasma drug concentrations
As pointed out, for most drugs concentration in the biophase determines the extent of drug action. Drug concentration in the biophase is related to drug concentration in plasma, as stated above. Plasma drug concentration should therefore provide a measure of drug action. Is there then a plasma drug concentration, or range of concentrations, which is associated with optimal therapeutic effects for each drug? Experience has shown that for many drugs, including most of the anticonvulsants, this is the case. However, plasma concentrations of a drug metabolite may sometimes correlate better with pharmacological effect that does concentration of the unchanged drug. The 'therapeutic' or 'optimal' range of plasma drug concentrations should be that range of plasma drug levels associated with the best chance of obtaining the desired therapeutic effect in the majority of patients, but without producing an unacceptable risk of unwanted effects of the type regarded as due to drug overdosage. Plasma drug levels below the therapeutic range are likely to be associated with an inadequate response to treatment. Idiosyncratic reactions, which by their nature are rare, may be associated with any plasma drug level. Such a concept of a therapeutic range should lend itself to statistical evaluation once sufficient data are available. However the therapeutic ranges for many drugs quoted in literature (including anticonvulsants) have usually been defined without rigorous statistical analysis. Nevertheless in practice the ranges prove useful as a guide to therapy.

The therapeutic range is a population parameter. It would be impractical, and possibly unethical, to determine the therapeutic range for every individual patient. In the majority of patients the individual therapeutic range should fall within the limits of the population therapeutic range. However, it is possible that in a minority of patients the individual therapeutic range may lie outside the range for the population. This point should be kept in mind when therapeutic ranges derived from populations of patients are used as a guide to therapy in individual patients.

Drug concentrations in other body fluids
Because of the various equilibria involved in drug distribution it would be possible to use drug concentration in body fluids other than blood plasma (e.g. CSF, urine or saliva) as an index of drug concentration at sites of biological activity. Such measurements largely avoid the problems which come from estimating a protein-bound drug fraction, in addition to the drug free in plasma water (since CSF, urine and saliva normally contain little protein). Unfortunately, in other ways drug levels in these fluids are often more remote measures of drug level at sites of biological activity than is the total drug level in plasma. Saliva and urine, though not CSF, are likely to be at a different pH from plasma, and these fluids are separated from plasma water by lipoidal cell membranes which do not permit the ready passage of ionized molecules. The amount of ionized drug may differ between plasma water and urine or saliva because of pH effects on drug ionization. Consequently total drug concentrations in the fluids also will differ. In urine the situation may be further complicated by the presence of active transport mechanisms. Therefore in most circumstances whole plasma drug concentration is likely to be a more satisfactory measure of drug concentration at sites of biological activity than is drug

level in urine or in saliva. CSF, though having advantages over saliva and urine from the point of view of pH differences, is not as readily available.

The blood-brain barrier

Certain drugs do not enter the brain as easily as they enter other tissues, due to so-called 'blood-brain barrier' effect. The cerebral capillaries appear to have endothelial cells with particularly tight intercellular junctions. Small inorganic ions and other small molecules (e.g. urea) may cross the blood-brain barrier, as can a few larger polar molecules for which specific transport mechanisms exist (e.g. levodopa). Otherwise only drugs which are sufficiently lipid-soluble to penetrate cell membranes fairly readily can cross the barrier and enter brain parenchyma.

The apparent volume of distribution (V_d)

One pharmacokinetic parameter that is widely used as a measure of a drug's extent of distribution in the body, is its apparent volume of distribution (V_d). The V_d (often expressed on a body weight basis, i.e. as litres kg^{-1}) is notionally determined by dividing the dose of a drug (e.g. in mg kg^{-1}) that actually enters the circulation by the maximum plasma drug concentration (e.g. in mg litre^{-1}) that would have applied if the whole dose had entered the circulation instantly. In practice the calculation is usually made in other ways, using numerical values that can be directly obtained from experimental data. However, because the calculation of V_d assumes that drug concentration in plasma is identical with drug concentration throughout the entire distribution of the drug, values for V_d in excess of the total volume of body water can be obtained if a drug is concentrated at some site, or sites, in tissues. A V_d of about 0·05 litres kg^{-1} suggests that a drug is distributed throughout the vascular compartment. V_d values around 0·15 litres kg^{-1} suggest that a drug distributes throughout extracellular water, and V_d values of 0·5 to 0·6 litres kg^{-1} suggest that a drug distributes throughout total body water. Higher V_d values than this imply that a drug is concentrated in tissues.

Sometimes mathematical analysis of the time course of a drug's plasma levels may indicate that the drug appears to distribute rapidly through a portion of its total volume of distribution (the central compartment) and more slowly through an additional volume of the body (the peripheral compartment). The volumes of each of these compartments may be calculated. The system is then referred to as a 'two-compartment model'. The pharmacokinetics of the two-compartment model are more complex than those of the one-compartment model, in which the drug is considered to distribute at the same rate throughout its whole volume of distribution.

DRUG ABSORPTION

Once a drug enters the circulation its plasma level rises (while absorption preponderates over elimination). The level reaches a peak when absorption and elimination become equal. Thereafter drug plasma levels decline as elimination exceeds absorption. The rate of absorption of a drug (from the alimentary tract or other administration site) relative to its elimination rate will determine the rate of rise of the plasma level of the drug after a dose is taken, and the time until the drug builds up an effective concentration at its sites of biological activity. While the time (T_{max}) to achieve a peak plasma level (C_{max}) is often regarded loosely as a measure of the rate of drug absorption, T_{max} also depends on drug elimination rate. If two drugs are absorbed equally rapidly, T_{max} will occur earlier for the drug which is more rapidly eliminated. Drug absorption is usually a passive diffusion process, mathematically following first order kinetics. Thus a constant proportion of the amount of a drug dose still to be absorbed will be absorbed each unit time. Mathematical analysis of the time course of drug plasma levels after a dose permits calculation of an absorption rate constant (k_{abs}) expressed as the proportion of the dose remaining to be absorbed which is absorbed each hour. Alternatively, the rate constant can be converted to an absorption half-life ($T_{1/2}$), the time for absorption of half the amount of material awaiting absorption at any time.

$$T_{\frac{1}{2}}(abs) = \frac{\log_n 2}{k_{abs}} = \frac{0 \cdot 693}{k_{abs}}$$

Although the rate constant is the primary measure of rate of drug absorption, the clinician is more likely to be interested in T_{max} and C_{max}, as these parameters provide a measure of the time and extent of maximum drug action.

Bioavailability

When drugs are given by any route other than intravenous injection, it is possible that the whole drug dose may never enter the general circulation. For various reasons part of the dose may fail to absorb. In addition, certain drugs may absorb completely from the intestine, but during the initial passage of drug molecules through the intestinal wall or during the first circuit of the drug through the liver in the portal blood a substantial proportion of the drug dose may be metabolized. In either circumstance (i.e. incomplete absorption, or extensive 'first-pass' metabolism) the drug is incompletely bioavailable. The term 'bioavailability' refers to the proportion of the dose of a drug which enters the general circulation, but also to its rate of entry (a drug may absorb completely, but too slowly for a desired effect).

DRUG ELIMINATION

The term 'elimination', used in relation to a drug, refers to the sum of two processes, biotransformation (or metabolism) and excretion. The rate of drug elimination is usually the chief determinant of the duration of action of a drug dose. The elimination rate of a drug is conveniently assessed in terms of the rate of fall of the plasma concentration of the drug (Fig. 2.1). Generally this rate of fall proves to be monoexponential, or biexponential in the case of a drug which follows two-compartment kinetics. An elimination rate constant, analogous to the absorption rate constant, may be calculated. When the decline in plasma level is monoexponential the elimination rate constant is usually signified by k, expressed as a decimal fraction per hour. When the decline is biexponential, the rate constant for the initial phase of the decline is usually termed a, and the rate constant for the terminal phase of decline is β. In these circumstances β is a hybrid constant, and not the true elimination rate constant. A terminal plasma half life may be calculated, analogous to the absorption half life, by dividing $\log_n 2$ by k, or β, as the

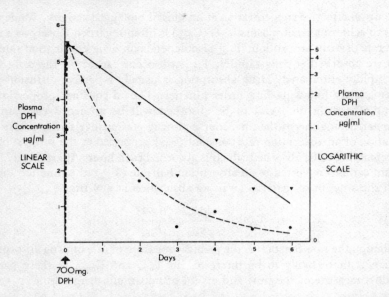

Fig. 2.1 The time-course of plasma phenytoin concentrations in a patient following a single oral 700 mg dose of the drug. Drug concentrations are expressed on a linear (solid circles: dotted line) and a logarithmic (solid triangles: continuous line) scale. Plasma phenytoin concentrations tend to fall exponentially with time.

case may be. The terminal half-life defines an important pharmacokinetic property with which the contemporary clinician needs to be familiar.

If a drug is given at constant dosage and at fixed intervals shorter than the elimination time of the drug, the drug concentration in plasma, and at receptor sites, will rise in a series of oscillating steps. A stage will be reached at which the amount of drug absorption equals the amount of drug elimination over each dosage interval. This is called the steady state. During each dosage interval plasma and receptor drug concentrations will then fluctuate about a constant plateau value until drug intake or drug elimination changes. For a given rate of absorption the longer the drug half-life relative to the dosage interval, the more rapidly the mean plasma level of drug will rise, the longer it will take to achieve a steady state and the smaller proportionately will be the fluctuations in plasma and receptor drug levels between doses when this state is reached (Fig. 2.2). The longer the half-life, the smaller is the dosage or the longer is the dosage interval necessary for a drug to achieve a particular steady-state concentration. It requires the passage of four half-lives for a drug, given in regular dosage, to achieve approximately 94 per cent, and five half-lives to achieve approximately 97 per cent, of its final steady state concentrations. Thus for practical purposes a steady state is attained after the expiry of four or five drug half-lives.

The rate of drug absorption from administration sites also will influence the extent of plasma drug level fluctuations in the steady state. To reduce fluctuations, drug absorption may be slowed or the individual doses reduced and dosage intervals shortened. In view of these considerations it is clear that the dosage interval for various drugs used on a long-term basis (e.g. anticonvulsants) should be worked out in terms of absorption and elimination half-life data and knowledge

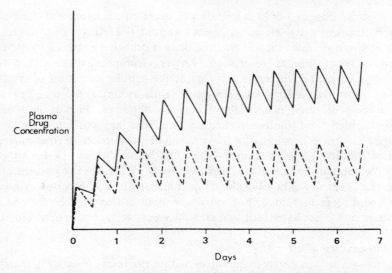

Plasma
Drug
Concentration

Fig. 2.2 Theoretical time-courses of the plasma levels of two drugs, one with twice the half-life of the other, each being given twice daily in identical molar dosage. The drug with the longer half-life (continuous line) reaches steady-state conditions more slowly than the drug with the shorter half-life, but its plasma levels are then higher and inter-dosage fluctuations in its plasma levels tend to be proportionately less.

of an acceptable range of plasma level fluctuations between doses. A sufficient dose should be given at suitable intervals so that, as far as possible, there is at all times a drug concentration at receptor sites which will provide an adequate biological action without producing over-dosage effects.

Anticonvulsants are nearly always given on a long-term basis. If they are given in constant dosage at fixed dosage intervals, and if overdosage is to be avoided, it would appear likely that there will be an initial period of delay before a sufficient drug concentration builds up at receptor sites to produce a useful anti-epileptic effect. This delay can be reduced by shortening the dosage interval in the first few days of therapy or by using larger initial loading doses.

Drug clearance
The elimination rate constant (k), the complex constant β (and the terminal half-lives derived from these values) have so far been the only parameters of drug elimination mentioned. However these are measures of the *rate* of drug elimination, and not of its *amount*. The product of the apparent volume of distribution (V_D) and the elimination rate constant (k), or β (i.e. $V_D \times k$ or $V_D \times \beta$), provides the so-called clearance value, which is a measure of amount of drug elimination. Drug elimination lowers drug concentrations throughout the body. However the concept of clearance interprets elimination as if the drug were completely removed (i.e. cleared) from a portion of its volume of distribution in the body, but as if its concentration were left unaltered in the remainder of the body. The concept of clearance is thus a mathematical device which describes a situation that does not exist in reality. Nevertheless, such notional clearance values may convey information about the pattern of a drug's elimination.

If most of the dose of a drug is found to be excreted unchanged in urine (so that little is biotransformed), clearance values around $0 \cdot 11$ litres kg^{-1} $hour^{-1}$ (the glomerular filtration rate) suggest that the drug is probably excreted by glomerular filtration, without tubular resorption. Lower clearances suggest that tubular resorption occurs, and higher values that active tubular secretion is involved in drug elimination. In the latter case clearance values as high as $0 \cdot 6$ litre kg^{-1} $hour^{-1}$ (i.e. the value of renal plasma flow) may be obtained. For drugs which are eliminated chiefly by biotransformation (i.e. the amount of drug excreted unchanged in urine accounts for only a small proportion of the bioavailable portion of the drug dose) clearance values can be as high as $1 \cdot 3$–$1 \cdot 4$ litres kg^{-1} $hour^{-1}$, the value of hepatic blood flow. If this is so, during the passage of blood through the liver, virtually all of the drug contained in that blood is extracted by the liver, and biotransformed. For a drug handled in this way the factor limiting drug elimination is not hepatic drug metabolising capacity, but hepatic blood flow.

Drug biotransformation

Many drugs are at least partly metabolized within the body. Most drug metabolism occurs in the liver. The chief pathway of drug metabolism is the non-specific hepatic microsomal mixed oxidase system which probably has the normal function of degrading various endogenous steroids (Oorenius, Das and Gnosspelius, 1969; Conney, 1971). There are other hepatic enzyme systems which reduce, hydrolyze or conjugate drugs (Parke, 1968). Sometimes drug metabolism may yield a product with equal or greater biological activity than the parent substance, but generally metabolism produces more polar molecules (Brodie, 1964). Usually increasing molecular polarity correlates with decreasing biological activity. On the whole, polar molecules are relatively water-soluble and lipid-insoluble, and do not pass readily through cell membranes, including the lipid membranes of the blood-brain barrier. Polar molecules thus do not easily gain access to sites where they might bond to brain receptors. Once such polar molecules enter the renal glomerular filtrate they are not readily resorbed passively across the membranes of the renal tubular cells. Hence they tend to be excreted in the urine. While biotransformation may sometimes yield biologically active products, the overall effect of drug metabolism is to reduce the biological activity of drugs, and to facilitate their excretion (Fig. 2.3).

Should a biologically-active drug produce a biologically-active metabolite the considerations regarding the body's handling of the drug will also apply to its metabolite. In this circumstance, in effect two drugs are present at the same time. The therapeutic situation must be interpreted in terms of the simultaneous presence of both drugs. If the metabolite is biologically inactive, for many pharmacological purposes its presence can be ignored. However it may complicate chemical estimations of the parent substance.

Drug excretion

Most drugs and drug metabolites are excreted via the urine. Some drugs and drug metabolites are excreted into bile. In this case, the drug, and possibly its metabolites, may subsequently be absorbed from the intestine, thus undergoing an entero-hepatic circulation.

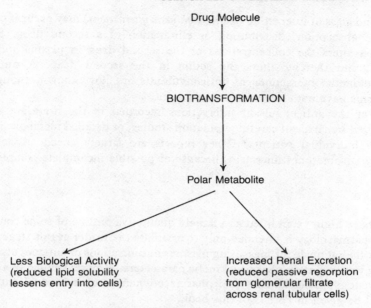

Fig. 2.3 Consequences of drug biotransformation.

Any drug or drug metabolite, with a molecular weight below 69 000 and not bound to plasma protein, is likely to be filtered from plasma into glomerular fluid. During passage down the renal tubules, non-polar drug and metabolite molecules will tend to resorb passively as water resorbs across the renal tubular epithelium. Adjustment of pH in the distal renal tubules may alter the ionization of drugs and their metabolites, and consequently alter their passive resorption, since ionization increases molecular polarity. There is also the possibility that certain acidic and basic drugs, and their metabolites (in particular their glucuronide conjugates), may be actively secreted into urine. Being relatively polar, such molecules tend not to undergo passive resorption from the renal tubules, and hence are excreted in urine.

Apart from volatile substances, which are excreted into expired air, the amount of drug excretion other than via the urine and faeces (often as a result of biliary excretion) is for practical purposes negligible, except during lactation or when there is pathological loss of a body fluid.

DRUG INTERACTIONS

Drug combinations are often used in human therapeutics. Whenever two drugs are taken concurrently it is possible that one drug may alter the action of the other. This interaction may take place at receptors, when one drug may act on the receptors of the second drug to alter its effects qualitatively or quantitatively. The concentration of the second drug in the biophase (or in plasma) is not altered. These are *pharmacodynamic interactions*. Anticonvulsants are often given concurrently, in the hope that additive or even synergistic pharmacodynamic interactions will occur, producing an increased overall anti-epilepsy effect.

A second class of interaction (*pharmacokinetic interactions*) may occur if one drug alters the absorption, distribution or elimination of a second drug. Such an interaction alters the concentrations of the second drug in plasma and in the biophase, and thereby alters the action of the second drug. A number of pharmacokinetic interactions of anticonvulsants are now known, though their mechanisms have not always been worked out.

Some of the anticonvulsant interactions recorded in the literature are well documented by virtue of careful population studies, or detailed metabolic investigations in individual patients. Other reports are largely anecdotal, and their reliability is sometimes uncertain, because of possible incomplete compliance by patients.

*   *   *

The above highly simplified and largely qualitative outline of some concepts of clinical pharmacology is intended only to orientate the reader at this stage. It aims to set out the rationale for measuring plasma concentrations of anticonvulsants and for citing values of their pharmacokinetic parameters. A more detailed treatment of the relevant pharmacokinetics and pharmacodynamics of individual anticonvulsants will be given in Part II of this book.

REFERENCES

Brodie, B. B. (1965) Of mice, microsomes and man. *Pharmacologist*, **6**, 12–26.

Conney, A. H. (1971) Environmental factors influencing drug metabolism in *Fundamentals of drug metabolism and drug disposition* ed. La Du, B. N., Mandel, G. H. & Way, E. L., Baltimore: Williams and Wilkins Co., 253–278.

Gibaldi, M. & Perrier, D. (1975) *Pharmacokinetics*. New York: Marcel Dekker.

Goldstein, A., Aronow, L. & Kalman, S. M. (1975) Principles of drug action. 2nd Edition. New York: Wiley.

Oorenius, S., Das, M. & Gnosspelius, Y. (1965) Overall biochemical effects of drug induction on liver microsomes in *Microsomes and drug oxidations* ed. Gillette, J. R., Conney, A. H., Cosmides, G. J., Estabrook, R. W., Fouts, J. R. & Mannering, G. J. New York: Academic Press, 251–277.

Parke, D. V. (1968) *The biochemistry of foreign compounds*. Oxford: Pergamon Press.

Rang, H. P. (1971) Drug receptors and their function. *Nature*, **231**, 91–96.

Wagner, J. G. (1975) *Fundamentals of clinical pharmacokinetics*. Hamilton: Drug Intelligence Publications.

3

Measurement of anticonvulsant concentrations in biological material

The previous chapter indicated the potential importance of measuring the concentrations of drugs in plasma and other biological fluids as an aid to the rational and efficient use of these drugs in man. Those who treat epilepsy have increasingly to interpret plasma anticonvulsant level measurements in the light of clinical situations. To do this adequately clinicians need not only be conversant with elementary pharmacokinetic principles and with their patients' clinical states, but should also be able to assess the reliability of the techniques used to carry out the measurements. Lack of assay accuracy, sensitivity or specificity may produce results which are clinically misleading.

PRINCIPLES OF DRUG CONCENTRATION MEASUREMENT

The following discussion relates particularly to measurements of anticonvulsant drugs. A more detailed consideration of the subject of drug assay in biological material is given by De Silva (1970). Basically, the measurement of drug concentration in a biological fluid involves two processes: firstly, the isolation of the drug from all other possible interfering substances present in the biological fluid and, secondly, the measurement of the quantity of drug that has been isolated. In practice, many of the devices used for measuring the quantity of a drug are also capable to some degree of isolating the drug from other substances. Thus the later stages of drug isolation and the quantitation may occur almost simultaneously in some measurement techniques. The less specific the measuring device, the more extensive should be the preliminary separation of the drug.

SEPARATION

1. Separation from particulate matter
If cells or particulate matter are present in the biological fluid (as in whole blood) they can be separated from the liquid portion by centrifuging. Most measurements of drug concentration are made on either plasma or serum. In the account that is to follow plasma alone will be discussed, though similar principles apply for other biological fluids (e.g. saliva, CSF).

2. Separation from plasma proteins
If drug in plasma water is to be measured, the aqueous components of plasma must

be separated from the plasma protein by a method gentle enough not to displace any bound drug from the plasma protein during the process of separation. Equilibrium dialysis, ultrafiltration or gel filtration, preferably at 37°C, will serve this purpose. On the other hand, if the drug in whole plasma is to be measured, the drug attached to plasma protein may have to be separated from binding sites prior to measurement. This may be done in some cases either by using organic solvents to dissolve the bound drug, or by altering the conformation of the plasma protein molecules with acids or salts so that the denatured protein precipitates and releases the bound drug.

3. Separation from other molecules to which the measuring device also responds

Depending on the specificity of the measuring device used, it may or may not be necessary to separate the drug molecules in which one is interested from other molecules to which the measuring device will also respond. The techniques used to effect such separation usually depend on solvent partitioning. Occasionally chemical reactions may be used to distinguish a drug from other molecules (e.g. the use of the Bratton-Marshall reaction for aromatic amines, which was employed in the classic assay for phenytoin devised by Dill, Kazenko, Wolf and Glazko, 1956).

In solvent partitioning techniques, all drug molecules present are converted either to their ionized or non-ionized forms by pH adjustment. The drug in solution is then allowed to come in contact (once, or more often) with an immiscible solvent which has a polarity such that the drug and other molecules to which the detecting device might respond are partitioned differentially between the solvents. In drug measurements, separation of the drug from its (structurally similar) metabolites is often a problem (and unfortunately sometimes a problem that is ignored). Drug metabolites are usually more polar than the parent drugs. Therefore if partitioning is carried out between the least polar solvent that will extract all the drug, and a more polar but immiscible solvent, there is a good chance that the metabolite will separate from the drug and appear in the more polar solvent (Brodie, Udenfriend and Baer, 1947). Solvent partitioning may be carried out between two fluids in a common container (e.g. a test tube) or in more complex apparatus (e.g. counter-current distribution equipment). In chromatography the separation system is arranged so that there are repeated partitionings between a mobile phase containing the drug and a stationary phase over which the mobile phase flows. The different classes of molecules in the mobile phase emerge from the system at different times. The stationary phase is maintained in position by the support of paper (paper chromatography), by a layer of silica gel or alumina (thin layer chromatography) or by some other inert material, while the mobile phase may be a liquid (as in high pressure liquid chromatography) or a gas (as in gas-liquid chromatography).

MEASUREMENT

Anticonvulsant drug concentration assays involve the capacity to measure quantities of drug ranging from a few nanograms (10^{-9} g) to several hundred micrograms (10^{-6} g) contained in 0·5 to 5 ml of body fluid. Measuring devices of appropriate sensitivity are required for the assays. Some of the techniques that have been used are indicated below.

1. Visual matching with standards

If the drug can be isolated, as on a chromatography plate, it can then be displayed by its fluorescence in ultraviolet light, or be seen in visible light after it is reacted with chemicals to yield a coloured product. By visual comparison with standards of known concentrations applied to the same plate and treated similarly an approximate quantitation of the drug can be effected.

2. Spectrophotometry

a. Visible light.

If the drug under consideration is isolated in solution as a coloured product, a spectrophotometer may be used to measure the light absorbed in passing through a layer of this solution of known thickness. This absorption, compared with the light absorption of standard solutions under identical conditions, provides a measure of drug concentration. The method is reasonably sensitive for quantities of drug in the microgram range. Since relatively few drugs are coloured, chemical reactions are usually necessary to produce coloured products before the method can be applied.

b. Ultraviolet spectrophotometry

Many chemical substances will absorb ultraviolet light. By measuring ultraviolet light absorption at the particular wave length at which the drug absorbs maximally, one can obtain a moderately sensitive measurement of drug concentration in the microgram range. Specificity depends largely on the preliminary separation procedures.

c. Fluorescence spectrophotometry (Udenfriend, 1969)

Some organic substances fluoresce, or can be made to fluoresce, by chemical manipulation. They will then absorb light over a specific range of wave lengths, and emit it at other (generally longer) wave lengths. This property allows an increase in specificity of fluorescence spectrophotometry over ultraviolet spectrophotometry. The absorption wave length band confers a degree of specificity, and the emission wave length band, which is not the same for all substances with identical absorptions, enhances the specificity. Fluorescence spectrophotometry is also more sensitive than ultraviolet spectrophotometry. Up to a point, fluorescence intensity increases with increasing strength of incident light. Ultraviolet spectrophotometry measures the relative energy difference between the entering and the departing light, and this relative difference does not increase with increased intensity of entering light. For certain compounds, fluorescence spectrophotometry is capable of measurements in the nanogram range. Unfortunately fluorescence spectrophotometry involves certain technical problems (e.g. the need to work in very dilute solution and to have highly purified solvents).

3. Measurement after chromatographic separation

When paper or thin layer chromatography has been used to separate drugs from other substances which might interfere in their assay, the quantity of drug present may be measured *in situ* by densitometric techniques. Alternatively the separated drug may be eluted into an appropriate solvent, and then measured by one of the spectrophotometric techniques mentioned above.

When separation has been achieved by gas-liquid chromatography or high pressure liquid chromatography, the groups of molecules emerging from the chromatographic systems are measured by various types of detector which are often built into the instrument itself. For high pressure liquid chromatography certain types of spectrophotometric detector are usually used. For gas-liquid chromatography the flame ionization detector, which measures all organic compounds as they emerge from the separation column, is widely employed. More specific and more sensitive detectors (e.g. the alkali flame ionization detector, the electron capture detector) are available. In general, high pressure liquid chromatography and gas liquid chromatography with flame ionization detection permit highly specific measurements of drug concentrations in the low microgram (μg) to high nanogram (ng) range. Gas liquid chromatography with electron capture detection permits measurement of as little as a few nanograms of drug, though preliminary chemical derivatization of the drug molecule may be necessary to achieve such sensitivity. Generally, gas liquid chromatography or high pressure liquid chromatography provides the optimal method for measuring biological concentrations of anticonvulsants.

The effluent from a gas chromatographic column can be introduced into a mass-spectrometer, for identification and measurements of the components of the effluent. Gas chromatography-mass spectrometry (GC-MS) offers the best available specificity and sensitivity of detection, but the apparatus required is very expensive to purchase and to operate.

4. Immune-assay techniques

In immune-assay methods the stages of the method which ensure specificity coincide with the stages which ensure sensitivity. An antibody to the drug in question is prepared and the ability of an unknown quantity of drug to bind to the antibody may be measured in a variety of ways. Most immune-assays depend on the principle of competitive protein binding. An unknown quantity of the drug which is to be measured is introduced to a system which contains the antibody with its binding sites already occupied by drug 'labelled' in some way. The unlabelled drug competes for these binding sites and displaces some of the 'labelled' drug, which is then measured. The assay is calibrated by introducing known quantities of drug to the system, and measuring the displacement of 'labelled' drug from the antibody. Three of the more commonly used techniques of 'labelling' the drug are 'labelling' with radioactive isotopes, with enzymes or with chemical (nitroso) groups.

In *radio-immune assay* (Hawker, 1973; Skelley, Brown and Besch, 1973) great sensitivity can be attained because of the ability to measure β or γ emission. Rather expensive counting apparatus is required and it is necessary to separate bound and unbound 'labelled' drug physically (e.g. by adsorption onto charcoal) before radiation measurement is carried out.

In *enzyme multiplied immune test (EMIT) assays* (Scharpe, Cooreman, Bloome and Laekeman, 1973) the active sites of an enzyme become unmasked when the drug-enzyme combination is displaced from the antibody. The enzyme can then catalyse a chemical reaction, the products of which can be measured by relatively simple techniques using conventional apparatus (e.g. a spectrophotometer). No separation procedure is necessary. If an enzyme 'label' with suitable kinetic properties is used, sensitivity equal to that of radio-immune assay e.g. measurement in the low nanogram or high picogram (10^{-12}g) range can be attained.

In *spin-immune assay* (Montgomery, Holtzman and Leute, 1975), displaced drug 'labelled' with a nitroso group shows different electron spin resonance (ESR) properties from the same 'labelled' drug bound to antibody. Quantitation is achieved by measuring changes in the ESR spectrum. Again great sensitivity is possible, and no separation stage is needed after the competitive binding step. However electron spin resonance spectrophotometers are very expensive.

Immune-assay techniques have the great virtue of relative simplicity and extreme sensitivity. They are capable of measurements in the nanogram and sub-nanogram range. Their specificity depends on the specificity of the antibody produced, which should be capable of distinguishing between the drug and its metabolites, as well as other substances. In fact some commercially available immune-assays do not meet this requirement. One assay kit for phenobarbitone will measure both methylphenobarbitone and phenobarbitone, without distinguishing between them. The two substances are usually present together in the body if methylphenobarbitone is taken. Another kit measures the phenobarbitone metabolite p-hydroxy-phenobarbitone as if it were the parent substance (Viswanathan, Booker and Welling, 1977). Further, since many drugs have metabolites which have not yet been identified, proving that an immune-assay differentiates between a drug and all known metabolites does not necessarily indicate that the assay is completely specific for the drug in question. Introduction of preliminary separation steps (e.g. solvent partitioning) into the assay would go some way to obviating these problems of insufficient specificity. Unfortunately at the same time it would remove one of the great advantages of immune-assay (*viz*. its simplicity).

ASSAYS USED IN PRACTICE

At the present time most anticonvulsant concentration measurements are made by means of gas liquid chromatography or enzyme-immune assays. Both techniques offer adequate sensitivity. Gas chromatography is rather more versatile and, as currently used, may be a little more specific. The technique, with its preliminary solvent partitioning stages and perhaps the preparation of chemical derivatives (to obtain adequate chromatograms), is more time-consuming than the immune-assay techniques. However, with suitable assay conditions several drugs may be measured simultaneously by gas liquid chromatography (Fig. 3.1). If the patient is taking several drugs, each must be measured in a separate procedure if currently available immune-assays are used.

Till satisfactory antibodies are available to all the anticonvulsants, immune-assays will be unable to displace gas chromatography completely. However, there can be little doubt that the advent of immune-assays, particularly EMIT assays which obviate the need for radioactivity counting, has considerably facilitated the

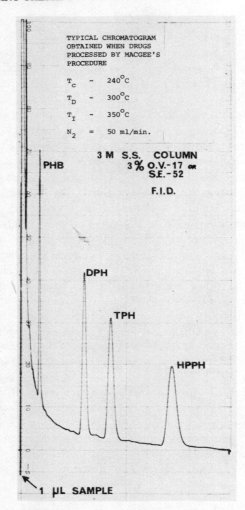

Fig. 3.1. Gas chromatogram showing solvent front and peaks for phenobarbitone (PHB), phenytoin (DPH), the internal standard 5-(p-methylphenyl)-5-phenylhydantoin (TPH) and 5-(p-hydroxyphenyl)-5-phenylhydantoin (HPPH). These substances have been chromatographed as methyl derivatives, prepared by flash methylation with tetramethylammonium hydroxide. Peak height ratios are proportionate to the quantities of the respective substances present (Eadie and Tyrer, 1973).

routine measurement of many of the more commonly used anticonvulsants.

In the first edition of this book the various available assays for the anticonvulsants were discussed. Over the ensuing five years there has been such a proliferation of assays, some novel, others merely minor variants of earlier methods, that any detailed consideration of the individual assays no longer seems appropriate to the main purposes of this book. Details of the available methods may be found in works such as Meijer, Meinardi, Gardner-Thorpe and van der Kleijn (1973) or Pippenger, Penry and Kutt (1978).

ACCURACY OF MEASUREMENTS

Now that the practice of measuring anticonvulsant concentrations in biological fluids has come into widespread use, the question of intra-laboratory and inter-laboratory variation in the results of the assays has arisen. A survey of the scatter of results produced by a number of laboratories when measuring drug concentrations in aliquots of the same sample of biological fluid gives cause for concern (Pippenger, Penry, White, Daly and Buddington, 1976). Many laboratories involved in measuring anticonvulsants are now participating in quality control schemes such as that operated from St. Bartholomew's Hospital, London (Richens, 1975). However, the situation regarding accuracy and reproducibility of assay results still does not appear entirely satisfactory. The clinician should be aware of this, and of the other technical limitations of the assays as intimated above, when he applies the results of anticonvulsant level measurements to the management of his patients.

REFERENCES

Brodie, B. B., Udenfriend, S. & Baer, J. E. (1947) The estimation of basic organic compounds in biological material. I. General principles. *J. Biol. Chem.*, **168**, 299–309.

de Silva, J. A. F. (1970) The analysis of drugs and their metabolites in biological specimens in *Current concepts in the pharmaceutical sciences: biopharmaceutics*, edited Swarbrick, J. Philadelphia. Lea and Febiger, 203–264.

Dill, W. A., Kazenko, A., Wolf, L. M. & Glazko, A. J. (1956) Studies on 5-5'-diphenylhydantoin (Dilantin) in animals and man. *J. Pharmacol. Exp. Therap.* **118**, 270–279.

Eadie, M. J. & Tyrer, J. H. (1973) Plasma levels of anticonvulsants. *Aust. N.Z. J. Med.* **3**, 290–303.

Hawker, C. D. (1973) Radioimmunoassay and related methods. *Anal. Chem.* **45**, 878A–890A.

Meijer, J. W. A., Meinardi, H., Gardner-Thorpe, C. & van der Kleijn, E. (1973) *Methods of analysis of anti-epileptic drugs.* Amsterdam. Excerpta Medica.

Montgomery, M. R., Holtzman, J. L. & Leute, R. K. (1975) Application of electron spin resonance to determination of serum drug concentrations. *Clin. Chem.* **21**, 1323–1328.

Pippenger, C. E., Penry, J. K. & Kutt, H. (1978) *Antiepileptic drugs: quantitative analysis and interpretation.* New York. Raven Press.

Pippenger, C. E., Penry, J. K., White, B. G., Daly, D. D. & Buddington, R. (1976) Interlaboratory variability in determination of plasma antiepileptic drug concentrations. *Arch. Neurol (Chic.)* **33**, 351–355.

Richens, A. (1975) Results of a phenytoin quality control scheme, in Schneider, H., Janz, D., Gardner-Thorpe, D., Meinhardi, H. & Sherwin, A. L. *Clinical pharmacology of anti-epileptic drugs.* Berlin: Springer. 293–303.

Scharpe, S. L., Cooreman, W. M., Blomme, W. J. & Laekeman, G. M. (1976) Quantitative enzyme immunoassay: current status. *Clin. Chem.* **22**, 733–738.

Skelley, D. S., Brown, L. P. & Besch, P. K. (1973) Radioimmunoassay. *Clin. Chem.* **2**, 146–186.

Udenfriend, S. (1969) *Fluorescence assay in biology and medicine.* Vol. 2. New York and London: Academic Press.

Viswanathan, C. T., Booker, H. E. & Welling, P. G. (1977) Interference by p-hydroxyphenobarbital in the ^{125}I-radioimmunoassay of serum and urinary phenobarbital. *Clin. Chem.* **23**, 873–876.

4

The study of anticonvulsant drug action

The action of anticonvulsant drugs may be studied at a number of different levels of biological complexity. In this book the mechanisms of action of the individual anticonvulsants are dealt with in Part II, where each drug is considered separately. However, it may be useful here to discuss in a general way how anticonvulsant drugs act, considering their effects on a number of biological systems ranked in order of decreasing complexity.

ACTIONS OF ANTICONVULSANTS ON THE WHOLE HUMAN BRAIN

To the clinician, the most important consideration regarding anticonvulsant drugs is their effectiveness in human epilepsy. Experience has shown that certain types of human epilepsy are more likely to respond to certain anticonvulsants than to others. If human epilepsy is subdivided on the basis of a simplified version of the classification of epileptic seizures proposed by the International League Against Epilepsy (Gastaut, 1969), one can correlate the type of epilepsy with the drugs likely to be effective in that type of epilepsy (Table 5.1). While these correlations between type of drug and type of epilepsy are not complete, they are reasonably close. This theme of relative specificity of anticonvulsant action is more fully developed in subsequent chapters of this book, when anticonvulsant therapy in epileptic patients is considered in detail.

Occasionally the actions of anticonvulsant drugs have been studied in non-epileptic patients who were undergoing electro-convulsive therapy for psychiatric disorders. Such studies do not appear to have shed much light on anticonvulsant drug action.

ACTIONS OF ANTICONVULSANTS ON THE BRAIN OF EXPERIMENTAL ANIMALS

The actions of anticonvulsant drugs have been studied in a number of whole animal models. The various experimental preparations have been reviewed by Naquet and Lanoir (1973) and Swinyard (1973). It is possible to divide the experimental animal models into several groups, and to discern analogies between these preparations and particular types of human epilepsy.

Animals with spontaneous seizures

The two animal models with spontaneous seizures that are usually studied are the photo-sensitive baboon, Papio papio (with photogenic seizures), and mice with hereditary audiogenic seizures. The analogy between the mice with audiogenic seizures and any particular form of human epilepsy is not clear, since there is uncertainty as to the correct interpretation of the electrographic features of the audiogenic seizures (Naquet and Lanoir, 1973). However, the photogenic seizures of Papio papio have obvious affinities to the variety of photogenic myoclonic epilepsy that occurs in children. In fact Papio papio serves as a reasonable model of human myoclonic epilepsy. The anticonvulsants effective in this type of epilepsy in man (e.g. clonazepam, diazepam, valproate, and phenobarbitone) are also effective in Papio papio.

Animals with evoked seizures

1. Models of generalised epilepsy

Electrical shocks applied to the heads of experimental animals, often mice, may produce seizures resembling human generalized tonic-clonic or clonic epilepsy. The most widely used variant of this epileptic model is the maximum electroshock seizure, usually taken as being equivalent to human generalized epilepsy with tonic-clonic fits. Maximum electroshock seizures in animals are prevented, or the seizure pattern is modified, by drugs which are useful in the analogous type of human epilepsy (viz. phenytoin, phenobarbitone, methylphenobarbitone, primidone, carbamazepine, clonazepam and suthiame). By employing less power-ful electrical fields, minimum electroshock seizures can be produced in animals. These seizures resemble mild human tonic-clonic seizures with a predominant bilateral tonic phase. Again, phenytoin, carbamazepine, phenobarbitone, and clonazepam are effective in man and in the experimental animals.

Chemical convulsants, administered systemically, may cause a generalized activation of cortico-reticular circuits, and produce generalized clonic seizures, with or without a tonic phase. The pattern of such seizures resembles myoclonic epilepsy, or clonic generalized epilepsy in man. However, such induced seizures in animals have sometimes been equated with absence attacks (petit mal) in man. One doubts whether this is appropriate. The most commonly used chemical convulsant is pentylenetetrazole, but many other substances have been used (e.g. strychnine, thiosemicarbazide, 2,4-dimethyl-5-hydroxy-methyl pyrimidine, local anaesthetics such as procaine, lignocaine or cocaine, bicuculline, bemegride, picrotoxin). It would appear that phenobarbitone, troxidone, clonazepam and valproate are probably the most effective agents against chemically-induced generalized convulsions in animals. These same agents, with the possible exception of troxidone, are also the most useful drugs for controlling human myoclonic seizures. There are some apparent inconsistencies in the correlations between therapeutic efficacy of anticonvulsants and the response of seizures produced by particular systemically administered convulsants. To some extent these discrepancies may be explained by an anticonvulsant acting as a specific antagonist to a particular convulsant agent but not to others (e.g. valproate in the case of seizures produced by bicuculline or picrotoxin, both of which diminish gamma aminobutyrate-mediated inhibition in the brain). In such circumstances the anticonvulsant may appear very much more effective than in chemically-induced seizures provoked through different biochemical mechanisms.

It would appear that there is no adequate animal model of human absence (*petit mal*) epilepsy that has found widespread use.

2. Models of partial epilepsy

Electrical fields applied to restricted volumes of the cerebral cortex, or to certain subcortical structures, may activate various patterns of partial seizure. With chronic repeated applications of sub-threshold localized electrical shocks a discharging focus may finally develop, and this may subsequently initiate 'mirror' foci. In many ways this 'kindling' model provides the best available analogy to human partial epilepsy (Wada, 1977). Though there are species differences, phenytoin, phenobarbitone, carbamazepine and diazepam appear to exert protective effects against such 'kindled' seizures.

Chemical convulsants (e.g. penicillin, strychnine, pentylenetetrazole), if applied locally to the cortex of experimental animals, may instigate a temporary epileptic focus which can produce partial seizures. A delayed but more enduring cortical epileptic focus can be induced by local application of cobalt, alumina gel, or tungstic acid. Injury due to local freezing can also set up a cortical epileptic focus. Drugs useful against seizures from these various induced cortical foci, and also useful in human partial epilepsy, include phenytoin, phenobarbitone, carbamazepine, clonazepam and valproate. However, the role of valproate in human cortical epilepsy is not well established.

In assessing the results of studies of anticonvulsant drug action on the various experimental animal models of epilepsy it is useful to bear in mind:

a. how analogous the animal model is to the various types of human epilepsy (Fig. 4.1)

b. whether an anticonvulsant action occurs at drug concentrations similar to those at which an effect occurs in man. This latter point has often been ignored, which makes the interpretation of some experimental work uncertain.

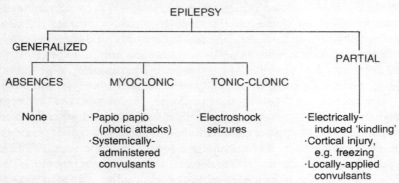

Fig. 4.1. Correlation between types of human epilepsy and animal models of epilepsy.

ACTIONS OF ANTICONVULSANTS ON NEURON POOLS

The actions of anticonvulsants on certain of the above-mentioned animal models of epilepsy may be studied at a more intimate level than by observing the response of the whole animal. Such studies are carried out mainly on models of partial epilepsy. However, it seems likely that conclusions drawn from these studies may also be applicable to generalized epilepsy, since all epilepsy appears to arise in hyperexcitable neuronal pools. Certain neuron pools are more often studied than others, largely because hyperexcitability is more easily produced in these pools. In man, monkey and cat post-stimulus after-discharging is more readily instigated in the hippocampus than in the motor cortex, amygdala and basal ganglia. After-discharge thresholds are even higher in the frontal and occipital cortices, and within the thalamus after-discharge thresholds are higher in the non-specific than in the specific nuclei (Naquet and Lanoir, 1973).

Krupp and Monier (1973) reviewed the effects of anticonvulsants on the electrical functioning of such neuron pools. The electrical phenomena that have been studied include:

1. the activity at the site of epileptogenesis,
2. the propagation of activity from the site,
3. transmission across synapses, and
4. local after-discharges, and secondary after-discharges set up in other neuron pools.

In general, anticonvulsants appear to have relatively little or no effect on cortical spike activity at epileptogenic foci. The drugs which have most effect on such activity are ethosuximide and valproate. Neither is of established value in human partial epilepsy. However, some of the anticonvulsants useful in human partial seizures (e.g. phenytoin, carbamazepine and clonazepam) inhibit the spread of epileptic activity from its focus of origin.

Some anticonvulsants alter transmission at various synapses. Phenytoin has the unusual property among anticonvulsants of depressing post-tetanic potentiation of synaptic transmission. This effect occurs even when phenytoin is present in concentrations that have no other detectable effect on neurological function (Esplin, 1957).

After-discharges reflect a neuron pool's continuing hyperexcitability and there-fore its potential for further epileptic discharging. After-discharges are suppressed (or the threshold for inducing after-discharges is raised) by phenytoin, phenobar-bitone, carbamazepine, troxidone, clonazepam and valproate. The effects of these anticonvulsants on after-discharges may differ from one brain region to another, and may also differ, depending on how the after-discharges are induced.

Studies of the electrical properties of experimental epileptic neuron pools thus suggest that anticonvulsants do not so much prevent the initiation of epileptic activity as limit its ease of spread, both within and outside these pools. The effects of anticonvulsants may differ, if neuron pools from different brain regions are studied, but this is a matter requiring more extensive investigation.

ACTIONS OF ANTICONVULSANTS ON SINGLE NEURONS

The effects of anticonvulsants on the electrical properties of single neurons do not appear to have been extensively studied. The literature on this subject, reviewed by Chalazonitis and Arvanitaki (1973), relates mainly to phenytoin. Several paramet-

ers of neuronal electrical function have been investigated. These include:
1. resting membrane potential
2. action potential
3. post-synaptic excitation
4. post-synaptic inhibition.
Such studies require exacting micro-electrode techniques. There may be problems in dissolving an anticonvulsant so that the drug, in an appropriate concentration contained in water at physiological pH, can be delivered in the vicinity of the neuron being studied.

Sufficient data are not available to permit generalizations about the effects of anticonvulsants on the electrical functions of single neurons. The available information will be discussed when individual anticonvulsants are considered in Part II of this book.

ACTIONS OF ANTICONVULSANTS ON BIOCHEMICAL MECHANISMS

A considerable amount of information is available regarding the effects of anticonvulsants on various biochemical mechanisms in neural tissue. How some of the described biochemical changes relate to anticonvulsant effect is obscure. However, other drug-induced alterations in biochemical function appear potentially capable of anti-epilepsy effects. These changes include:
1. alterations in energy production in neurons (necessary to maintain cell structure and the polarization of cell membranes, and to permit the synthesis of synaptic transmitter molecules).
2. alterations in ionic concentration gradients across cell membranes
3. alterations in synaptic transmitters
4. alterations in folates, and
5. alterations in macromolecule synthesis.

Alterations in energy production
A number of anticonvulsants have effects on biochemical processes related to the production of high energy phosphate, which provides energy for the various activities of neurons. Details of these biochemical effects will be provided when the individual drugs are considered in Part II. The general tendency is for anticonvulsants (notably phenytoin and phenobarbitone) to have biochemical effects which would restrict the availability of cellular energy. Whether this has an anticonvulsive effect, and how such an effect might be mediated biochemically, are uncertain.

Alterations in ionic concentration gradients across cell membranes
The existence of ionic concentration gradients across neuronal cell membranes is responsible for the resting membrane potential, and also for action potential initiation and propagation. Alterations in the concentration gradients of Na^+, K^+, Ca^{++} and Cl^- ions across neuronal cell membranes could change neuronal excitability, and thus have anticonvulsant effects.

Several anticonvulsants (phenytoin, phenobarbitone and troxidone) cause a fall in intracellular Na^+ concentration. The effects of the newer anticonvulsants (clonazepam, valproate) do not appear to have been studied in this regard. The mechanisms involved in this fall in Na^+ concentration are controversial, and will be discussed in detail later. Phenytoin and phenobarbitone also impair Ca^{++} flux across cell membranes.

Alterations in synaptic transmitters

Whether or not altered synaptic transmitter concentrations have an anticonvulsant effect would seem to depend on whether the transmitter has an inhibitory or excitatory function in the pathway in question. Certain anticonvulsants are known to alter brain concentrations of several known or putative neurotransmitters including acetylcholine, dopamine, noradrenaline, serotonin and γ-aminobutyrate (GABA). However, it is only for the latter two substances, and perhaps for noradrenaline, that there is evidence that the altered transmitter concentration has an anti-epileptic role.

Anderson, Markowitz and Bonnycastle (1962) found a relation between protection against maximum electroshock seizures in rats and phenytoin-induced elevation of brain serotonin levels. In mice, drugs which lower brain serotonin or noradrenaline levels reduce protection against electrically-induced convulsions (Meyer and Frey, 1973). In man, therapeutic (but not subtherapeutic) plasma levels of phenytoin and phenobarbitone are associated with raised CSF levels of the serotonin metabolite 5-hydroxyindoleacetic acid (Chadwick, Jenner and Reynolds, 1975). This raised serotonin metabolite level is probably due to increased serotonin release in the brain, with subsequent metabolic degradation. Phenytoin, phenobarbitone and clonazepam raise brain serotonin levels. These drugs, and diazepam, also raise brain noradrenaline levels.

GABA is an inhibitory central synaptic transmitter, deficiency of which is a rare cause of myoclonic epilepsy in infancy. Brain GABA levels in experimental animals are increased by phenytoin, phenobarbitone, ethosuximide, diazepam and valproate.

Alterations in folates

There are several reports of an association between use of anticonvulsant drugs and folate deficiency in man. Continued intake of phenytoin, phenobarbitone or primidone leads to reduced serum, red blood cell or CSF folate levels in 27–91 per cent of epileptic patients (Reynolds, 1976). Carbamazepine therapy may also produce folate deficiency (Reizenstein and Lund, 1973). Folate deficiency may have an anticonvulsant effect, though the mechanism involved is uncertain. In animals, folates are cerebral excitants. Obbens (1973) found that folate administration increased seizure activity arising from an experimental epileptic focus produced by local cobalt application. If rats are given large intravenous injections of folate, convulsions may ensue (Hommes, Obbens and Wijffels, 1973). Tetrahydrofolate, dihydrofolate, 5-formyltetrahydrofolate and 5-methyltetrahydrofolate all act as convulsants in rats (Obbens and Hommes, 1973). Folate and folinate increase the firing rates of single cortical neurons of cats (Davies and Watkins, 1973).

While anticonvulsant-induced folate deficiency may contribute to an anti-epileptic effect, this is unlikely to be the chief mode of biochemical action of the anticonvulsants. These drugs protect against epilepsy long before there has been time for their use to cause folate deficiency in the individual.

Alterations in macromolecule synthesis

Phenytoin is known to have several effects on the synthesis of different biological macromolecules. There have been suggestions that altered macromolecule structure may alter neuronal membrane properties, and ionic conductance across these membranes (Shanes, 1958). Such alterations might lead to an anti-epileptic effect.

*   *   *

The available information does not permit the development of any general hypothesis as to the electrophysiological or biochemical mechanisms of action of anticonvulsant drugs. Certain actions of the drugs are known which appear likely to contribute towards an anticonvulsant effect. However, some of these actions are not possessed by some anticonvulsants. The relevant available facts are discussed in more detail in relation to individual drugs in Part II of this book.

REFERENCES

Anderson, E. G., Markowitz, S. D. & Bonnycastle, D. D. (1962) Brain 5-hydroxytryptamine and anticonvulsant activity. *J. Pharmacol. Exp. Therap.*, **136**, 179–182.

Chadwick, D., Jenner, P. & Reynolds, E. H. (1975) Amines, anticonvulsants and epilepsy. *Lancet* i, 1425–1426.

Chalazonitis, N. & Arvanitaki, A. (1973) Convulsants and anticonvulsants on single neurons, in Mercier, J. Anticonvulsant Drugs. *International Encyclopaedia of Pharmacology and Therapeutics, Section 19*, Vol. 2. Oxford: Pergamon Press. 401–424.

Davies, J. & Watkins, J. C. (1973) Facilitatory and direct excitatory effects of folate and folinate on single neurons of cat cerebral cortex. *Biochem. Pharmacol.* **22**, 1667–1668.

Esplin, D. W. (1957) Effect of diphenylhydantoin on synaptic transmission in cat spinal cord and stellate ganglion. *J. Pharmacol. Exp. Therap.* **120**, 301–323.

Gastaut, H. (1969) Clinical and electroencephalographical classification of epileptic seizures. *Epilepsia* (Amst.) **10**, Suppl: 2.

Hommes, O. R., Obbens, E. A. M. T. & Wijffels, C. C. B. (1973) Epileptogenic activity of sodium folate and the blood-brain barrier in the rat. *J. Neurol. Sci.* **19**, 63–71.

Krupp, P. & Monnier, M. (1973) Action of anticonvulsants on cerebrospinal systems, in Mercier, J. Anticonvulsant Drugs. *International Encyclopaedia of Pharmacology and Therapeutics. Section 19, Vol. 2.* Oxford. Pergamon Press. 371–400.

Meyer, H. & Frey, H. H. (1973) Dependence of anticonvulsant drug action on central monoamines. *Neuropharmacology*, **12**, 939–947.

Naquet, R. & Lanoir, J. (1973) Essay on antiepileptic drug activity in experimental animals: special tests, in Mercier, J. Anticonvulsant Drugs. *International Encyclopaedia of Pharmacology and Therapeutics. Section 19, Vol. 1.* Oxford: Pergamon Press. p. 67–122.

Obbens, E. A. M. T. (1973) Experimental epilepsy induced by folate derivatives. Thesis. Nijmegan, cited by Reynolds, E. H. (1976). *loc. cit.*

Reizenstein, P. & Lund, L. (1973) Effect of anticonvulsive drugs on folate absorption and the cerebrospinal fluid folate pump. *Scand. J. Haemat.* **11**, 158–165.

Reynolds, E. H. (1976) Folate and epilepsy, in Bradford, H. F. and Marsden,C. D. *Biochemistry and Neurology*. London: Academic Press. p. 247–252.

Shanes, A. M. (1958) Electrochemical aspects of physiological and pharmacological action in excitable cells. *Pharmacol. Rev.* **10**, 59–273.

Swinyard, E. A. (1973) Assay of antiepileptic drug activity in experimental animals: standard tests, in Mercier, J. Anticonvulsant Drugs. *International Encyclopaedia of Pharmacology and Therapeutics. Section 19, Vol. 1.* Oxford: Pergamon Press. p. 47–65.

Wada, J. A. (1977) Parmacological prophylaxis in the kindling model of epilepsy. *Arch. Neurol.* (Chic) **34**, 389–395.

Obbens, E. A. M. T. & Hommes, D. R. (1973) The epileptogenic effects of folate derivatives in the rat. *J. Neurol. Sci.* **20**, 223–229.

5

Principles of anticonvulsant therapy

As stated in Chapter 1, epilepsy is usually treated by drugs prescribed with the intention of continuously suppressing epileptic activity in the brain for a sufficiently long period that seizures do not recur in the patient's lifetime, even after treatment is ceased. Before treatment for epilepsy is prescribed certain questions should have been asked and answered. These questions are:

1. Are the patient's attacks in fact epileptic and not due to some other disorder?
2. Is the epilepsy caused by any cerebral or extracerebral pathological condition which requires treatment in its own right?
3. Are there removable or reversible factors which aggravate the epilepsy or precipitate individual attacks?
4. Is there a significant risk of further epilepsy is the patient is left untreated?

The diagnosis of epilepsy
Clearly a patient's disorder must be correctly diagnosed before appropriate treatment can be prescribed on rational grounds. The detailed differentiation of epilepsy from disorders such as syncope, paroxysmal positional vertigo, 'hemiplegic' migraine, consequences of overbreathing, or the drop attacks of vertebrobasilar arterial insufficiency or cataplexy will not be considered here. However the reader will be well aware that all transient disturbances of cerebral function are not epileptic in nature.

The diagnosis of the cause of epilepsy
In many instances the pathological condition causing epilepsy will have reached a stationary phase in its evolution before clinical seizures appear. The cause may have ceased to act directly, though it may have damaged the brain (e.g. temporal lobe damage from hypoxia at birth). Sometimes epilepsy may occur during the acute phases of pathological conditions which require treatment in their own right. On other occasions such acute pathological conditions (e.g. bacterial meningitis) may elevate a pre-existing latent epileptic tendency to a clinically apparent level. If such conditions can be treated effectively and promptly the chance of residual brain damage may be lessened. Consequently the risk of any enduring epileptic tendency is reduced. Epilepsy may also develop during the course of chronic progressive conditions which require treatment (e.g. gliomas). Disturbances of extracerebral origin (e.g. hypoxia, hypoglycaemia, hypocalcaemia, over-hydration, pyrexia, alkalosis, uraemia, withdrawal of alcohol or of barbiturates such as

amylobarbitone) may produce epileptic disturbances in persons who have not had epilepsy in the past. Further, such extracerebral disturbances may activate pre-existing known or latent epileptic tendencies. If these extracerebral disorders are corrected the risk of continuing epileptic attacks is lessened. However, even if a causative cerebral or extracerebral pathological condition is totally removed, its previous presence may have set up an enduring epileptic potentiality in a brain which had never before been the site of epileptic activity.

The risk of further epilepsy

The question of significant risk of subsequent epilepsy if no treatment is given is one which has been discussed in Chapter 1 of this book. Here it suffices to repeat the view expressed there: that everyone who has had a single proven epileptic manifestation should be treated except for those in whom the risk of further epileptic manifestations is assessed as remote. Such an assessment can be made when one has determined the factor that precipitated the solitary epileptic seizure, knows that this precipitating factor is most unlikely to recur, and knows that there is no predisposing factor (hereditary or acquired) which would favour the recurrence of epilepsy.

The prevention of further seizures consists of the use of appropriate drugs, in adequate dosage, for a sufficient length of time to abolish the presumptive epileptic process.

APPROPRIATE DRUGS FOR TREATING EPILEPSY

Experience has shown that particular types of epilepsy in man respond best to particular anticonvulsant drugs. The correlation between type of epileptic seizure and type of effective drug is set out in Table 5.1. Correlations between type of drug

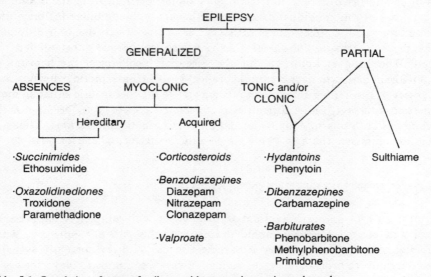

Table. 5.1. Correlation of types of epilepsy with appropriate anticonvulsant drugs.

and type of epilepsy are not absolute. Sometimes a patient's type of epilepsy may appear to overlap two adjacent columns of the Table. Families of drugs in one column often have a useful degree of effect on the type of epilepsy in the immediately adjacent columns, though usually not in more distant columns, except in the cases of clonazepam and valproate.

If a patient has one type of epilepsy, one drug from the appropriate column should be selected. However, one patient may have two types of epilepsy and these may require different types of drugs (e.g. drugs for tonic-clonic seizures and *petit mal* absences). If so, a drug from each of the appropriate columns may be prescribed. If the patient's two types of epilepsy are represented in adjacent columns of the Table it may be reasonable to use a single drug likely to be effective against the more troublesome kind of seizure. It is possible that this drug will also have a sufficient degree of action against the less troublesome kind of epilepsy represented in the adjacent column.

The primary anticonvulsant may fail to control epilepsy after dosage has been taken to the limit of tolerance. If so, a drug from a different chemical family within the same column should be introduced. There are two reasons for preferring combinations of chemically different families of drugs to combinations of drugs from the same chemical family. Drugs from the one chemical family may produce a common biologically active metabolite. Therefore combining two drugs with similar chemical structures at times may merely prove equivalent to increasing the dose of the primary drug, yet this dose should have already been taken to its limit of tolerance. Diversity of chemical structure in anticonvulsant combination increases the possibility that the drugs may have separate inhibitory actions on different aspects of epileptogenesis, whereas structurally similar chemicals are more likely to have a common mode of action. It is therefore conceivable that chemically different anticonvulsants may act additively, each drug interfering with a different aspect of epileptogenesis. This raises the question of whether combinations of chemically different anticonvulsants should be used from the outset. So long as doses of the individual drugs are sufficient, such combinations may offer increased therapeutic effectiveness with less risk of side-effects due to overdosage. In the present state of knowledge this view can neither be substantiated nor refuted. Too little is known about the essential biochemical mechanisms of anticonvulsant action to have a sure theoretical basis for interpreting this possibility. However, combining anticonvulsants may make the therapeutic situation more complex to interpret if any difficulties or unwanted effects arise, because of the possibility of both pharmacodynamic and pharmacokinetic interactions. Thus one prefers to commence therapy with a single anticonvulsant, whenever possible.

ADEQUATE ANTICONVULSANT DOSAGE

The ideal dose of an anticonvulsant is that which will completely suppress all clinical and electroencephalographic evidence of the patient's epilepsy, while producing no immediate or delayed adverse effects. With the currently available anticonvulsants this desirable state cannot always be attained. Nevertheless it should always be sought before a less perfect therapeutic situation is accepted.

If a patient has frequent epileptic manifestations, and the individual manifestations are not very disturbing to the patient (as is often the case in *petit mal* absences), it is usually comparatively easy to adjust anticonvulsant doses on clinical grounds. Dosage increases are made at intervals until the epilepsy ceases, or unwanted effects appear. Dosage increases should be made at long enough intervals to allow plasma and brain levels of the drug to attain steady-state conditions between dose increments. Too frequent an increase in dose may lead to excessive dosage. This may not be recognised until a few days later when overdosage manifestations appear. The dose would then need to be reduced and control of the epilepsy sought again. However, should a rapid therapeutic effect be desired, it is sensible to use loading doses of anticonvulsants, bearing in mind the pharmacokinetic parameters of the individual anticonvulsant, as discussed in Part II.

In the more commonly encountered clinical situation when the patient's epilepsy is less frequent, but the individual attacks are more disrupting to the quality of life (e.g. tonic-clonic fits), adjustment of anticonvulsant dosages on clinical grounds often proves less satisfactory. Standardized anticonvulsant dosages yield a wide range of plasma levels of drug, and very different degrees of biological effect, in different patients (Eadie, 1971). One may prescribe a conventional dose of an anticonvulsant, wait for weeks or months, and then when a seizure occurs realize the dose has been inadequate. After a further period of several weeks or months, an increased dose may also be proved inadequate when there is a further seizure. In such situations measurement of plasma anticonvulsant concentration at an early stage of therapy is valuable. Enough experience has accumulated to indicate what ranges of plasma anticonvulsant concentrations are likely to correlate with the best prospects of control of epilepsy in the individual, with a minimal risk of unwanted effects due to drug overdosage. Higher or lower plasma levels may be associated with therapeutic effectiveness in an individual patient with epilepsy, though levels above the 'therapeutic' ('desirable' or 'optimal') range are likely to be associated with overdosage effects. In types of epilepsy which occur infrequently, or when the patient is treated after his first seizure before the natural history of his epilepsy has had time to reveal itself, dosages of an appropriate anticonvulsant should be adjusted in the light of the plasma anticonvulsant concentration until a concentration in the 'therapeutic' range is achieved. Dosage adjustment should be made at long-enough intervals to allow plasma and brain levels of the drug to achieve steady state conditions between dosage changes. A plasma anticonvulsant concentration in the therapeutic range does not guarantee a patient immunity from epilepsy. However, it does offer the average patient his best chance of control of epilepsy while using the drug prescribed. Consequently it should reduce the patient's uncertainty in facing life.

Unwanted effects of therapy may limit anticonvulsant use and dosage increase. These unwanted effects fall into four groups: (1) local, often irritant, effects at the site of administration (commonly the alimentary tract); (2) hypersensitivity or idiosyncratic effects; (3) effects due to overdosage; (4) dysmorphogenic effects in the fetus. Hypersensitivity and idiosyncratic effects may occur unpredictably. If they are severe enough, or carry sufficient potential hazard (e.g. bone marrow depression), the drug must be withdrawn. The drug or its congeners should never be used again in that patient. Overdosage effects will ultimately occur in every patient if the dosage is sufficiently increased. Overdosage with many of the anticonvulsants produces drowsiness and ataxia of gait, but each drug also has its own particular effects. The clinician should be familiar with the side-effects of each anticonvulsant, and should specifically seek out the possible presence of these effects in all patients undergoing treatment. If the clinician relies on the patient's spontaneous complaints, unwanted effects may reach an advanced stage before they are detected. Patients (or their relatives) should be made aware of unwanted effects, particularly those which may appear soon after a dosage change or the addition of a second drug. Then, if these effects occur, appropriate action may be taken quickly. The question of dysmorphogenesis from anticonvulsants is discussed at length in Chapter 6.

If epilepsy continues to occur with plasma anticonvulsant concentrations in the 'therapeutic' range for the drug used, the patient may still tolerate further cautious dosage increments. Control of the epilepsy may still be obtained before overdosage effects preclude any further dosage increase. Once an anticonvulsant is taken to its limit of tolerance without controlling a patient's epilepsy, a second appropriate anticonvulsant should be introduced following the principles indicated above. The dose of the second drug is thereafter adjusted as the dose of the primary drug was adjusted. It could be argued that the primary anticonvulsant should be withdrawn after the second drug has had time to exert its effects. Such a policy would depend on the belief that the primary drug had no beneficial effect on the epilepsy. One can rarely be certain that this is so. An apparent failure to control seizures completely may represent the partial control of severe or worsening epilepsy. Therefore it is probably safer to continue the primary anticonvulsant after a second drug is added. However, the dose of the primary drug should be reduced to just below the threshold at which its unwanted effects begin to appear.

When a combination of two anticonvulsants fails, a third appropriate drug should be added, and its dosage adjusted as suggested above. This policy of combining drugs is continued either until the epilepsy is controlled, or until all available therapy is exhausted if used in doses which leave the patient free from unwanted effects. In the latter circumstance one must decide if the patient's epilepsy disturbs him sufficiently to warrant his accepting some drug side-effects as a price for full (or at least better) control of epilepsy when drug dosages are increased. The situation has then become one of compromise between the disadvantages of therapy and the consequences of the epilepsy for the life of the individual, his family and the community. It is often a therapeutically and psychologically brittle situation but one which, it is hoped, will become less frequent with earlier and more efficient treatment of epilepsy.

DURATION OF ANTICONVULSANT THERAPY

If epilepsy is partly but not fully controlled, anticonvulsant therapy should be continued indefinitely. Full control of epilepsy means that the patient shows no clinical or EEG evidence of any epileptic manifestation, however minor. Full control does not mean merely that the patient is free from severe seizures. If anticonvulsants are withdrawn while the epileptic process remains active, however minor its expressions, there is risk of worsening of the epilepsy and of greater future difficulty in controlling it.

After epilepsy has been fully controlled, many neurologists believe that anticonvulsants should be continued in full dosage for between 2 and 4 years before a withdrawal of treatment is contemplated. Juul-Jensen (1964) found that, in 200 patients whose epilepsy was fully controlled for 2 years, there was a 36·5 per cent risk of recurrence in the 4 years after therapy was withdrawn. Holowach, Thurston and O'Leary (1972) studied a group of 148 children suffering from epilepsy. They showed that, if the disorder has been totally suppressed for four years, there were about 3 chances in 4 of freedom from subsequent seizures for at least five years after the anticonvulsant therapy was withdrawn. However, the more delay there had been in obtaining initial control of the epilepsy, even though seizures were subsequently totally suppressed for 4 years, the less were the chances of lasting cure. Rabe (1972) and Loiseau, Henry and Prissard (1972) both stated that the recurrence rate for epilepsy after ceasing anticonvulsants varied for different seizure types. Generalized convulsive seizures tended to have a better prognosis than the more common forms of partial epilepsy.

If epilepsy can be fully controlled with anticonvulsant doses which produce no appreciable unwanted effects, there is usually little to be gained by early cessation, or reduction, of therapy. In the presence of complete control there is much to commend a policy of at least four years continuous treatment with full dosage of anticonvulsants. After this time treatment should be ceased only if the EEG is free from paroxysmal activity and if the patient is not likely to be subjected to factors which tend to activate epilepsy (e.g. exposure to flickering light in the course of employment of persons with the myoclonic type of generalized epilepsy).

It is often recommended that the withdrawal of anticonvulsants be gradual, over a period of months (Livingstone, 1972). Whether this is really necessary after 3 or 4 years complete control of epilepsy is uncertain. However the policy is a safe one and is not likely to be abandoned readily.

Once the diagnosis of epilepsy is made, any treatable causative or precipitating factors should be dealt with. Thereafter, the use of appropriate anticonvulsant drugs in adequate dosage (as determined by the clinical response and suggested by the plasma drug concentration), prescribed as soon as possible after the first known epileptic manifestation, and continued in full dosage for at least 3 or 4 years, appears to offer the patient the best chance of lasting future freedom from all manifestations of epilepsy.

REFERENCES

Eadie, M. J. (1971) Blood levels of anticonvulsants, in Geigy Symposium on Epilepsy, ed. Winton, R. R., Australasian Medical Publishing Co., 81–87.
Holowach, J., Thurston, D. L. & O'Leary, J. (1972) Prognosis in childhood epilepsy. Follow-up study of 148 cases in which therapy had been suspended after prolonged anticonvulsant control. *New Eng. J. Med.*, **286,** 169–174.
Juul-Jensen, P. (1964) Frequency of recurrence after discontinuance of anticonvulsant therapy in patients with epileptic seizures. *Epilepsia* (Amst.) **5,** 352–363.

Livingstone, S. (1972) *Comprehensive management of epilepsy in infancy, childhood and adolescence.* Springfield: Charles C. Thomas.

Loiseau, P., Henry, P. & Prissard, A. (1972) Considerations sur l'arret des traitments antiepileptiques. *Bordeaux Med.* **5,** 2631–2642.

Rabe, E. F. (1972) Anticonvulsant therapy. To stop or not to stop. *New Eng. J. Med.* **286,** 213–214.

Pharmacology of the anticonvulsants

Introduction to Part II

The clinical pharmacology of individual anticonvulsant drugs is discussed in the following nine chapters. Only those drugs which are, and which appear likely to remain, in fairly widespread use in man have been considered in detail. Some other drugs in occasional use are dealt with briefly. The data set out are, wherever possible, obtained from studies on man. Animal work is cited only if human data are unavailable or inadequate and if the animal results throw light on some aspect of anticonvulsant pharmacology likely to be important in man.

For simplicity, each anticonvulsant, or family of anticonvulsants, is dealt with in the same order, as follows:

1. History and use. A brief account of the history of the drug, and of its use in clinical medicine.

2. Chemistry. An outline of the chemical properties of the drug which are relevant to its pharmacological use.

3. Pharmacodynamics
  a. the actions and uses of the drug in man
  b. the actions of the drug in certain experimental animals
  c. mechanisms of anticonvulsant action: as far as possible mechanisms of action are discussed in terms of:
     (i) electrophysiological effects (on neuron pools, and on single neurons)
     (ii) biochemical effects.

4. Pharmacokinetics
  a. absorption and bioavailability
  b. distribution, including plasma protein binding and the concentrations of the drug in different body fluids
  c. elimination considered as the overall process, and in terms of the pattern of
     (i) drug biotransformation
     (ii) drug excretion
  d. clinical pharmacokinetics, taking in matters such as the time course of the presence of the drug in the body, the therapeutic range of plasma levels of the drug, the relation between drug dose and steady-state plasma level in the individual and in the population, and the effect on this relationship of body weight, age, sex and concurrent disease.

5. Interactions. Principally interactions between the drug and other drugs given concurrently. However, for convenience, interactions between the drug and certain exogenous and endogenous substances are also considered. Interactions

may be classified as:
   a. pharmacodynamic
   b. pharmacokinetic

   6. *Toxicity.* The toxicity of the drug, including:
   a. local effects at sites of administration
   b. dose-dependent systemic unwanted effects. However the frequency of these effects usually correlates better with plasma levels of the drug than with the drug dose administered
   c. side-effects due to idiosyncrasy or hypersensitivity. These effects are uncommon. However there are some side-effects which occur rather too frequently to be due to hypersensitivity and yet which are not clearly dose-dependent. In the present work these effects have generally been tentatively classed with the dose-dependent ones, as a matter of convenience
   d. effects on the fetus and neonate (including dysmorphogenic effects).

   7. *Preparations available.* A range of commercially available preparations is given, not intended to be exhaustive.

*   *   *

The reader may find it helpful to refer to the two tables on the inside back cover of the book. These give the pharmacokinetic parameters of, and the therapeutic ranges, average doses and times to achieve steady state for the more commonly used anticonvulsants.

*   *   *

The material contained in this part of the book provides the factual basis on which the principles set out in Part I can be applied to the concrete situations of patients with epilepsy, to be discussed in Part III.

6

Hydantoin anticonvulsants

A number of substances containing the heterocyclic hydantoin ring have anticonvulsant activity. This class of compound was discovered by Baeyer (1861). Ware
(1950) discussed their chemistry and uses. For a variety of reasons, mostly toxicity
or relative ineffectiveness, only a few of the hydantoin anticonvulsants have come
into clinical use. Of these, phenytoin is widely used and its clinical pharmacology
has been extensively studied.

PHENYTOIN

Common proprietary names: 'Dilantin', 'Epanutin'
Phenytoin (diphenylhydantoin) was synthesized by Biltz (1908). According to
Gruhzit (1939) phenytoin was first tested as a possible hypnotic. Its anticonvulsant
properties were discovered by Merritt and Putnam (1938). Phenytoin has since
been widely used in clinical practice for treating all varieties of epilepsy except *petit
mal* absences and myoclonic seizures. The drug is occasionally used to treat cardiac
arrhythmias, tic douloureux, certain types of central pain and occasional varieties
of migraine.

CHEMISTRY

Phenytoin (5,5-diphenylhydantoin) is a white crystalline bitter-tasting powder. Its
molecular weight is 252·26. It is sparingly soluble in water and almost insoluble in
acids, but it will dissolve in aqueous bases and in organic solvents such as ethanol,
acetone and chloroform. It is a weak acid with a pKa value formerly stated to be 9·2
(Dill, Kazenko, Wolf and Glazko, 1956), but more recently said to be 8·3 (Agarwal
and Blake, 1968) or 8·06 (Schwartz, Rhodes and Cooper, 1977). Orally, phenytoin
is often administered as its more water-soluble sodium salt. Allowance should be
made for the difference in molecular weights between acid phenytoin (M.W.
252·26) and sodium phenytoin (M.W. 274·25) when a patient's treatment is
changed from one substance to the other.

PHARMACODYNAMICS

ACTIONS IN MAN

1. Anticonvulsant actions

Phenytoin is an effective anticonvulsant for all varieties of partial epilepsy in man, whether or not the seizures proceed to secondary generalization. Some clinicians consider that phenytoin is more effective in preventing the secondary generalization of partial seizures than in controlling the manifestations of the local cortical discharge itself. Phenytoin also appears useful in primary generalized epilepsy which presents as tonic-clonic or clonic seizures. However some think that it is less effective in this variety of epilepsy than the barbiturate anticonvulsants, particularly when the patient also experiences epileptic myoclonic jerks. Phenytoin is of little use in preventing absence attacks or myoclonic seizures.

2. Other actions

Phenytoin has been used to treat tic douloureux (Pennybacker, 1961). In this regard it appears less effective than carbamazepine. However it may be useful when patients cannot tolerate the latter substance. Phenytoin has sometimes proved useful in treating central pain (Cantor, 1972; Agnew and Goldberg, 1976) and also for treating the painful crises of Fabry's disease (Lockman, Hunninghake, Krivit and Desnick, 1973). Childhood migraine is sometimes prevented by regular phenytoin intake. The drug may also protect against 'hemiparaesthetic' and basilar artery migraine (Eadie and Tyrer, 1979). Phenytoin has been used in treating myotonia (Munsat, 1967), though the efficacy of the drug in this disorder is somewhat uncertain.

In cardiology, phenytoin has been used as an anti-arrhythmic agent with some success (Bigger, Schmidt and Kutt, 1968). The drug has been used to decrease insulin secretion in patients with insulinomas (Cudworth and Cunningham, 1974). It inhibits antidiuretic hormone release (Fichman, Kleeman and Bethune, 1970). A literature has developed (Bogoch and Dreyfus, 1970) suggesting that phenytoin is of benefit in a number of ill-defined disorders (e.g. overactive brain syndromes, sleep disturbances and miscellaneous somatic symptoms). The validity of these latter claims is uncertain.

ACTIONS IN ANIMALS

1. Models of generalized epilepsy

Phenytoin protects against photomyoclonic seizures in the baboon Papio papio, but only when given in doses that are toxic to the animals (Meldrum, Horton and Toseland, 1975). The drug is relatively ineffective against seizures due to the following systemically administered convulsants: pentylenetetrazole (Woodbury and Esplin, 1959), strychnine (Blum, Haefely, Jalfre, Polc and Scharer, 1973), thiosemicarbazide and 2,4-dimethyl-5-hydroxymethylpyrimidine (Banziger and Hane, 1967), bicuculline (Blum, Haefely, Jalfre, Polc and Scharer, 1973), strychnine and picrotoxin (Loescher and Frey, 1977), penicillin (Guberman, Gloor and Sherwin, 1975) and various local anaesthetics, e.g. procaine, cocaine, lignocaine (Eidelberg, Neer and Miller, 1965).

Phenytoin protects against maximum electroshock seizures in various species (mostly mice) and raises the threshold for evoking minimum electroshock seizures (Woodbury and Esplin, 1959).

In brief, phenytoin appears effective in animal models of generalized convulsive epilepsy, but relatively ineffective in models of myoclonic epilepsy.

2. Models of partial epilepsy

At plasma concentrations in the therapeutic range, phenytoin is effective against amygdaloid 'kindled' seizures in cats and baboons, though possibly not in other species (Wada, 1977). Racine, Livingstone and Joaquin (1975) found that the drug was more efficient in controlling seizures kindled by stimulating the neocortex than in controlling seizures produced by amygdaloid kindling.

Phenytoin has been shown to prevent clinical seizures in cats with penicillin-induced cortical foci (Louis, Kutt and McDowell, 1968). At therapeutically relevant concentrations (7–20 μg/ml) it appeared less effective against seizures arising from an alumina-induced focus in cats (Majkowski, Sobieszek, Bilinska Nigot and Karlinski, 1976).

Thus phenytoin appears reasonably effective as an anticonvulsant drug in animal models of partial epilepsy.

MECHANISMS OF ACTION

Neuron pools

Phenytoin failed to suppress (Louis, Kutt and McDowell, 1968), or only briefly suppressed (Dow, Fortar and McQueen, 1973), spike activity at experimental epileptic foci in the cortex. However, phenytoin did limit the propagation of epileptogenic activity from these foci (Musgrave and Purpura, 1963; Louis, Kutt and McDowell, 1968). After-discharges, reflecting residual local electrical instability, have their threshold for electrical induction increased by phenytoin (Schallek and Kuehn, 1963). This increase in threshold occurs to a greater extent in the frontal and parietal cortex than in the thalamus. Not only does the drug raise the after-discharge threshold, it also reduces the amplitude and duration of any after-discharges that are induced. Phenytoin also reduces the repetitive after-discharges that follow maximum electroshock generalized seizures in mice (Woodbury and Esplin, 1959). However, phenytoin failed to decrease after-discharges that arose in penicillin-induced cortical epileptogenic foci in rats (Edmonds, Stark and Hollinger, 1974).

The above findings suggest that phenytoin may limit the spread of epileptogenic activity rather than prevent the initiation of such activity. The effect of phenytoin in profoundly depressing the post-tetanic potentiation of nerve impulse transmission (Esplin, 1957) may explain its limiting effect on seizure spread. This action on post-tetanic potentiation occurs at phenytoin doses which have no other detectable effect on neural function. Other anticonvulsants appear to have relatively little effect on post-synpatic potentiation. Largely on this basis, Sherwin (1973) proposed the hypothesis that phenytoin acts mainly on responses which depend on repetitive activity in polysynaptic neural circuits.

In mice with congenital cerebellar damage the anticonvulsant action of phenytoin is reduced (Julien, 1972). However, phenytoin does not alter cerebellar Purkinje cell activity (Pieri and Haefely, 1975; 1976).

Single cells

Phenytoin has no action on the resting potential or on the conductance across the cell membrane of skeletal muscle. The drug alters membrane conductance in certain invertebrate neurons without altering their resting membrane potentials (Ayala, Lin and Johnston, 1977). Woodbury (1955) has stated that phenytoin increased the resting membrane potential. The effect of phenytoin on action potentials differs in different experimental preparations (Ayala and Johnston, 1977). The drug produces little change in the action potential of squid giant axons (Korey, 1951), or muscle cells (Carnay and Grundfest, 1974). Phenytoin decreases post-synaptic excitatory potentials in neurons of the lamprey (Selzer, 1978) and of the invertebrate Aplysia (Ayala and Johnston, 1977). In the latter animal the drug had little effect on Cl^- dependent post-synaptic inhibitory potentials. However phenytoin prolonged gamma-aminobutyrate mediated inhibitory post-synaptic potentials in the crayfish stretch receptor.

It is a little difficult to relate these findings in non-human excitable cells to the effects of phenytoin in human epilepsy.

Biochemical effects

Effects on energy production

Phenytoin inhibits beef heart terminal mitochondrial NADH dehydrogenase at drug concentrations (10^{-3} M) comparable to those which have an anticonvulsant effect in man (Cowger and Laabe, 1967). 'Therapeutic' concentrations of phenytoin were said to reduce oxygen consumption in a microsomal-synaptosomal preparation made from rat brain (Spector, 1972). This phenytoin-induced decrease in oxidative metabolism could be reversed if tetrahydrofolate or noradrenaline was added to the preparation.

There have been some studies of the effects of phenytoin on enzymes involved in oxidative metabolism. Leznicki and Dymecki (1974) found that long term phenytoin administration to rats caused a fall in brain succinate dehydrogenase activity. However, Green, Halpern, Thomas and Amick-Corkill (1973) showed that the drug had no effect on succinate dehydrogenase activity in chronically isolated cerebral cortex of the cat. Karkos (1975) and Hitchcock and Gabra-Sanders (1977) failed to find any change in rat cerebellar succinate dehydrogenase activity after prolonged phenytoin therapy. The drug did not alter 'resting' levels of redox enzymes in the cortex or spinal cord (LaManna, Lothman, Rosenthal, Somjen and Younts, 1977). While phenytoin probably does not influence the activity of the Krebs cycle enzyme succinate dehydrogenase, the drug might reduce brain oxygen consumption (and energy availability) by an inhibitory effect on terminal mitochondrial oxidation. Phenytoin has another biochemical effect which might increase energy availability for the neuron. The drug increases the conversion of a glutamate to Krebs cycle intermediates via a-ketoglutaric acid (Woodbury, 1969a).

It is difficult to see how these effects of phenytoin on energy metabolism relate to the anticonvulsant effect of the drug. However they might correlate with a general depression of brain function which may occur at higher drug doses.

Effects on inorganic ions

Na^+. Woodbury's (1955) finding that phenytoin caused a fall in brain intracellular Na^+ concentration has been generally accepted by subsequent workers. However, the mechanisms involved in this effect remain unsettled. There appear to be two main possibilities.

1. there may be an increase in the active extrusion of Na^+ from cells
2. there may be impaired entry of Na^+ into cells.

Increased Na^+ extrusion would most probably be due to increased activity of the sodium pump (Woodbury, 1955), the membrane-bound enzyme Na^+, K^+-linked adenosine triphosphatase (Skou, 1965; Askari, 1971). The literature concerning the effects of phenytoin on this enzyme contains apparently conflicting findings. Some workers have found that phenytoin produced no activation of the enzyme and indeed have noted inhibition of the enzyme (Pincus and Giarman, 1967; Pincus and Rawson, 1969; Formby, 1970; Deupree, 1976; Gilbert and Wyllie, 1976). In lobster nerve, phenytoin-mediated changes in intracellular Na^+ concentration still occurred when energy yielding reactions were inactivated, e.g. by cyanide (Pincus, Grove, Marino and Glaser, 1970). This finding would make it unlikely that the Na^+ shifts were mediated by an enzyme using adenosine triphosphate as its substrate. However other workers have obtained evidence suggesting that phenytoin does activate the enzyme, though often only at certain critical $Na^+ : K^+$ ratios (Festoff and Appel, 1967; Escueta and Appel, 1971; Siegel and Goodwin, 1972). In experimental epileptic cortex (produced by means of local freezing) phenytoin activated Na^+, K^+ adenosine triphosphatase, but only at certain crucial $Na^+ : K^+$ concentration ratios (Escueta and Appel, 1972). The current consensus appears to be that phenytoin does not reduce brain intracellular Na^+ concentrations by activation of Na^+, K^+ adenosine triphosphatase (Ayala and Johnston, 1977; Deupree, 1977; La Manna, Lothman, Rosenthal, Somjen and Younts, 1977). It is possible that phenytoin could have its effect on Na^+ by increasing the efficiency of Na^+, K^+ adenosine triphosphatase, without activating this enzyme. However, this would be almost impossible to prove experimentally (Deupree, 1977). The latter author proposed an explanation for the discrepant findings regarding the effects of phenytoin on Na^+, K^+ adenosine triphosphatase. He suggested that those workers who found apparent activation of the enzyme may have allowed some K^+ contamination of their reaction media to occur, because of the difficulty in dissolving phenytoin in aqueous media at neutral pH. When Escueta and Appel (1972) studied freeze-damaged epileptogenic cortex it is possible that injured cells may have released K^+ into their incubation media.

If phenytoin does not enhance Na^+ extrusion from cells by activating Na^+, K^+ adenosine triphosphatase, or some other energy-dependent enzyme, it seems likely that the drug lowers intracellular Na^+ concentrations by restricting Na^+ influx. The studies of Pincus and Rawson (1970), Pincus, Grove, Marino and Glaser (1970) and Pincus (1972) favour this latter possibility. Impeded Na^+ influx would lower intracellular Na^+ concentration, and consequently reduce the stimulus for active extrusion of Na^+. It is believed that increased Na^+ extrusion, following neuronal activity, is responsible for the phenomenon of post-tetanic hyperpolarisation. Phenytoin reduces the extent of post-tetanic hyperpolarisation.

K^+. The transport of K^+ into synaptosomes is stimulated by phenytoin, but only under ionic concentrations which simulate the depolarized state (Escueta and Appel, 1971). In synaptosomes from epileptogenic cortex (produced by local freezing) still higher environmental concentrations are required before phenytoin will stimulate K^+ uptake (Escueta and Appel, 1972). The latter authors considered it possible that some K^+ uptake in these circumstances may have been mediated by a mechanism other than activation of the sodium pump. In a further study Escueta, Davidson, Hartwig and Reilly (1975) again used nerve terminals from a cortical freezing focus. They showed that phenytoin increased K^+ uptake at environmental K^+ concentrations of 10^{-2} M, but not at the physiological K^+ concentration of 5×10^{-3} M.

It is difficult to know whether these effects of phenytoin on K^+ transport would apply to a significant extent under the circumstances in which the drug is used clinically.

Ca^{++}. Phenytoin reduces Ca^{++} influx into rat neurones (Pincus and Lee, 1973). Hasbani, Pincus and Lee (1974) showed that phenytoin decreased Ca^{++} flux across the membrane of resting lobster axons. Possibly the drug decreased membrane permeability to Ca^{++}. In the cat soleus nerve Dretchen, Standaert and Raines (1977) found that phenytoin blocked the cyclic nucleotide–mediated influx of Ca^{++} that occurs when neurotransmitters are released. The influx of Ca^{++} in these circumstances controls the slow K^+ current that may contribute to the phenomenon of post-tetanic hyperpolarization. Sohn and Ferrendelli (1976) showed that a therapeutic concentration of phenytoin (0.8×10^{-4} M) inhibited Ca^{++} influx into depolarized synaptosomes. However, Ferrendelli and Kinscherf (1977) demonstrated that supratherapeutic phenytoin concentrations (above 20 μg/ml) increased Ca^{++} influx into such synaptosomes, but decreased K^+ influx. There thus seems to be general agreement that phenytoin reduces Ca^{++} influx across neuronal cell membranes. Goldberg (1977) found that phenytoin (10^{-4} M) increased the binding of Ca^{++} to phospholipids.

Phenytoin would seem to alter the properties of neuronal cell membranes in relation to the flux of small inorganic cations. The mechanisms involved in this effect are incompletely understood. The altered ionic concentrations produced by phenytoin do not appear to change the resting membrane potential or the action potential of neurons. However, the altered ion concentrations may explain how phenytoin reduces post-tetanic hyperpolarization at nerve terminals. This in turn may relate to the way in which phenytoin inhibits post-tetanic potentiation of synaptic transmission, the mechanism by which phenytoin appears to exert much of its anticonvulsant effect.

Effects on synaptic transmitters

Acetylcholine. Phenytoin alters acetylcholine release in the brain (Woodbury, 1969). Low drug doses increase, and high doses or chronic administration decrease, the release of this neurotransmitter. The drug decreases acetylcholine biosynthesis (Mori, 1974). However, Bianchi, Beani and Bertelli (1975) showed that phenytoin increased the concentration of acetylcholine in the forebrain of the guinea pig.

Acetylcholine is a neurotransmitter in certain pathways which ascend from the mid-brain (Lewis and Shute, 1967; Shute and Lewis, 1967). To some extent these pathways may correspond with the centrencephalic integrating system of Penfield and Jasper (1954). Altered acetylcholine function in these pathways might conceivably affect primary generalized epilepsy.

Serotonin. As mentioned in Chapter 4, raised brain serotonin levels appear to correlate with protection against epilepsy. Phenytoin raises brain serotonin levels (Bonnycastle, Paasonen and Giarman, 1956; Bonnycastle, Giarman and Paasonen, 1957; Chase, Katz and Kopin, 1969), probably because the drug increases serotonin synthesis (Green and Graham Smith, 1975). Monoamine oxidase, the enzyme which mediates serotonin degradation, is said to be inhibited by phenytoin (Azzaro, Gutrecht and Smith, 1973). This action of the drug would tend to increase brain serotonin levels. However Leznicki and Dymecki (1974) failed to find monoamine oxidase inhibition when working with only slightly supratherapeutic phenytoin concentrations.

Noradrenaline. There is some correlation between raised brain noradrenaline concentrations and protection against epilepsy (Chapter 4). Phenytoin, at therapeutic concentrations (10^{-5} to 10^{-4} M) increases noradrenaline uptake into rat cerebral cortical slices (Azzaro, Gutrecht and Smith, 1963), but inhibits the uptake of this catecholamine into rat brain synaptosomes (Weinberger, Nicklas and Berl, 1976). Snider and Snider (1977) showed that phenytoin increased noradrenaline concentrations in rat hindbrain, but slightly decreased concentrations of this amine in the forebrain. Phenytoin inhibition of monoamine oxidase, mentioned above, would tend to raise brain noradrenaline levels. Deitrich and Erwin (1975) showed that phenytoin, at a slightly supratherapeutic concentration, inhibited brain aldehyde dehydrogenase. This action could delay the further biotransformation of metabolic intermediates formed from noradrenaline, but it is not known whether this would raise brain noradrenaline concentrations.

Dopamine. The evidence relating altered brain dopamine concentrations to an anti-epileptic effect is not strong. Phenytoin is known to be a brain dopamine antagonist (Mendel, Cotzias, Mena and Papavasilou, 1975). The drug blocks dopamine uptake into the striatum (Azzaro, Gutrecht and Smith, 1973). However Snider and Snider (1977) showed that the intake of phenytoin produced little change in dopamine concentrations in rat brain. This dopamine blocking action of phenytoin may be responsible for the very occasional development of dyskinesia when an overdose of the drug is given (see later).

Gamma-aminobutyrate (GABA). Phenytoin raises brain GABA concentrations, according to Vernadakis and Woodbury (1960), Saad, El Masry and Scott (1972) and Mori (1974). However in the rat cerebellum, Hitchcock and Gabra-Sanders (1977) showed that phenytoin decreased GABA concentrations. The drug reduces brain concentrations of glutamate, the metabolic precursor of GABA (Mori, 1974). Sawaya, Horton and Meldrum (1975) showed that phenytoin did not inhibit mouse brain GABA transaminase, the enzyme immediately responsible for GABA degradation. Phenytoin inhibited the next enzyme in the GABA breakdown pathway, succinate semialdehyde dehydrogenase, but only at drug concentrations at least 20 times those found therapeutically. Increased brain GABA concentrations related to phenytoin intake are therefore likely to be due to increased GABA synthesis.

Tappaz and Pacheco (1973) found that phenytoin (2×10^{-4} M) increased the intensity of the potassium chloride-stimulated release of GABA from rat cerebral cortical slices. The drug increased the uptake of GABA and its precursor glutamate by rat brain synaptosomes (Weinberger, Nicklas and Berl, 1976). However Olsen, Lamar and Bayless (1977) found that phenytoin did not alter the uptake or release of GABA by mouse brain synaptosomes.

The above findings raise the possibility that phenytoin may increase concentrations of the inhibitory transmitter GABA at synapses, but the data are somewhat equivocal. GABA is a metabolic intermediate as well as a synaptic transmitter, and local regional concentrations of the substance may not necessarily parallel GABA concentrations in the synaptic cleft.

Effects on folates

Phenytoin is one of the anticonvulsants which may cause folate deficiency (Klipstein, 1964; Malpas, Spray and Witts, 1966; Reynolds, 1976). As indicated in Chapter 4, low folate concentrations may contribute toward an anti-epileptic effect.

It has been suggested that phenytoin interferes with the absorption of dietary folates (Hoffbrand and Necheles, 1958; Rosenberg, Godwin, Strieff and Castle, 1968). However certain other findings make this action unlikely (Baugh and Krumdieck, 1969; Fehling, Jagerstand, Lindstrand and Westesson, 1973). Folate deficiency might occur if folate metabolism were inhibited prior to synthesis of biologically active folate derivatives. However, Hamfelt and Wilmanns (1965) stated that phenytoin did not inhibit dihydrofolate reductase, N^5, N^{10}-methylenetetrahydrofolate dehydrogenase or N^5, N^{10}-methylenetetrahydrofolate formylase. Narisawa, Honda, Yoshida and Arakawa (1972) found that phenytoin (50 μg/ml) did not inhibit any of the following enzymes involved in folate metabolism in rat liver: histidase, urocanase, formyliminotransferase, N^{5-10}-methylenetetrahydrofolate reductase, formyltetrahydrofolate synthetase, serine hydroxymethylase and glycine cleavage enzyme. Subsequently Arakawa, Honda and Narisawa (1973) appeared to find that phenytoin did decrease hepatic histidase activity in rats. In man they showed that phenytoin treatment caused an increased proportion of an oral dose of histidine to be excreted in urine as formiminoglutamic acid. How phenytoin produces reduced folate concentrations in man remains unclear. The clinical effects of this drug-induced folate deficiency are discussed in the section on the unwanted effects of phenytoin (p. 102).

Effects on macromolecules

Phenytoin alters macromolecule biosynthesis. If such an action alters the properties of protein molecules in cell membranes, it may conceivably change the properties of cell membranes towards the passage of small inorganic cations (Shanes, 1958). If so, this may explain how the effects of phenytoin on intracellular ion concentrations occur. Carnay and Grundfest (1974) raised the possibility that phenytoin may have an anti-epileptic action by a different type of effect on neuronal cell membranes. The drug appears to stabilize the hydrophobic configuration of macromolecules in the resting cell membrane of the frog neuromuscular junction, yet the macromolecules retain the capacity to assume the hydrophilic configuration of the excited membrane.

Phenytoin enhances the incorporation of orotic acid into ribosenucleic acid (Kemp and Woodbury, 1971). The drug at concentrations of $2-10 \times 10^{-4}$ M causes diminished ^{14}C leucine incorporation into proteins of the immature rat brain (Swaiman and Spright, 1973). At a plasma concentration of 10 μg/ml phenytoin also reduced leucine incorporation into rat cerebral cortical proteins (Jones and Woodbury, 1976). The drug at therapeutic concentrations decreased the net phosphorylation of two rat brain synaptosomal proteins of MW 60 000–63 000, and 49 000–52 000 respectively (De Lorenzo, Emple and Glaser, 1977). This effect occured irrespective of adenosine triphosphate concentration. Therefore it was unlikely to be a consequence of phenytoin having reduced the energy production in neurons. De Lorenzo and Freedman (1977) suggested that this altered synaptosomal protein phosphorylation might permit altered neurotransmitter release into the synaptic cleft. Izquierdo and Nasello (1973) showed that phenytoin prevented the increase in formation of RNA that occurs in the hippocampus following afferent stimulation in rats. However, in rat brain the drug does not inhibit DNA-dependent synthesis of RNA, catalyzed by RNA polymerase (Steinberg and Doctor, 1976).

In the present state of knowledge it is uncertain whether the various recorded effects of phenytoin on macromolecules are related to the anti-epileptic actions of the drug.

PHARMACOKINETICS

ABSORPTION AND BIOAVAILABILITY

Oral administration

Phenytoin is usually given orally, and much less frequently by intramuscular or intravenous injection. In 6 subjects Gugler, Manion and Azarnoff (1976) calculated the oral absorption rate constant to be $0 \cdot 569 \pm 0 \cdot 134$ hour^{-1}, giving an absorption half-time of $1 \cdot 62 \pm 0 \cdot 29$ hours. These authors quoted a T_{max} of $6 \cdot 0 \pm 0 \cdot 9$ hours. Gibberd and Webley (1975) quoted the T_{max} as 8–12 hours, whereas Glazko (1975) gave a figure of 4–12 hours for this parameter. Earlier figure for the T_{max} were 2–8 hours (Triedman, Fishman and Yahr, 1960), or 5 hours (O'Malley, Denckla and O'Doherty, 1969).

Absorption of the drug from the alimentary tract is reasonably complete, usually less than 5 per cent of an oral dose being passed in the faeces (personal unpublished data). Inadequate absorption of the drug is comparatively rare, if there is no excipient interaction with the drug (Tyrer, Eadie, Sutherland and Hooper, 1970; Bochner, Hooper, Tyrer and Eadie 1972). However, the papers of Kutt, Haynes and McDowell (1966) and Ramsay, Strauss, Wilder and Willmore (1978) each reported single instances of apparent impaired alimentary absorption of the drug. Booker (1975) mentioned a patient who passed apparently intact phenytoin capsules in faeces. The level of the alimentary tract at which phenytoin absorbs is not known. As the drug is a weak acid (pKa $8 \cdot 3$) it should be virtually non-ionized in the acid environment of the stomach and therefore might be expected to absorb, as other non-ionized drugs do, across the gastric mucosa. However, Woodbury (1969) pointed out that phenytoin is so insoluble at acid pH as to virtually preclude its absorption from the stomach. At small gut pH, the drug would be rather more soluble and still largely non-ionized. Therefore, orally-administered phenytoin probably absorbs at small gut level. It has been shown that phenytoin absorbs faster from the gut when the drug is in its free acid form than when given as sodium salt. However, this effect is thought due to particle size differences only (Dill, Kazenko, Wolf and Gazko, 1956). Speed of absorption, in contradistinction to amount of absorption, is probably of little significance in connection with the long-term oral use of the drug.

There have been a number of studies of phenytoin bioavailability reported since the Australasian outbreak of phenytoin intoxication alluded to above (Tyrer, Eadie, Sutherland and Hooper, 1970) was traced to a bioavailability problem (see page 96). Such studies include those of Albert, Sakmar, Hallmark, Weidler and Wagner (1974), Arnold, Gerber and Levy (1970), Gugler, Manion and Azarnoff (1976), Lund (1974), Lund, Alvan, Berlin and Alexanderson (1974), Manson, Beal, Magarey, Pollar, O'Reilly and Sansom (1975), Neuvonen, Pentikainen and Elfving (1977), Pentikainen, Neuvonen and Elfving (1975), Sansom, O'Reilly, Wiseman, Stern and Derham (1975), Stewart, Ballinger, Devlin, Miller and Ramsay (1975), Tammisto, Kauro and Viukari (1976) and Weiss, Heffelfinger and Buchanan (1969). These studies will not be discussed in detail. They have sometimes shown differences in the rate and extent of phenytoin bioavailability between different preparations. However these conclusions may apply only for the particular batches of the particular preparations studied. Further, in many of the studies, extent of bioavailability has been assessed by comparison of areas under the plasma level curves. Jusko, Koup and Alvan (1976) have pointed out the fallacies inherent in area under the curve comparisons for a drug such as phenytoin which is not eliminated by processes which follow first order kinetics. If mathematical refinements are not employed, comparisons of areas under the curves will tend to magnify differences in bioavailability of phenytoin.

The clinician should be aware that phenytoin is poorly soluble in water at physiological pH, and that its bioavailability after oral administration is just adequate in ordinary circumstances. Should anything reduce the solubility of the drug, or should gastro-intestinal transit time shorten, it is possible that the bioavailability of phenytoin may decrease to an unsatisfactory level.

Intramuscular administration
Phenytoin solutions for parenteral use are made up at a pH of approximately 12 to dissolve the drug in an acceptably small volume of fluid. When such solutions encounter a more physiological pH it seems possible that some of the drug may not remain in solution. Data are available suggesting that the absorption of phenytoin from sites of intramuscular administration is slow and unpredictable (Wallis, Kutt and McDowell, 1968), and that intramuscular injection is less efficient than oral administration in producing adequate plasma levels of the drug. Dam and Olsen (1966) found that serum phenytoin levels rose at least twice as fast when the same subjects were given the same phenytoin dose orally than when they were given it

intramuscularly. These authors also showed that serum phenytoin levels fell for a few days after oral administration was replaced with the same phenytoin dosage, given intramuscularly. Serrano, Roye, Hammer and Wilder (1973), Wilensky and Lowden (1973) and Wilder, Serrano, Ramsay and Buchanan (1974) obtained essentially similar results. Wilder and Ramsay (1976) found that it was necessary to increase phenytoin dose by about 50 per cent to maintain plasma drug levels at the same values when patients previously given phenytoin orally had to be given the drug by intramuscular injection. However, in the longer term, the same phenytoin dose given orally or intramuscularly, is said to produce the same blood level of the drug (Cantu, Schwab and Timberlake, 1968).

Serrano and Wilder (1974) showed that phenytoin crystallized out at intramuscular injection sites in rats examined 24 hours after drug administration. There also was local muscle necrosis. Wilensky and Lowden (1973) had previously demonstrated phenytoin crystals at intramuscular injection sites. On a basis of this knowledge Kostenbauder, Rapp, McGovren, Foster, Perrier, Blacker, Hulon and Kinkel (1975) developed a pharmacokinetic model for phenytoin absorption from intramuscular injection sites. This model considered the possibility of the drug crystallizing out of solution and then redissolving. These workers found the T_{max} for phenytoin absorption from intramuscular sites had a broad range of 15–25 hours, and that the ultimate bioavailability of the drug, given in this way, would be about 95 per cent.

Thus it appears that phenytoin is not very suitable for intramuscular use, because of its slow absorption.

Intravenous administration

As mentioned above, phenytoin preparations for parenteral use are made up at alkaline pH (around 12) because of the poor solubility of the drug at lower pH values. If such solutions are introduced into drip bottles containing larger volumes of fluid at more physiological pH, there is risk of the phenytoin precipitating out in the drip bottle, or in the drip tubing. Consequently, the amount of drug administered may be uncertain. If phenytoin solution is given directly into a vein, the dose that can be given safely is sometimes limited by the fact that too large a volume of undiluted solvent (propylene glycol) may produce hypotension (Wallis, Kutt and McDowell, 1968).

DISTRIBUTION

V_d

A number of values for the apparent volume of distribution of phenytoin are available. These include the following:

0.52 ± 0.04 litres kg^{-1} (Lund, Alvan, Berlin and Alexanderson, 1974)

0.52 ± 0.01 litres kg^{-1} (Gugler, Manion and Azarnoff, 1976)

0.65 litres kg^{-1*} (Kostenbauder, Rapp, McGovren, Foster, Perrier, Blacker, Hulon and Kinkel, 1975)

0.78 ± 0.11 litres kg^{-1} (Crawford, Leppik, Patrick, Anderson and Kostick, 1977)

0·9 litres kg^{-1}* (Mawer, Mellen, Rodgers, Robins and Lucas, 1974), and
in children
0·78 litres kg^{-1} (Garrettson and Jusko, 1975)
in neonates
0·80 litres kg^{-1} (Loughnan, Greenwald and Purton, 1977)
1·19±0·19 litres kg^{-1} (Painter, Pippinger, Carter and Pitlick, 1977)

*assuming 70 kg body weight.

The lowest of the values quoted corresponds reasonably with total body water. The higher values raise the possibility that phenytoin in man is not only distributed through body water but may also be bound to some tissue components.

Plasma protein binding
Published figures indicating the extent to which phenytoin is bound to plasma protein vary, e.g. 42–45 per cent (Viukari and Tammisto, 1968); 60 per cent (Vapaatalo and Lehtinen, 1971; Barlow, Firemark and Roth, 1962); 83 per cent (Eadie, Tyrer and Hooper, 1970); 88 per cent (Ehrnebo and Odar-Cederlof, 1975); 87·4 per cent (Porter and Layzer, 1975); 90 per cent (Triedman, Fishman and Yahr, 1960); 92 per cent (Lund, Lunde, Rane, Borga and Sjoqvist, 1971); 93 per cent (Kristensen, Hansen and Skovsted, 1969; Lunde, Rane, Yaffe, Lund and Sjoqvist, 1970; Barth, Alvan, Borga and Sjoqvist, 1976); 92–95 per cent (Conard, Haavik and Finger, 1971).

Some of the discrepancies in the figures may be due to the different techniques used for separating protein-bound drug from free drug in plasma, and for measuring the drug. However, the main source of the apparent discrepancies may be that different workers have carried out their measurements at different environmental temperatures. As Lunde, Rane, Yaffe, Lund and Sjoqvist (1970) and Hooper, Sutherland, Bochner, Tyrer and Eadie (1973) have shown, phenytoin binding to plasma protein lessens as temperature rises (Fig. 6.1). When correction is made for temperature effects, or when binding is measured at 37°C, the data available suggest that 80–85 per cent (Hooper, Sutherland, Bochner, Tyrer and Eadie, 1973), 89 per cent (Hooper, Bochner, Eadie and Tyrer, 1974), or 90 per cent (Lund, Berlin and Lunde, 1972) of the drug is bound to plasma protein at body temperature in man. Binding also varies with pH, increasing from 73 per cent at pH 7·0 to 82 per cent at pH 7·6 (Pruitt, Zwiren, Patterson, Dayton, Cook and Wall, 1975). Differing ages of patients in the various studies also may contribute to the discrepancies in the protein binding figures. Hooper, Bochner, Eadie and Tyrer (1974) and Hayes, Langman and Short (1975) have shown that phenytoin binding to plasma proteins decreases with advancing age.

Phenytoin binding is also proportionately less in the neonate (Ehrnebo, Agurell, Jalling and Boreus, 1971), and in children below 3 months of age (Loughnan, Greenwald and Purton, 1977). There is evidence that the extent of phenytoin binding to plasma protein is reduced by low plasma albumin levels (Hooper, Bochner, Eadie and Tyrer, 1974; Fredholm, Rane and Persson, 1975; Olsen, Bennett and Porter, 1975), and raised bilirubin (Rane, Lunde, Jalling, Yaffe and Sjoqvist, 1971; Hooper, Bochner, Eadie and Tyrer, 1974) and raised free fatty acid

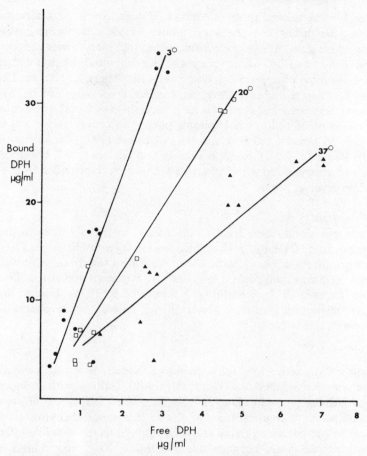

Fig. 6.1 The effect of environmental temperature on the *in vitro* binding of phenytoin to human plasma protein, studied by an equilibrium dialysis technique. Phenytoin binding decreased as temperature rose (Hooper, Sutherland, Bochner, Tyrer and Eadie, 1973).

levels (Rudman, Bixler and Del Rio, 1971; Fredholm, Rane and Persson, 1975).

The effect of other drugs on the plasma protein binding of phenytoin is discussed later (page 88).

Drug concentrations in various body fluids

Phenytoin concentrations in various body fluids, relative to the simultaneous concentration of the drug in plasma, reflect differences in the protein contents of the various fluids. Differences in pH are usually unimportant, since the pKa of phenytoin is not close enough to physiological pH.

Whole blood

Phenytoin levels in whole blood, and in plasma, were said to be similar (Dill, Kazenko, Wolf and Glazko, 1956). More recently Dill and Glazko (1972) found that their fluorimetric assay yielded considerably lower phenytoin levels for whole blood than for the plasma from this blood. Wilder, Streiff and Hammer (1972) obtained similar differences between whole blood and plasma, using a gas chromatographic assay. It seems clear that phenytoin is at a lower concentration in red blood cells than in whole plasma. The unbound phenytoin in plasma equilibrates with the phenytoin that enters red cells (Sherwin, Harvey, Leppik and Gonda, 1976). Over the plasma phenytoin concentration range of 5 to 55 μg/ml the ratio between unbound and total plasma phenytoin was found to be constant and the ratio of red blood cell to whole plasma phenytoin concentration was 0·23 : 1·0 (Kurata and Wilkinson, 1974). Hansotia and Keran (1974) found the ratio to be 0·27 : 1·0. Borondy, Dill, Chang, Buchanan and Glazko (1973) observed that the red blood cell phenytoin to whole plasma phenytoin ratio provided a good measure of phenytoin level in plasma water.

Cerebrospinal fluid
Since phenytoin should be virtually non-ionized at the pH of both plasma and cerebrospinal fluid, the latter with its low protein level might be expected to be in effect an ultrafiltrate of blood plasma with respect to the drug. It proves to be so (Triedman, Fishman and Yahr, 1960; Barlow, Firemark and Roth, 1962; Lund, Berlin and Lunde, 1972; Schmidt and Kupferberg, 1975; Troupin and Friel, 1975). CSF phenytoin levels are about 10 per cent of whole plasma phenytoin concentrations.

Saliva
After absorption, phenytoin is found in saliva (Noach, Woodbury and Goodman, 1958; Svensmark, Schiller and Buchthal, 1960). Saliva, with a mean protein content of 262 mg per cent (Drevon and Donikian, 1956), would appear to be virtually equivalent to an ultrafiltrate of plasma in so far as phenytoin is concerned. Differences in pH between plasma and saliva should have negligible effects on the distribution of phenytoin between the two fluids. The drug should be almost non-ionized in both fluids, since the pH of each fluid is significantly more acid than the pKa of phenytoin. The study of Bochner, Hooper, Sutherland, Eadie and Tyrer (1974) confirmed the expected finding of a close correlation (almost a 1:1 ratio) between plasma water and salivary phenytoin concentrations (Fig. 6.2). These workers suggested using salivary phenytoin levels as a convenient measure of plasma water phenytoin concentration.

The findings of Bochner, Hooper, Sutherland, Eadie and Tyrer (1974) have been confirmed by a number of workers (Cook, Amerson, Poole, Lesser and O'Tauma, 1975; Schmidt and Kupferberg, 1975; Troupin and Friel, 1975; Horning, Brown, Nowling, Letratanangkoon, Kellaway and Zion, 1977; McAuliffe, Sherwin, Leppik, Fayle and Pippinger, 1977; Paxton, Rowell, Ratcliffe, Lambie, Nanda, Melville and Johnson, 1977). These workers' result have been in close agreement *viz.* that salivary phenytoin level is 10–12 per cent of the simultaneous whole plasma phenytoin level, providing that plasma protein binding of the drug is normal.

Milk
Human milk has a protein content of about 1 gram per cent, which is appreciably

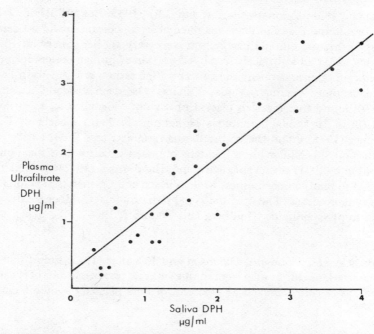

Fig. 6.2 The correlation between the simultaneous concentrations of phenytoin in plasma ultrafiltrate and in saliva in 26 patients (Bochner, Hooper, Sutherland, Eadie and Tyrer, 1974).

higher than that of cerebrospinal fluid or saliva. Therefore, on the basis of plasma protein binding data for the drug, one might anticipate that phenytoin levels in milk would be about 20–25 per cent of simultaneous plasma levels of the drug, so long as phenytoin entered milk mainly by passive diffusion, as appears to be the case. For one patient Svensmark, Schiller and Buchthal (1960) found a phenytoin concentration in milk of 6 μg/ml when the drug concentration in plasma was 28 μg/ml. Mirkin (1971) stated that phenytoin levels in milk were approximately 25–50 per cent of those in plasma. Rane, Garle, Borga and Sjoqvist (1974) found the concentration of phenytoin in the milk of a single patient was 45 per cent of her plasma phenytoin concentration.

Concentrations in tissues
The distribution of phenytoin in the body of the rat was described by Noach, Woodbury and Goodman (1958). For at least the first four hours after administration, drug concentrations were highest in liver, salivary gland and kidney, and lower in fat, muscle and brain, the levels in the latter organ being slightly above the plasma phenytoin concentration. Illustrations of whole body autoradiographs of the distribution of phenytoin in the squirrel monkey have been published (van der Kleijn, Guelen, van Wijk and Baars, 1975).

Brain
In experimental animals, brain phenytoin levels are similar to, or a little higher than, simultaneous phenytoin levels in whole plasma or serum (Noach, Woodbury

and Goodman, 1958; Firemark, Barlow and Roth, 1963; Lee and Bass, 1970). The latter authors found that simultaneous phenytoin concentrations in rat cerebrum, basal ganglia, brain stem and cerebellum were very similar. Sherwin, Eisen and Sokolowski (1973), in a surgically removed portion of human epileptogenic brain, found the brain to plasma phenytoin concentration ratio was 1·5 : 1·0. In 12 human temporal lobectomy specimens Vajda, Williams, Davidson, Falconer and Brecken-ridge (1974) found that brain to plasma phenytoin concentration ratios averaged 0·75±0·19 : 1·0. In similar specimens Houghton, Richens, Toseland, Davidson and Falconer (1975) found the brain : plasma ratio averaged 1·04 : 1.

In studies on subcellular brain fractions obtained by ultracentrifugation Kemp and Woodbury (1971) and Yanagihara and Hamburger (1971) showed that the drug tended to bind to microsomes, while Nielsen and Cotman (1971) found that it bound to synaptosomes. The drug binds to brain proteins (Goldberg and Todoroff, 1973) and to phospholipids (Goldberg and Todoroff, 1976).

Other tissues
Houghton, Richens, Toseland, Davidson and Falconer (1975) found that pheny-toin concentrations in human temporalis muscle averaged 60 per cent, and concentrations in skin averaged 53 per cent, of total plasma phenytoin concentra-tions.

Concentrations in the fetus
Phenytoin concentrations are similar in neonatal umbilical cord plasma and in maternal plasma (Mirkin, 1971). Harbison, Olubadewo, Dwivedi and Rama Sastry (1975) claimed the human placenta concentrated phenytoin by means of an energy-dependent mechanism.

ELIMINATION

Pharmacokinetic Parameters

Elimination rate
In the past the elimination of phenytoin was analyzed as if it followed first order kinetics. Suzuki, Saitoh and Nishihara (1970) collected much of the information on phenytoin half-life that was then available. One of the more extensive studies was that of Arnold and Gerber (1970) who found that the drug in man had a mean half-life of 22± 9 hours. More recent figures for phenytoin elimination, expressed in terms of the drug's half-life, are 14·5± 1·2 hours (Lund, Alvan, Berlin and Alexanderson, 1974); 18·3 hours (Kostenbauder, Rapp, McGovren, Foster, Perrier, Blacker, Hulon and Kinkel, 1975) and 16·8± 1·3 hours for a β phase half-life (Gugler, Manion and Azarnoff, 1976).

Dayton, Cucinell, Weiss and Perel (1967) noted that the plasma half-life of phenytoin in dogs was dose-related, being longer at higher drug doses than at lower doses. Subsequently Garrettson and Kim (1970) showed that the rate of decline of plasma phenytoin levels in two overdosed children was not monoexponential. (An example of this phenomenon in an adult is shown in Fig. 6.3). Urinary excretion of the main phenytoin metabolite, p-hydroxyphenytoin was virtually unaltered in the two overdosed children while plasma drug levels fell from 43·8 and 47·6 μg/ml to, respectively, 11·8 and 25·2 μg/ml. These findings suggested that the rate of phenytoin elimination in humans could become saturated under conditions encountered in treatment. Dayton and Perel (1971) obtained evidence that the half-life of phenytoin in man was dose-dependent. Bochner, Hooper, Tyrer and

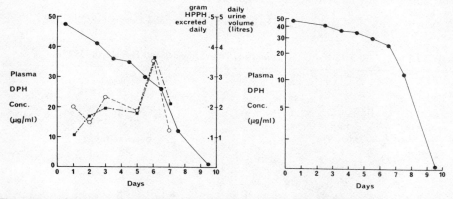

Fig. 6.3 Rate of decline in plasma phenytoin (DPH) concentration (solid line) in an overdosed patient in whom therapy was ceased on day 0. Data are plotted on a linear and on a logarithmic scale. Daily urinary excretion (solid squares; broken line) of the phenytoin metabolite p-hydroxyphenytoin (HPPH) is relatively constant despite the fall in plasma phenytoin level. Excretion of this metabolite appears dependent on urine volume (open circles; broken line). The findings are consistent with capacity-limited formation of HPPH when plasma phenytoin levels are above 20 μg/ml.

Eadie (1972a) showed that the relation between steady-state plasma phenytoin level and drug dose in the individual was not linear (see page 81), whereas linearity would be expected if monoexponential kinetics applied. These authors also showed that the stage of disproportionate rise in steady-state plasma phenytoin concentration was associated with saturation of capacity to metabolize the drug to p-hydroxyphenytoin.

In recent years it has been increasingly appreciated that the elimination of phenytoin is more appropriately described in terms of Michaelis-Menten than of first order kinetics. Thus it is not strictly appropriate to speak of a half-life for the drug's elimination, though conclusions drawn from the phenytoin half-lives cited above are not likely to lead to gross errors so long as phenytoin levels in plasma do not exceed the therapeutic range. In the exact sense, phenytoin elimination almost certainly follows simultaneous mixed first-order and Michaelis-Menten kinetics. As will be discussed later, a small proportion of a phenytoin dose is eliminated by simple renal excretion, which is a first-order process. Some published values for the Michaelis-Menten kinetic parameters of phenytoin are given below.

Clearance
Cranford, Lepkik, Patrick, Anderson and Kostick (1977) obtained a mean value of 0·0157±0·9132 litres kg^{-1} hour^{-1} for phenytoin clearance, and Gugler, Manion and Azarnoff (1976) a mean value of 0·022±0·002 litres kg^{-1} hour^{-1}. Hayes,

Published values for the Michaelis-Kinetic parameters of phenytoin.

K_m (μg/ml)	V_{max} (mg/kg/day)	Author
6·77	6·1	Gerber and Wagner (1972)
14·4	16·3	Atkinson and Shaw (1973)
3·8	8·0	Mawer, Mullen, Rodgers, Robins and Lucas (1974)
4·0	—	Richens (1974)
5·8 (adults)	8·1	Eadie, Tyrer, Bochner and Hooper (1976)
5·3 (children)	12·5	
11·5±5·0	10·3±2·1	Martin, Tozer, Sheiner and Riegelman (1977)

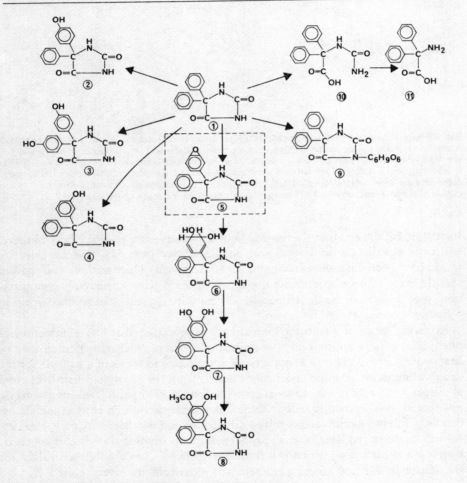

Fig. 6.4 First stage-biotransformation products of phenytoin.
1. phenytoin (DPH-diphenylhydantoin).
2. 5-(p-hydroxyphenyl)-5-phenylhydantoin (p-HPPH), the main metabolite in man (Butler, 1957; Noach, Woodbury and Goodman, 1958; Maynert, 1960).
3. 5-5-bis(4-hydroxyphenyl) hydantoin, a minor metabolite found in rat urine (Woodbury, 1969) and human urine (Thompson, Beghin, Fife and Gerber, 1976).

Langman and Short (1975) showed that phenytoin clearance in persons under 45 years (0.0422 ± 0.0056 litres kg^{-1} $hour^{-1}$) was greater than its clearance in persons over 65 years (0.0261 ± 0.037 litres kg^{-1} $hour^{-1}$). Guelen (1975) published figures showing a progressive decline in phenytoin clearance from 0.064 litres kg^{-1} $hour^{-1}$ in children younger than 5 years, to 0.021 litres kg^{-1} $hour^{-1}$ in adults aged 26 to 35 years.

Percentage excreted unchanged

Only about 5 per cent of phenytoin dose is excreted unchanged in urine (Glazko, Chang, Baukema, Dill, Goulet and Buchanan, 1969).

Biotransformation

Biotransformation pattern

The liver is the only known site of phenytoin biotransformation. Phenytoin oxidation occurs in the liver microsomes, utilizing the non-specific mixed oxidase pathway (Kutt and Verebely, 1970). A number of metabolites have been described in animals and man, the pattern of metabolism differing to some extent from species to species (see Fig. 6.4, in which those metabolites thus far found in man are indicated). The major metabolite in man is the para isomer of 5-hydroxyphenyl-5-phenylhydantoin (p-HPPH). Pharmacologically it is thought to be relatively inactive (Butler, 1957). However, there is some evidence that at least one phenytoin metabolite present in plasma inhibits the leucocyte enzyme transketolase (Markkanen, Peltola, Himanen and Riekkinen, 1971). Most of the hydroxylated metabolites are conjugated with glucuronic acid in the liver and then enter the blood or the bile. Direct glucuronide conjugation of the hydantoin ring also occurs (Smith, Daves, Lynn and Gerber, 1977). The conjugated metabolites in bile may undergo an entero-hepatic circulation, probably after some of the conjugates are hydrolyzed in the gut by the enzyme β-glucuronidase (Smith and Williams, 1966). The metabolites are then resorbed from the gut into the blood

---

4. 5-(m-hydroxyphenyl)-5-phenylhydantoin (m-HPPH) found in human urine in small amounts (Atkinson, MacGee, Strong, Garteiz and Gaffney, 1970; Dill, Baukema, Chang and Glazko, 1971; Butler, Dudley, Johnson and Roberts, 1976). It may not be a natural metabolite, but may form as a result of acid hydrolysis of metabolite 6 during isolation of metabolites from urine (Atkinson, MacGee, Strong, Garteiz and Gaffney, 1970; Chang, Savory and Glazko, 1970; Gerber, Weller, Lynn, Rangno, Sweetman and Bush, 1971).
5. a postulated, short-lived epoxide metabolite (Glazko, 1973).
6. a dihydrodiol metabolite [5-(3,4-dihydroxyl-1,5-cyclohexadiene-1-yl)-5-phenylhydantoin], probably occurring in man (Atkinson, MacGee, Strong, Garteiz and Gaffney, 1970; Chang, Savory and Glazko, 1970; Gerber, Weller, Lynn, Rangno, Sweetman, and Bush, 1971; Horning, Stratton, Wilson, Horning and Hill, 1971)
7. a catechol metabolite [5-(3,4-dihydroxyphenyl)-5-phenylhydantoin] found in rat urine (Woodbury, 1969; Chang, Okerholm and Glazko, 1972-a; Borga, Garle and Gutova, 1973; Gerber, Seibert and Thompson, 1973) and in human urine (Midha, Hindmarsh, McGilveray and Cooper, 1977).
8. a methylated catechol metabolite [5-(4-hydroxy-3-methoxyphenyl)-5-phenylhydantoin], found in rats (Chang, Okerholm and Glazko, 1972b; Gerber, Seibert and Thompson, 1973) and in man (Midha, Hindmarsh, McGilveray and Cooper, 1977).
9. an N-glucuronide of phenytoin, found in rat and human urine, and apparently formed without prior hydroxylation (Smith, Daves, Lynn and Gerber, 1977).
10 & 11. diphenylhydantoic acid and α-amino-diphenylacetic acid, possible metabolites described in early studies in man (Kozelka and Hine, 1943), but not confirmed since. The former has been identified in rat urine (Chang, Savory and Glazko, 1970).

stream. The main metabolite, p-HPPH, in conjugated form can be found in plasma in measurable concentrations between 30 and 60 minutes after the drug is taken by mouth for the first time (Fig. 6.5). In biochemical systems *in vitro* there is evidence that p-HPPH exerts a product inhibition on the liver enzymatic reaction by which it is formed from phenytoin (Ashley and Levy, 1972, 1973; Borondy, Chang and

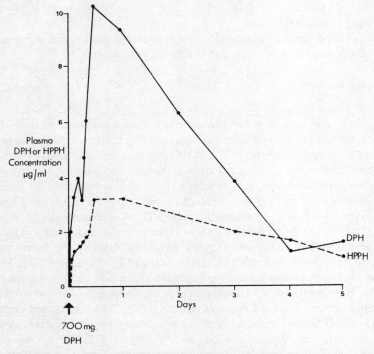

Fig. 6.5 Time-courses of plasma phenytoin (DPH) and 5-(p-hydroxyphenyl)-5-phenylhydantoin (HPPH) levels in a patient following his first oral dose of phenytoin (700 mg).

Glazko, 1972). Batt, Ziegler and Siest (1975) showed that HPPH is also a competitive inhibitor of various glucuronidations which occur in rat liver. Glazko (1973, 1975) stated that the catechol and methylated catechol metabolites of phenytoin also inhibited the drug's biotransformation to p-HPPH. Albert, Hallmark, Sakmar, Weidler and Wagner (1974), on the basis of plasma concentrations of unconjugated p-HPPH, expressed the view that significant product inhibition of phenytoin metabolism was unlikely in man if therapeutic doses of phenytoin were taken.

In man, plasma concentrations of unconjugated p-HPPH are less than 6 per cent (Albert, Hallmark, Sakmar, Weidler and Wagner, 1974), or about 1 per cent (Hoppel, Garle, Rane and Sjoquist, 1977) of simultaneous whole plasma phenytoin levels. Most of the p-HPPH in plasma is present in conjugated form and is excreted as such in urine (Maynert, 1960) though small amounts can be found in faeces (Bocher, Hooper, Tyrer and Eadie, 1972b). Plasma levels of conjugated p-HPPH are in the range 1·2 to 4·5 μg/ml when whole plasma phenytoin levels lie between 5 and 30 µg/ml (Hoppel, Garle, Rane and Sjoqvist, 1977). Total plasma levels of p-HPPH are not closely related to total plasma phenytoin levels (Bochner, Hooper, Sutherland, Eadie and Tyrer, 1973; Wilson, Hojer and Rane, 1976; Fig. 6.6). If anything, the relation between the two is an inverse one. Data from *in vitro* studies are available suggesting that 81–84 per cent of p-HPPH in plasma is bound to

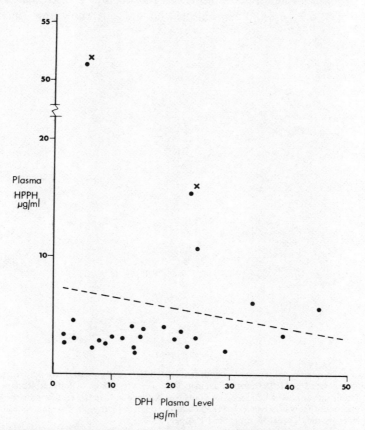

Fig. 6.6 The lack of correlation between plasma concentrations of 5-(p-hydroxyphenyl)-5-phenylhydantoin (HPPH) and phenytoin (DPH) in 26 subjects. The two points with the x superscript are from patients with uraemia (Bochner, Hooper, Tyrer and Eadie, 1973).

plasma protein (Conard, Haavik and Finger, 1971), but in this work p-HPPH itself, rather than p-HPPH glucuronide, was used. The latter is the form in which most of metabolite is present in plasma. Ultrafiltration data suggest that a mean of 44 per cent of HPPH conjugate in human plasma is protein-bound (Bochner, Hooper, Sutherland, Tyer and Eadie, 1973).

Quantitative aspects

Figures for the percentage of a given phenytoin dose excreted in urine as conjugated and unconjugated p-HPPH vary, e.g. 60 per cent (Maschner and Bernhardt, 1973), 75 per cent (Glazko, Chang, Baukema, Dill, Goulet and

Buchanan, 1969), 81 per cent (Karlén, Garle, Rane, Gutova and Lindborg, 1975), 59–88 per cent (Borofsky, Louis and Kutt, 1973). Eadie, Tyrer, Bochner and Hooper (1976) correlated steady-state plasma phenytoin levels with drug doses and daily urine p-HPPH output in four closely studied subjects. In three of the four, the proportion of the phenytoin dose that was excreted as p-HPPH decreased as phenytoin dose rose, though the subjects still remained in a steady state as regards the drug (Figs. 6.7, 6.8). The subject who did not show this phenomenon

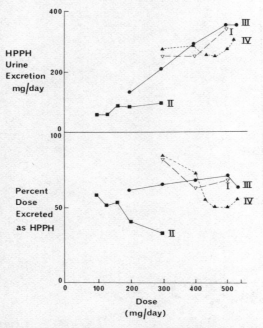

Fig. 6.7 Mean daily urinary excretion of p-hydroxyphenytoin (HPPH), and mean percentage of daily phenytoin dose excreted as HPPH plotted against daily phenytoin dose in four subjects in whom steady-state conditions applied when measurements were carried out. In the steady-state the proportion of the phenytoin dose that was excreted as HPPH tended to fall as phenytoin dose increased in three of the four subjects (Eadie, Tyrer, Bochner and Hooper, 1976).

progressively accumulated the drug once his plasma phenytoin level exceeded 12 μg/ml, despite an unaltered phenytoin dose (Fig. 6.9). These findings suggest that biotransformation of phenytoin to metabolites other than p-HPPH may become increasingly important as a means of eliminating the drug as its dose is increased.

Excretion
Small amounts of a phenytoin dose leave the body in faeces, unchanged or as p-HPPH, according to the findings of Bochner, Hooper, Tyrer and Eadie (1972b). Most of a given phenytoin dose is finally excreted in urine as the p-HPPH glucuronide conjugate, and about 5 per cent is present in urine as unmetabolized drug (Glazko, Chang, Baukema, Dill, Goulet and Buchanan, 1969). There is a

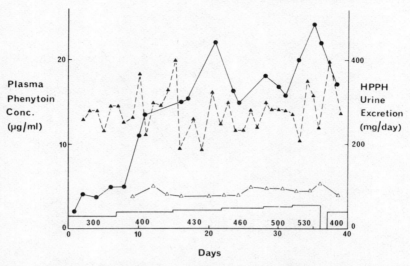

Fig. 6.8 In one subject urinary excretion of p-hydroxyphenytoin (HPPH: solid triangles) and plasma levels of this substance (open triangles) remained virtually constant despite phenytoin dosage increments which produced substantial changes in plasma phenytoin concentrations (solid circles). It seems likely that an increasing proportion of the phenytoin dose was converted to metabolites other than HPPH as phenytoin dose was increased (Eadie, Tyrer, Bochner and Hooper, 1976).

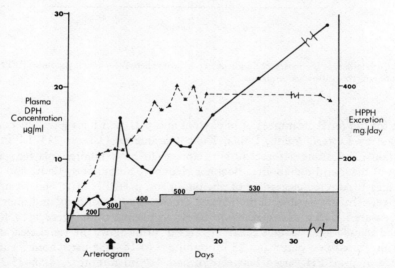

Fig. 6.9 In one subject plasma phenytoin level (solid circles) and daily urinary excretion of p-hydroxyphenytoin (p-HPPH: solid triangles) increased in proportion as phenytoin dose was increased from 200 mg per day to 500 mg per day. However, a further phenytoin dose increase to 530 mg per day produced no further increase in urinary excretion of p-HPPH and, over a 6 week period, a slow progressive rise in plasma phenytoin concentration occurred.

linear relation between urine p-HPPH excretion rate and plasma p-HPPH concentration in an individual (Dill, Baukema, Chang and Glazko, 1971; Fig. 6.10).

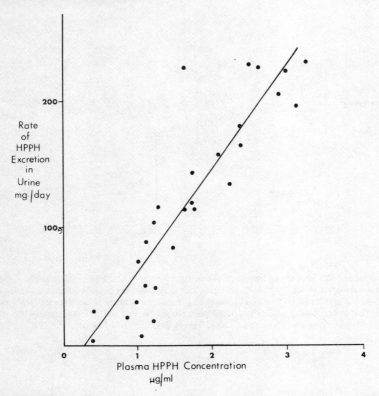

Fig. 6.10 Correlation between urine excretion of 5-(p-hydroxyphenyl)-5-phenylhydantoin (HPPH) and concentration of this substance in plasma.

Data for the renal clearances of phenytoin and p-HPPH for a few subjects were published by Letteri, Mellk, Louis, Kutt, Durante and Glazko (1971). In their calculation of clearances these authors appear to have ignored plasma protein binding of drug and metabolite. Bochner, Hooper, Sutherland, Eadie and Tyrer (1973) measured renal clearances of phenytoin and p-HPPH in 16 and 14 subjects respectively. In these subjects the plasma protein binding of drug and metabolite were measured. Drug and metabolite levels in plasma water were used for the clearance calculations. Over a range of rates of urine flow, the renal clearance of phenytoin varied between 3 and 23 ml minute^{-1} ($0·18–1·38$ litres hour^{-1}) and the clearance of p-HPPH varied between 76 and 420 ml minute^{-1} ($4·56–25·2$ litres hour^{-1}) in persons whose simultaneous creatinine clearances were in the range 83 to 148 ml minute^{-1} ($4·98–8·88$ litres hour^{-1}). The clearances varied with rate of urine excretion, as shown in Figs. 6.11 and 6.12. The data suggest that phenytoin is handled by the kidney in the manner of a lipid-soluble substance which is filtered through the glomeruli and then passively resorbed across the renal tubules when water is resorbed. The more water-soluble p-HPPH glucuronide would appear to undergo active secretion into tubular urine (as do other glucuronides), but also some resorption from urine.

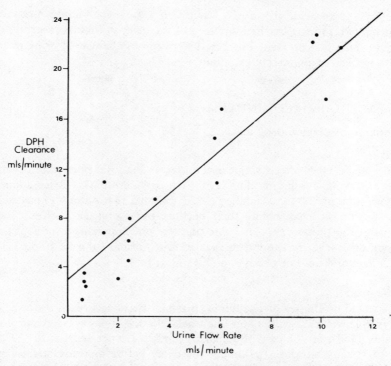

Fig. 6.11 The relation between renal clearance of phenytoin (DPH) and urine flow rate (Bochner, Hooper, Tyrer and Eadie, 1973).

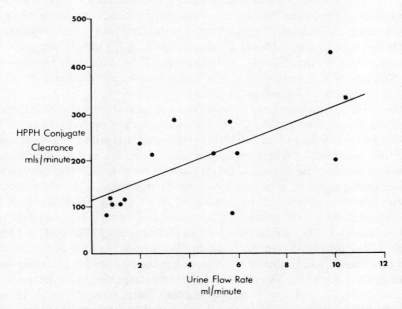

Fig. 6.12 The relation between renal clearance of 5-(p-hydroxyphenyl)-5-phenylhydantoin (conjugated to glucuronic acid) and urine flow rate (Bochner, Hooper, Tyrer and Eadie, 1973).

Phenytoin is an acid with a pK_a value above 8. Urine should rarely become alkaline enough to increase the ionization of the drug so that its resorption across the renal tubule is decreased. For practical purposes changes of urine pH should have little effect on phenytoin excretion.

CLINICAL PHARMACOKINETICS

Time-course of plasma drug levels

Single dose

As mentioned earlier, after a single oral dose (see Fig. 6.5) phenytoin plasma level rises to a peak in 2–8 hours. The level then declines slowly. After a single oral phenytoin dose of 700 mg, Handley (1970) claimed that plasma phenytoin levels showed a biphasic peak before their decline, but Siersbaek-Nielsen, Skovsted, Hansen and Kristensen (1971) failed to find this phenomenon. A monophasic peak in plasma drug level was found in each of four normal subjects studied in detail after a single oral dose of phenytoin (Figs. 2.1, 6.5).

Repeated doses

With repeated oral doses of phenytoin, plasma drug levels reach a steady state in 2–7 days (Svensmark, Schiller and Buchthal, 1960), 4–8 days (Triedman, Fishman and Yahr, 1960), or 7–8 days (Buchanan, Kinkel, Goulet and Smith, 1972). The higher the phenytoin dose the longer the delay before a steady state is attained (Buchthal, 1960). This is understandable since phenytoin elimination rate is dose dependent, the half-life appearing to be longer at higher doses. (It requires the passage of five half-lives to attain 97 per cent of final steady state plasma levels). Bearing in mind the limitations of parenteral phenytoin therapy mentioned earlier, this behaviour of plasma phenytoin level with time after oral administration suggests the need to use oral loading doses of the drug if a rapid therapeutic effect is desired. Thus Wilder, Serrano and Ramsay (1973) found that an oral loading dose of 1 gram of phenytoin produced plasma phenytoin levels above 7·5 μg/ml in 14 out of 15 subjects within 8 to 24 hours.

In the steady state, Loeser (1961) showed that the same daily phenytoin dose gave similar blood levels of the drug, whether this dose was taken once or twice daily. Svensmark, Schiller and Buchtal (1960) found that with twice daily dosages, steady-state plasma phenytoin levels fluctuated through a ±10 per cent range throughout the day. Buchanan, Kinkel, Goulet and Smith (1972) compared the effects of giving the drug once daily, and three times a day. They showed that the different dosage intervals had no significant effect on the fluctuations in blood phenytoin level, which varied through a range of 2–3 μg/ml during the day. Haerer and Buchanan (1972), Strandjord and Johannessen (1972) and Wilder and Serrano (1973) obtained similar findings. Buchanan, Turner and Heffelfinger (1973) confirmed these results in children in a cross-over study. They showed that the change from multiple to single daily phenytoin doses caused no deterioration in control of epilepsy, and that plasma phenytoin levels were the same 12 and 24 hours after a single daily drug dose. Cocks, Critchley, Hayward, Owen, Mawer and Woodcock (1975) in another cross-over study obtained very similar results.

Vajda, Merory and Bladin (1975) illustrated clinically insignificant fluctuations in steady-state plasma phenytoin concentration over 24 hours in patients after once daily phenytoin dosage. At first sight it may appear surprising that steady-state plasma phenytoin levels should vary so little over 24 hours, when the level shows a definite peak after a single oral dose (Fig. 6.5). However single dose studies are often carried out on fasting subjects. In such circumstances the drug may reach the small intestine comparatively quickly, and may therefore absorb more rapidly than when taken by non-fasting patients during routine therapy. In the latter circumstance phenytoin absorption rate may be close to phenytoin elimination rate over much of a 24 hour dosage interval. This is particularly likely when plasma phenytoin levels are above 10 μg/ml, since the elimination of the drug is then more a zero order than a first order process. Instances such as those illustrated in Figs. 6.13 and 12.3 show how little steady-state plasma phenytoin concentrations change in the hours following an oral phenytoin dose. It would appear that oral phenytoin need not be taken more often than once a day if steady-state plasma drug levels are above 10 μg/ml and are producing a satisfactory clinical effect. As Strandjord and Johannessen (1974) pointed out, this conclusion may not be valid for lower plasma phenytoin levels. Here phenytoin will be eliminated more rapidly and plasma phenytoin levels will show greater proportionate fluctuations over 24 hours. It would also appear that so-called 'delayed action' preparations of phenytoin are unnecessary. On a molar dosage basis one of these preparations (containing phenytoin as the free acid rather than the sodium salt) did not produce higher blood phenytoin levels than ordinary preparations of the drug (Bochner, Hooper, Tyrer and Eadie, 1972c).

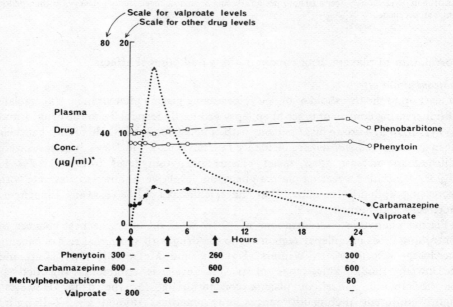

Fig. 6.13 Time-courses of steady state plasma concentrations of phenytoin, phenobarbitone and carbamazepine over a 24 hour period in a patient given a single oral dose of sodium valproate. Plasma levels of the first three anticonvulsants remained reasonably constant over the duration of the study.

Phenytoin absorbs slowly from sites of intramuscular administration (see page 54). This makes it difficult to achieve plasma phenytoin levels above 10 g/ml in previously untreated patients within 24 hours of commencing intramuscular phenytoin therapy when using volumes of the injection material which can be tolerated. The injected phenytoin may subsequently be released into plasma for several days, maintaining plasma phenytoin levels for some time after therapy is ceased. These points are illustrated in Fig. 6.14.

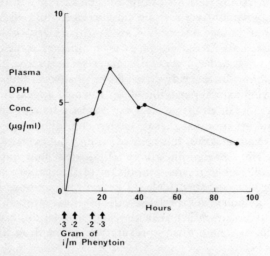

Fig. 6.14 Time course of plasma phenytoin (DPH) concentrations in a 48 kg patient given 1000 mg of the drug in divided doses over a 20 hour period. Plasma phenytoin levels did not achieve the therapeutic range at any stage.

Correlation of plasma drug concentrations and clinical effects

Anticonvulsant effects
At least up to the threshold of toxicity, increasing plasma phenytoin levels correlate with increasing control of types of epilepsy ordinarily responsive to the drug. Lund (1974) followed a group of 32 persons with epilepsy for 3 years. He found that their mean annual *grand mal* seizure incidence rate fell from 5·8 to 1·6 as drug doses were adjusted to increase their mean plasma phenytoin level from 6·1 ± 2·9 to 15·0 ± 2·5 μg/ml. Increasing plasma phenytoin levels were shown to correlate with decreasing epileptiform activity in the telemetered EEG (Rowan, Pippenger, McGregor and French, 1975).

Plasma phenytoin concentrations of 10 to 20 μg/ml offer the best chances of controlling types of epilepsy responsive to the drug with a minimal risk of causing overdosage effects (Kutt, Winters, Kokenge and McDowell, 1964; Kutt and McDowell, 1968). This range of plasma levels is commonly regarded as the 'therapeutic range' of plasma concentrations for the drug. However, slightly different therapeutic ranges are sometimes quoted e.g. 7–15 μg/ml (Loiseau, Brachet Liermain, Legroux and Jogeix, 1977); 5–15 μg/ml (Van Meter, Buckmaster and Shelley, 1970); 12–15 μg/ml (Van der Kleijn, Guelen, Van Wijk and Baars, 1975); 12–25 μg/ml (Norell, Lilienberg and Gamstorp, 1975); 15–25 μg/ml (Buchthal and Lennox-Buchthal, 1972); 5–22 μg/ml (Winek, 1976). Lund, Jorgensen and Kuhl (1964) found that plasma phenytoin levels below 10 μg/ml did not control frequently occurring major convulsions. Buchthal, Svensmark and Schiller (1960) found that 96 per cent of epileptics obtained significant benefit once the plasma phenytoin level was above 15 μg/ml, while EEG abnormalities began to improve once the plasma drug level exceeded 10 μg/ml. Norell, Lilienberg and Gamstorp (1975) found that plasma phenytoin levels above 13 μg/ml always controlled mild epilepsy, levels above 19 μg/ml controlled severe epilepsy and that the most severe grades of epilepsy could not be controlled, regardless of plasma phenytoin level.

For most purposes a plasma phenytoin therapeutic range of 10–20 μg/ml proves satisfactory. Thus, Reynolds, Chadwick and Galbraith (1976) used phenytoin as the sole anticonvulsant in 31 previously untreated epileptic patients who had types of seizures which were likely to respond to the drug. By adjusting drug doses to achieve plasma phenytoin levels between 10 and 20 μg/ml they attained satisfactory seizure control in 90 per cent of these patients.

It is clear that some patients achieve seizure control with plasma phenytoin levels below 10 μg/ml. It is also known that plasma phenytoin levels above the therapeutic range are sometimes associated with worsening control of epilepsy. In these latter circumstances dosage reduction, with lower plasma drug levels, leads to better seizure control (Levy and Fenichel, 1976; Perlo and Schwab, 1969; Lascelles, Kocen and Reynolds, 1970; Troupin and Ojemann, 1976).

The therapetutic range for plasma water phenytoin levels might be expected to be 1–2 μg/ml, i.e. 10 per cent of the value of the range in whole plasma. As pointed out above, plasma water and salivary phenytoin levels are similar. Reynolds, Ziroyanis, Jones and Smith, 1976) quoted a salivary phenytoin therapeutic range of 1–2·5 μg/ml.

Other therapeutic effects

Bigger, Schmidt, and Kutt (1968) showed that 80 per cent of the cardiac arrhythmias which will respond to phenytoin do so at plasma phenytoin levels below 18 μg/ml. Pain in 8 cases of Fabry's disease was controlled by plasma phenytoin levels above 4 μg/ml (Lockman, Hunninghake, Krivit and Desnick, 1973). Eadie (in press) noted that plasma phenytoin levels between 2 and 10 μg/ml often sufficed to prevent attacks of both 'hemiparaesthetic' and basilar artery migraine.

Unwanted effects

Some information is available correlating plasma phenytoin levels with toxic effects of the drug on the nervous system and on the gums.

Neurotoxicity. Horizontal nystagmus tends to appear when plasma phenytoin levels reach 20 μg/ml, though in some patients this sign may be absent even at much higher plasma drug levels (Perlo and Schwab, 1969). Haerer and Grace (1969) stated that 90 per cent of patients with plasma phenytoin levels above 25 μg/ml showed nystagmus. Livingstone, Berman and Pauli (1975) commented that most patients tolerate plasma phenytoin levels below 25 μg/ml, that levels of

30 μg/ml are likely to be associated with nystagmus, diplopia and ataxia, and levels of 50 μg/ml with extreme lethargy and coma. These conclusions are in general agreement with the earlier views of Kutt and McDowell (1968) and Buchthal and Svensmark (1959). However the former authors set a plasma phenytoin level of 40 μg/ml as the threshold for drowsiness. Wilder, Buchanan and Serrano (1973) studied plasma drug levels in phenytoin-intoxicated patients. They found that depression of consciousness was relieved when plasma phenytoin levels fell below 40 μg/ml.

Booker and Darcey (1973) studied the correlation between phenytoin levels in plasma water and manifestations of drug toxicity. They found no toxic effect with plasma water phenytoin levels below 1·5 μg/ml. Mild toxicity occurred at plasma water phenytoin concentrations of 1·5–3·0 μg/ml, and definite clinical intoxication at higher phenytoin concentrations. These authors considered that toxicity correlated more closely with plasma water drug levels than with whole plasma drug levels. However, Riker, Downes, Olsen and Smith (1978) failed to find a correlation between phenytoin concentrations in plasma water and the presence of nystagmus.

Undesirable effects of phenytoin may develop insidiously even with plasma phenytoin levels in the therapeutic range, and these effects become more obvious as the plasma drug levels rise further. Thus Reynolds and Travers (1974) showed a statistical correlation between increasing plasma phenytoin levels (within the therapeutic range) and psychomotor slowing, intellectual deterioration, personality change and the development of psychiatric illness. Unwanted effects of phenytoin, of a type usually associated with drug overdosage, may occasionally occur with therapeutic or even subtherapeutic plasma phenytoin levels. Eadie and Tyrer (1977) described a ballerina whose dancing performance was affected by ataxia when her plasma phenytoin levels exceeded 5 μg/ml, and a patient with old brain stem damage who developed ataxia of gait at a plasma phenytoin concentration of 6 μg/ml. In such instances drug concentrations insufficient to disturb balance in ordinary persons were sufficient to impair balance in circumstances where severe functional demands were made on the body's balance mechanism, or where the balance mechanism was already defective.

Rarely phenytoin intoxication may cause dyskinesia, usually choreiform. This phenomenon has been noted at plasma phenytoin concentrations of 40 μg/ml and 56 μg/ml (Kooiker and Sumi, 1974), at 51·0 μg/ml, 42·5 μg/ml, 30·0 μg/ml and 26·5 μg/ml (Ahmad, Laidlaw, Houghton, and Richens, 1975), and in another two cases at levels above 30 μg/ml (McLellan and Swash, 1974).

Plasma phenytoin levels above 30 μg/ml are occasionally associated with depression of mood rather than with the more common triad of nystagmus, diplopia and ataxia (Eadie, in press). In one patient Spector, Davidoff and Schwartzman (1976) found total external ophthalmoplegia in the presence of unimpaired consciousness, associated with a plasma phenytoin level of 36 μg/ml. Direkze and Fernando (1977) noted widespread fasciculation in one patient with plasma phenytoin levels of 12–14 μg/ml. These involuntary movements stopped when phenytoin was ceased.

Birket-Smith and Krogh (1971) described slowing in the motor conduction velocity of the deep peroneal nerve in patients with plasma phenytoin levels above

30 μg/ml. Chokroverty and Rubino (1973) and Chokroverty and Sayeed (1975) found that plasma phenytoin levels above 20 μg/ml were associated with slowed impulse conduction in motor nerves.

Gingival hypertrophy. Gum hypertrophy was at one time considered unrelated to plasma phenytoin level (Merritt, 1958; Kutt and McDowell, 1968). However, Kapur, Girgis, Little and Masotti (1973), Conard, Jeffay, Boshes and Steinberg (1974) and Little, Girgis and Masotti (1975) found that the incidence of gum hypertrophy rose as plasma phenytoin levels increased. Kapur, Girgis, Little and Masotti (1973) saw gum hypertrophy in 93 per cent of a group of chronic epileptics with plasma phenytoin levels in the range 10–20 μg/ml.

Plasma level—dose correlations in treated populations

In a population of persons chronically treated with phenytoin the steady-state plasma drug level tends to increase in linear fashion with increasing dosage (Plaa and Hine, 1960; Stensrud and Palmer, 1964). Whether or not dose is expressed on a body weight basis there is a very wide scatter of plasma levels in different people for any particular phenytoin dose (Fig. 6.15; Svensmark, Schiller and Buchthal, 1960; Triedman, Fishman and Yahr, 1960; Husby, 1963; Buchthal and Svensmark, 1959; Viukari and Tammisto, 1969; Lasselles, Kocen and Reynolds, 1970; Eadie, 1971). The correlation between plasma level and dose is appreciably improved in adults by expressing daily doses on a body weight basis, rather than by dealing with them merely as total doses (Fig. 6.16; Houghton, Richens and Leighton, 1975). Conventional phenytoin doses often produce plasma phenytoin levels below the therapeutic range (Fig. 6.15).

Effects of age

Svensmark and Buchthal (1964) analysed the effects of phenytoin dose on plasma phenytoin levels in groups of children corresponding in age to 1–6 years, 6–11 years and 10–14 years. They considered that the same phenytoin dose per unit body weight tended to produce higher plasma levels the older the child was. Jalling, Boreus, Rane and Sjoqvist (1970) found that comparable phenytoin doses on a body weight basis produced lower plasma phenytoin levels in infants below 3 months in age than in adults. Borofsky, Louis, Kutt and Roginsky (1972) examined the relation between serum phenytoin level and drug dose in 53 persons between 0 and 20 years of age. It is difficult to evaluate some of their findings as they included in their analysis multiple serum phenytoin measurements at different doses in some individuals. This introduced a complicating factor, since plasma phenytoin level is not linearly related to drug dose in the individual (page 81). Hooper, Eadie and Tyrer (1973) analyzed initial steady-state measurements of plasma phenytoin concentrations in 125 children divided into age groups 0–5 years, 6–10 years and 11–13 years. They showed that children under 11 years behaved as a reasonably homogeneous group which differed from adults in the relation between plasma drug level and dose. The children aged below 11 years required higher phenytoin doses (on a body weight basis) to attain the same plasma drug levels as compared with adults (Fig. 6.17). The older children (11 to 13 years) did not differ from adults to a statistically significant extent in relation to dosage requirement. This change in the body's handling of phenytoin around the age of

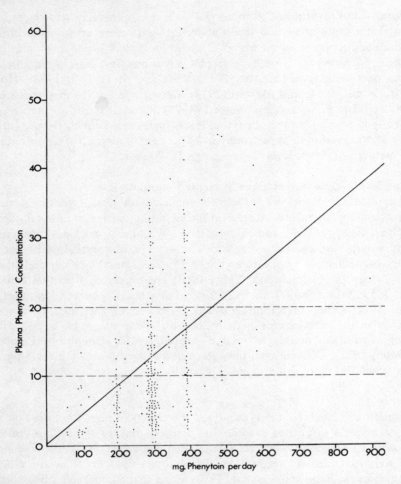

Fig. 6.15 Correlation between steady-state plasma phenytoin (DPH) levels and daily drug dose in 292 adults. The wide scatter of plasma level values around the therapeutic range of 10–20 μg/ml is shown (Eadie and Tyrer, 1973).

puberty may possibly be due to the increased output of steroidal sex hormones at this time competing with phenytoin for a common metabolic pathway.

Subsequent work (Sherwin, Loynd, Bock and Sokolowski, 1974) confirmed the effect of age on the relation between steady state plasma phenytoin level and drug dose. Berlet (1975) noted that the ratio of plasma phenytoin level to daily phenytoin dose increased as children increased in age from 4 to 16 years. Nolte and Brugmann (1975) noted that mean daily phenytoin dose to maintain mean plasma phenytoin level in the range 10–12 μg/ml fell from 9·5 to 5·8 mg/kg/day when children weighing 10–20 kg were compared with older children weighing 30–55 kg.

As pointed out above (page 56), the plasma protein binding of phenytoin decreased with age after puberty (Hooper, Bochner, Eadie and Tyrer, 1974).

Hayes, Langman and Short (1975) found that phenytoin clearance increased with age. They attributed this finding to the consequences of decreased protein binding of the drug. This finding forms a basis for the suggestion that phenytoin dosage

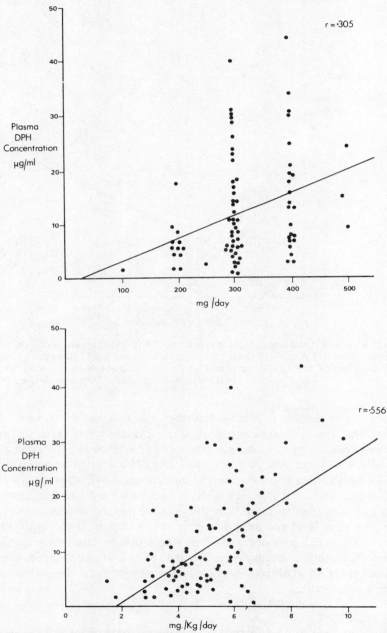

Fig. 6.16 Correlation between steady-state plasma phenytoin (DPH) levels in 92 adults and total daily drug dose expressed in mg (upper figure) and as mg per kg (lower figure). The correlation coefficient increased from 0·305 to 0·556 when dose was expressed on a body weight basis.

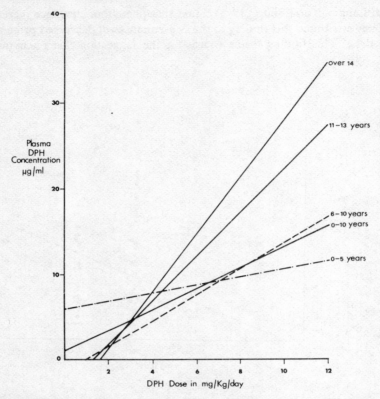

Fig. 6.17 Regressions for steady-state plasma phenytoin (DPH) concentrations on drug dose in persons in the age groups 0–5 years, 6–10 years, 11–13 years and over 14 years. There was no statistically significant difference between the regressions for the two youngest age groups. Hence a common regression line for children under 11 years has been drawn (Eadie, Tyrer and Hooper, 1973).

may need to be reduced in elderly. However, Eadie, Tyrer and Hooper (1973) did not find that the relation between whole plasma phenytoin level and drug dose changed after puberty. In a more recent study of a different population of patients aged between 15 and over 70 years, De Leacy, McLeay, Eadie and Tyrer (1979) again found no effect of age on the relation between steady-state plasma phenytoin concentration and drug dose. However, in view of the reduction in plasma protein binding of phenytoin with age, it is still possible that the relation between plasma water phenytoin level and drug dose may alter with age. If this is the case, toxic effects of phenytoin may occur at lower whole plasma drug levels than in young persons. Phenytoin doses may therefore need to be lower in the aged, even though the effect of age on whole plasma phenytoin levels relative to dose is too small to be detected statistically.

Effect of sex
The data of Eadie, Tyrer and Hooper (1973) and of Fig. 6.18 indicate that sex had no statistically significant effect on the relation between steady-state plasma phenytoin level and drug dose. Travers, Reynolds and Gallagher (1972) had earlier

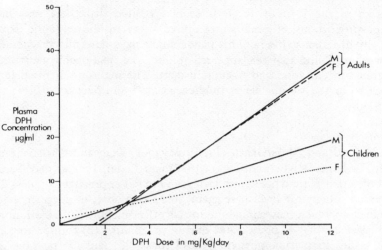

Fig. 6.18 The effects of sex on the regressions for steady-state plasma phenytoin (DPH) level on drug dose in adults (persons over 13 years), and in children. Sex had no statistically significant effect on the regressions for either age group.

suggested that sex did have an effect on the relationship, females tending to have lower plasma phenytoin levels than males for a given drug dose. However, these authors failed to provide statistically significant evidence for their assertion. Sherwin, Loynd, Bock and Sokolowski (1974) found that adult females had statistically significantly lower plasma phenytoin levels than adult males. Richens (1975) stated that females tended to have slightly lower plasma phenytoin levels than males. This finding was significant at the 1 per cent level of confidence. In another paper published in the same year Houghton, Richens and Leighton (1975) again mentioned this finding but indicated that it was not significant at the 5 per cent level of confidence. De Leacy, McLeay, Eadie and Tyrer (1979) reinvestigated the question, and again found no statistically significant effects of sex on the relationship between plasma phenytoin level and phenytoin dose in their patients. However, they found that use of oral contraceptives tended to cause higher plasma phenytoin levels relative to drug dose (Fig. 6.19). This finding was

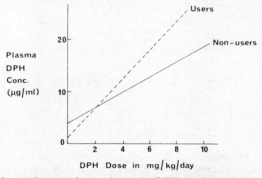

Fig. 6.19 Regressions for steady-state plasma phenytoin (DPH) level on drug dose in females taking oral contraceptives, and in females not taking oral contraceptives. The difference between the regression lines is statistically significant (DeLeacy, McLeay, Eadie and Tyrer, 1979).

significant at the $P = 0.06$ level. It seems possible that there may have been different proportions of oral contraceptive users in the epileptic populations studied by different workers. This factor might have determined whether or not these workers found that sex appeared to alter the relationship between plasma phenytoin concentration and phenytoin dose. The inclusion of pregnant females (see below) in the various series might also have an effect on different authors' conclusions.

Effect of pregnancy

Dam, Mygind and Christiansen (1976), Mygind, Dam and Christiansen (1976), Lander, Edwards, Eadie and Tyrer (1977) and Eadie, Lander and Tyrer (1977) have shown that plasma phenytoin levels tend to fall in pregnancy unless drug dose is increased. Phenytoin levels rise again, relative to dose, in the puerperium (Fig. 6.20). Factors which may contribute to this effect include (1) the dilutional effect of increased volume of body water during pregnancy, (2) routine folate therapy causing a fall in plasma phenytoin level (page 95) and (3) possible increased phenytoin biotransformation in foetal tissues and in the maternal liver, where there may be enzyme induction. One instance of proven phenytoin malabsorption during pregnancy has been reported (Ramsay, Strauss, Wilder and Willmore, 1978). The effect of pregnancy on epilepsy is more fully considered in Chapter 16.

The plasma protein binding of phenytoin is not altered by pregnancy (Hooper, Bochner, Eadie and Tyrer, 1974).

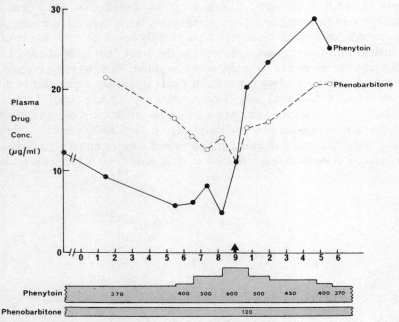

Fig. 6.20 Time courses of plasma levels of phenytoin and phenobarbitone in a patient during pregnancy, and in the six post-natal months. Plasma levels of both anticonvulsants fell during pregnancy despite increased dosage of phenytoin and constant dosage of phenobarbitone. After childbirth plasma levels of both drugs rose, necessitating serial reductions in phenytoin dose (Lander, Edwards, Eadie and Tyrer, 1977).

Effects of Tobacco and Alcohol

De Leacy, McLeay, Eadie and Tyrer (1979) found no statistical evidence that tobacco smoking or mild or moderate alcohol intake altered the relation between steady-state plasma phenytoin levels and phenytoin dose in persons aged over 14 years.

Plasma level—dose relationship in treated individuals

In individual patients the relation between increments of dose and increased steady-state plasma phenytoin level is not linear (Fig. 6.21; Remmer, Hirschmann and Greiner, 1969; Bochner, Hooper, Tyrer and Eadie, 1972a; and Richens and

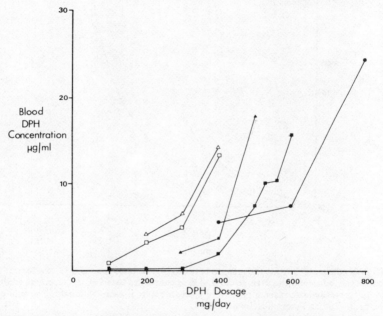

Fig. 6.21 The effect of two or more dose increments on steady-state blood phenytoin (DPH) concentrations in five patients. Sequential dose increments of equal size tend to produce increasingly large rises in blood phenytoin level (Bochner, Hooper, Tyrer and Eadie, 1972-a).

Dunlop, 1975). When the plasma phenytoin level is above the range of 6–9 μg/ml a given dosage increment produces a much greater rise in plasma level of the drug than does an equal dosage increment if the initial plasma level is below this range. This type of behaviour of plasma phenytoin level with dose increment in the individual is a consequence of the drug's chief mode of elimination being a saturable process and thus following Michaelis-Menten kinetics (page 61).

Similar behaviour of steady-state plasma level with dose increment occurs in children. However, in this age group there is a wider range of phenytoin dosage and a higher mean dosage necessary to raise plasma drug levels from zero to 6–9 μg/ml than in adults. With levels over 6–9 μg/ml the slopes of the curves for children and adults are similar, if doses are expressed relative to body weight (Fig. 6.22). These findings are consistent with the hypothesis that, as phenytoin

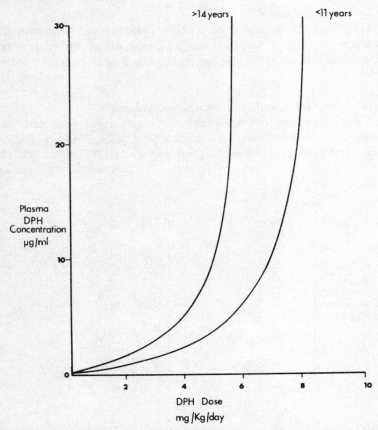

Fig. 6.22 Calculated curves showing the relation between plasma phenytoin (DPH) level and phenytoin dose for the average adult and the average child. These curves are based on data from 38 adults and 30 children who had steady-state plasma phenytoin levels measured, each while taking several different doses of the drug (Eadie, Tyrer and Hooper, 1973).

elimination capacity becomes saturated, the drug accumulates in the body in proportion to its volume of distribution, and body weight provides a measure of the latter.

The non-linear relation between plasma (and tissue) drug level and phenytoin dose in the individual is of considerable therapeutic importance. The phase of rapid rise in plasma level occurs through the 'therapeutic range' of 10–20 μg/ml. Thus if phenytoin dose increments are made in the expectation that in this range the relation between plasma level and dose is linear, many patients will become overdosed. Small alterations in phenytoin elimination may have profound effects on a plasma drug level in the therapeutic range. Equal changes in phenytoin elimination may have little effect on plasma drug levels which are below 6 μg/ml.

Effects of disease

Liver disease
Since hepatic biotransformation is the main avenue of phenytoin elimination, liver

disease might be expected to alter the pharmacokinetics of the drug. Phenytoin clearance appeared unaltered in cases of acute viral hepatitis (studied by Blaschke, Meffin, Melmon and Rowland, 1975). However, in severe impairment of liver function phenytoin levels may rise (Kutt, Winters, Kokenge and McDowell, 1964). A family with an apparent hereditary, selective relative deficiency of the enzyme system that hydroxylates phenytoin has been reported (Kutt, Wolk, Scherman and McDowell, 1964). Gerber, Lynn and Oates (1972) investigated another patient who metabolized phenytoin slowly, but who had no other manifestation of altered liver function. Bochner, Hooper, Eadie and Tyrer (1975) described a patient with a greatly reduced capacity to eliminate both phenytoin (average plasma half-life of 4·4 days) and warfarin, though not phenobarbitone (Fig. 6.23). Over a 6 day period this subject excreted considerably less pHPPH

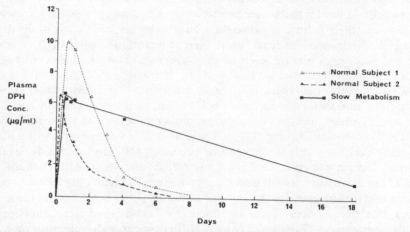

Fig. 6.23 Time-courses of plasma phenytoin (DPH) concentrations after a single oral 600 mg phenytoin dose in a slow metabolizer of the drug (solid circles and solid line), and after single oral 700 mg doses in two normal subjects (Bochner, Hooper, Eadie and Tyrer, 1975).

relative to dose, than did two control subjects. The only other indication of altered liver function in this patient was mildly increased bromsulphthalein retention. Engel, Cruz and Shapiro (1971) claimed that phenytoin therapy may have precipitated porto-systemic encephalopathy in one patient with alcoholic hepatitis but their data were open to other interpretations. Evidence has been obtained that the phenytoin binding capacity of plasma protein is reduced in liver disease (Hooper, Bochner, Eadie and Tyrer, 1974). This altered binding capacity appeared to correlate with changes in plasma albumin and bilirubin levels. In control plasma $10·77 \pm SD\ 2·26$ per cent of the drug was unbound, while in liver disease plasma $15·91 \pm SD\ 6·00$ per cent was unbound.

Renal disease
In uraemia it is known that the plasma proteins have a decreased capacity to bind phenytoin (Odar-Cederlof, Lunde and Sjoqvist, 1970; Blum, Riegelman and Becker, 1972; Reidenberg, Odar-Cederlof, Von Bahr, Borga and Sjoqvist, 1971; Shoeman and Azarnoff, 1972; Shoeman, Benjamin and Azarnoff, 1973; Odar-

Cederlof and Borga, 1976). Phenytoin half-life in plasma is reduced in uraemia (Letteri, Mellk, Louis, Kutt, Durante and Glazko, 1971; Shoeman, Benjamin and Azarnoff, 1973; Odar-Cederlof and Borga, 1974). The mechanism of this shortened half-life is not yet fully worked out. The apparent V_d of the drug is increased (Odar-Cederlof and Borga, 1974).

Normal persons taking phenytoin excrete about 5 per cent of their dose unchanged in urine. This would suggest that a patient with anuria taking 400 mg of the drug daily would retain about 20 mg extra phenytoin each day. Therefore after 2 or 3 days of anuria one might expect a significant rise in plasma and tissue levels of the drug if drug dosage and biotransformation are unaltered. In chronic renal insufficiency without anuria the considerations are more complex. Because of reduced plasma protein binding one would expect more free drug in plasma and therefore in glomerular filtrate. There might also be less resorption of the drug from the tubular fluid if there were polyuria. Hence plasma phenytoin levels might fall. However, there is little information as to whether tissue binding of the drug is also changed in uraemia. In renal failure there is retention of p-HPPH glucuronide in the body and high plasma levels of this substance (Dill, Baukema, Chang and Glazko, 1971; Letteri, Mellk, Louis, Kutt, Durante and Glazko, 1971). The accumulation of this metabolite might slow phenytoin biotransformation. Slowing of phenytoin biotransformation due to p-HPPH occurs *in vitro* (Ashley and Levy, 1972), and in the rat occurs *in vivo* when glucuronide formation is inhibited by salicylamide (Levy and Ashley, 1973). There appear to be no data relating plasma phenytoin levels to induced changes in plasma p-HPPH-glucuronide levels in individual human patients. Gerber, Lynn, Bush and Oates (1972) found that p-HPPH excretion rate was not directly proportional to plasma phenytoin concentration in a group of patients. In another group of patients, including some with uraemia, Bochner, Hooper, Tyrer and Eadie (1973) also found no relation between these two parameters (Fig. 6.6). Thus p-HPPH glucuronide retention may have little or no effect on plasma phenytoin level in the individual. Irrespective of what is predicted to happen to plasma phenytoin levels in patients with renal failure, it would seem wise to monitor phenytoin concentrations in plasma water (or saliva) periodically in uraemic patients. This should be done particularly if possible side-effects are occurring or if control of the patient's epilepsy is becoming impaired.

In one uraemic patient Adler, Martin, Gambertoglio, Tozer and Spire (1975) showed that a 6 hour period of haemodyalysis removed only 43·6 mg of phenytoin. Plasma phenytoin levels were scarcely altered. This is not surprising since the great majority of the phenytoin in plasma is bound to protein, and therefore not dialysable.

There has been a report of a solitary instance in which a ureterosigmoidostomy led to phenytoin intoxication, allegedly because the drug excreted by the kidney was resorbed from the colon (Savariyan and Dixey, 1969).

Alimentary disease
Although the possibility of alimentary malabsorption of phenytoin is sometimes mentioned, its actual occurrence has rarely been reported (Kutt, Haynes and McDowell, 1966). Peterson and Zweig (1974) found that higher than usual oral

doses of phenytoin were needed to achieve therapeutic plasma levels of the drug in patients with jejuno-ileal by-passes.

Brain disease
Viukari (1969) found some evidence that cases of Vogt-Spielmeyer neurolipoidosis tolerated phenytoin less well than did some other oligophrenic epileptics. There was no proof that this finding was due to altered phenytoin pharmacokinetics.

Surgery
Elfstrom (1977) found that the plasma protein binding of phenytoin was reduced after abdominal or cranial surgery, possibly because of the post-operative fall that may occur in plasma albumin levels.

INTERACTIONS

PHARMACODYNAMIC INTERACTIONS
Phenytoin is often given in combination with other anticonvulsants in the hope that an additive or synergistic interaction will occur, improving the control of epilepsy. Unwanted effects (e.g. drowsiness, mental dulling) may also be increased by the combination of two anticonvulsant drugs. These phenomena probably represent pharmacodynamic interactions. However, this has rarely been proved since the possibility of pharmacokinetic type interactions usually has not been fully excluded in these circumstances. Exclusion of a pharmacokinetic type interaction would require demonstration that there was no increase in the plasma water levels of either of the interacting drugs.

PHARMACOKINETIC INTERACTIONS

Phenytoin affecting other substances

Plasma protein binding
Markkanen, Himanen, Pajuta and Moenar (1973) found that phenytoin increased the binding of folic acid to serum proteins and in particular to transferrin. Phenytoin displaces thyroxine from its plasma protein binding sites (Schussler, 1971). *In vitro*, phenytoin displaces tricyclic antidepressants from plasma protein binding sites (Borga, Azarnoff, Forshell and Sjoqvist, 1969).

Physiological substances
Corticosteroids. Choi, Thrasher, Werk, Sholiton and Olinger (1971) showed that phenytoin shortened the half-life of cortisol in man without altering plasma cortisol concentrations. Probably there was increased synthesis and also increased biotransformation of cortisol. This increased biotransformation of cortisol was not seen in neonates exposed to phenytoin *in utero* (Renyolds and Mirkin, 1973). Fujii, Hayashi and Murata (1975) found that children receiving phenytoin had normal plasma concentrations of 11-hydroxycorticosteroids and corticotrophin, but that there was decreased suppression of 11-hydrocorticosteroid levels after dexamethasone or metopyrone (metyrapone) was given. Jubiz, Meikle, Levinson,

Mizutani, West and Tyler (1970) showed that phenytoin increased the hepatic conjugation of the synthetic steroid dexamethaxone. It also shortened the half-life and increased the metabolic clearance of prednisolone (Petereit and Meikle, 1977).

Thyroid hormones. Chronic phenytoin intake causes a fall in plasma protein-bound iodine level (Cantu and Schwab, 1966) and in total serum thyroxine (T_4) concentration. There is an increase in unbound thyroxine level but no alteration in triiodothyronine concentration (Finucane and Griffiths, 1976). These effects probably occur because the drug displaces thyroxine from plasma proteins, increasing the thyroxine clearance. Other workers (Larsen, Atkinson, Wellman and Goldsmith, 1970; Yeo, Bates, Howe, Ratcliffe, Schardt, Heath and Evered, 1978) have shown reduced serum free thyroxine levels during phenytoin therapy, and also decreased tri-iodothyronine levels (Yeo, Bates, Howe, Ratcliffe, Schardt, Heath and Evered, 1978).

Folates. It has been demonstrated (Jensen and Olesen, 1970; Davis and Woodliff, 1971; Korczyn, Elian, Don and Bornstein, 1974) that phenytoin therapy is associated with reduced serum folate concentrations (see page 52), and reduced CSF levels of N^5-tetrahydrofolate (Mauguiere and Karlin, 1975).

Lipids. Foster, Nagaswami and Reimer (1974) found some slender evidence for a relation between phenytoin intake and high plasma lipid levels, while Pelkonen, Fogelholm and Nikkila (1975) demonstrated a 6–48 per cent rise in serum cholesterol levels in patients on long-term phenytoin therapy. Livingstone (1976) commented that he had not seen any such incidence of hypercholesterolaemia in his treated epileptics.

Caeruloplasmin. Phenytoin therapy is associated with raised serum caeruloplasmin levels (Cantu and Schwab, 1966; Taylor, Krahn and Higgins, 1974; Vasiliades and Sahawneh, 1975). Serum copper levels are also raised (Taylor, Krahn and Higgins, 1974).

Sex hormone binding globulin. Phenytoin appears to cause raised levels of sex-hormone-binding globulin in women (Victor, Lundberg and Johansson, 1977).

Immunoglobulins. Phenytoin therapy sometimes is associated with reduced IgA concentrations in serum (Aarli and Tonder, 1975; Seager, Wilson, Jamison, Hayward and Soothill, 1975; Yabuki and Nakaya, 1976; Shakir, Behan, Dick and Lambie, 1978) and in saliva (Aarli, 1976). Less often serum Ig M and Ig G (Yabuki and Nakaya, 1976), and CSF Ig G (Fossan, 1976) concentrations are reduced. Fontana, Grob, Sauter and Holler (1976) claimed that reduced immunoglobulin levels were associated with constitutional types of epilepsy rather than with drug treatment of epilepsy. The mechanisms involved in producing the altered immunoglobulin concentrations are uncertain.

Enzymes. Phenytoin therapy in children is associated with increased serum levels of γ-glutamyl transpeptidase (Abe, Tamagawa, Eguchi, 1973; Gauchel, Lehr, Gauchel and von Harnack, 1973).

Other anticonvulsants

Phenobarbitone. Rizzo, Morselli and Garattini (1972) and Lambie, Nanda, Johnson and Shakir (1976) found that phenytoin therapy caused raised plasma phenobarbitone levels. Eadie, Lander, Hooper and Tyrer (1977) failed to find evidence of such an interaction in a population study.

Primidone. Phenytoin therapy appears to increase the biotransformation of primidone to phenobarbitone, leading to higher plasma phenobarbitone levels relative to primidone dose (Fincham, Schottelius and Sahs, 1974; Reynolds, Fenton, Fenwick, Johnson and Laundy, 1975; Schmidt, 1975; Eadie, Lander, Hooper and Tyrer, 1977; Garrettson and Gomez, 1977).

Carbamazepine. Christiansen and Dam (1973), Hooper, Dubetz, Eadie and Tyrer (1974), Johannessen and Strandjord (1975), Schneider (1975) and Lander, Eadie and Tyrer (1975; 1977) have demonstrated a consistent interaction in which phenytoin therapy causes a fall in plasma carbamazepine concentrations. Schneider (1975) found that the interaction led to raised plasma epoxycarbamazepine levels, but this has not been the present authors' experience. This interaction is discussed further in Chapter 7.

Clonazepam. Hvidberg and Sjo (1975) found that phenytoin therapy led to reduced plasma clonazepam concentrations in all of the 5 patients they studied.

Miscellaneous substances

Phenytoin therapy has been reported as associated with reduced plasma levels and/or reduced plasma half-lives of the following substances:

dicophane metabolites   (Davies, Edmundson, Carter and Barquet, 1969)

digitoxin   (Solomon, Reich, Spirt and Abrams, 1971)

dicumarol   (Hansen, Siersback-Nielsen, Kristensen, Skovsted and Christensen, 1971)

antipyrine   (Petruch, Schuppel and Steinhilber, 1974)

doxycycline, but not other tetracyclines   (Penttila, Neuvonen, Aho and
Lehtovarra, 1974; Neuvonen, Penttila, Lehtovarra and Aho, 1975)

nortriptyline   (Braithwaite, Flanagan and Richens, 1975)

phenazone   (Schuppel, Petruch and Steinhilber, 1973)

pyridoxine   (Reinken, 1973)

The mechanism of action of phenytoin in the various interactions described above is not established, except in the instances of drug displacement from plasma protein binding sites. In the great majority of these interactions the effect of phenytoin is to reduce plasma levels of the other substance involved. Sometimes increased elimination of the interacting substance has been demonstrated. It might reasonably be anticipated that phenytoin has induced hepatic enzymatic mechanisms, which increase the rate of metabolic degradation of the interacting substances. In rats Eling, Harbison, Becker and Fouts (1970) showed that phenytoin induced the hepatic enzymes which metabolize p-nitroanisole, hexobarbitone and aminopyrine. However, it is not yet proven that similar induction occurs in man.

Other substances affecting phenytoin

Many substances have been reported to alter plasma phenytoin levels. The number of interactions described may be explained in part by the fact that phenytoin has been in widespread use for over 35 years. It is also relevant that the therapeutic range of plasma phenytoin levels is attained only when the drug's elimination mechanism is nearly saturated. Therefore many substances which slow phenytoin elimination even slightly may have a significant effect on plasma phenytoin concentrations already in the therapeutic range, and thus produce clinically apparent phenytoin intoxication. On the other hand, interactions which are of equal magnitude in enhancing phenytoin elimination may cause only a slight fall in plasma phenytoin level. Such interactions may easily go unnoticed clinically, unless plasma phenytoin levels are measured.

Kutt, Haynes, Verebely and McDowell (1969) suggested that phenobarbitone may have two different effects on phenytoin biotransformation. Phenobarbitone may induce the hepatic mixed-oxidase system which catalyses phenytoin biotransformation. This effect would reduce plasma phenytoin levels. However, phenobarbitone may also act as an inhibitor of the enzyme system it induces. This inhibitory action tends to slow phenytoin biotransformation and raise plasma phenytoin levels. The overall effect of phenobarbitone on plasma phenytoin levels depends on which of these two mechanisms preponderates in the individual. Should other drugs have similar 'bidirectional' effects on phenytoin biotransformation, the interactions are most likely to be clinically apparent when they raise plasma phenytoin levels and produce toxic manifestations. Therefore small numbers of reported instances of particular interactions which produce raised plasma phenytoin levels may not necessarily indicate interactions which are consistently present. On the other hand, population studies may fail to detect 'bidirectional' interactions which may be of real significance in a small number of individuals. When plasma phenytoin levels in groups of individuals are studied, levels in some subjects may rise, and in some may fall, when there are 'bidirectional' interactions. Mean levels in the population may then show little change. The following account of interactions which alter plasma phenytoin levels should be read critically in the light of the above comments. It should also be appreciated that, when single instances of interactions have been described, incorrect compliance with prescribed dosage may not have always been excluded.

Altered plasma protein binding
The possibility that competition by other drugs for plasma protein binding sites might displace phenytoin has been assessed by *in vitro* studies. It appears that the following substances may displace phenytoin:

salicylic acid   (Lunde, Rane, Yaffe, Lund and Sjoqvist, 1970; Ehrnebo and Odar-Cederlof, 1977)
phenylbutazone   (Lunde, Rane, Yaffe, Lund and Sjoqvist, 1970)
halofenate   (Karch and Wardell, 1977)
diazoxide   (Roe, Podosin and Beaskovics, 1975)
tolbutamide   (Wesseling and Mols-Thurkow, 1975)
valproate   (Patsalos and Lascelles, 1977)
possibly sulthiame   (Hooper, Sutherland, Bochner, Tyrer and Eadie, 1973)

The effects of diazoxide and tolbutamide were shown to occur *in vivo* in man. *In vitro* studies suggest that the following substances if given to man are unlikely to compete with phenytoin for plasma protein binding sites:

phenobarbitone   (Kristensen, Hansen and Skovsted, 1969; Lunde, Rane, Yaffe, Lund and Sjoqvist, 1970; Hooper, Sutherland, Bochner, Tyrer and Eadie, 1973)
ethosuximide   (Lunde, Rane, Yaffe, Lund and Sjoqvist, 1970; Hooper,

Sutherland, Bochner, Tyrer and Eadie, 1973; Patsalos and Lascelles, 1977)

carbamazepine (Hansen, Siersboek-Nielsen and Skovsted, 1971; Hooper, Sutherland, Bochner, Tyrer and Eadie, 1973)

aspirin (Hooper, Sutherland, Bochner, Tyrer and Eadie, 1973)

acetazolamine (Lunde, Rane, Yaffe, Lund and Sjoqvist, 1970)

chlorothiazide (Lunde, Rane, Yaffe, Lund and Sjoqvist, 1970)

disulfiram (Lunde, Rane, Yaffe, Lund and Sjoqvist, 1970)

para-amino-salicyclic acid (Lunde, Rane, Yaffe, Lund and Sjoqvist, 1970)

Other anticonvulsants

Phenobarbitone. Phenobarbitone is a well known inducer of the hepatic microsomal drug metabolizing enzyme system (Conney, 1967). Cucinell, Conney, Sansur and Burns (1965) noted that the mean plasma phenytoin level was lower in epileptics treated concurrently with phenytoin and phenobarbitone than in those taking phenytoin alone. Similar findings have subsequently been reported by others (Sotaniemi, Arvela, Hakkarainen and Huhti, 1970). Cucinell, Conney, Sansur and Burns (1965) showed that phenobarbitone significantly shortened the half-life of phenytoin in dogs. Kristensen, Hansen and Skovsted (1969) found that phenobarbitone reduced the half-life of phenytoin in 11 of 12 patients. However, subsequent studies of the effect of phenobarbitone on plasma phenytoin concentrations have shown that the latter may rise, fall, or remain unaltered: any changes in phenytoin level are relatively small (Kutt, Hayes, Verebely and McDowell, 1969; Diamond and Buchanan, 1970; Garrettson and Dayton, 1970; Booker, Tormey and Touissaint, 1971; Buchanan and Allen, 1971; Morselli, Rizzo and Garattini, 1971; Sherwin, Loynd, Bock and Sokolowski, 1974; Richens and Houghton, 1975; Lander, Eadie and Tyrer, 1975). Mascher and Bernhardt (1973) found that phenobarbitone treatment did not alter p-HPPH production in persons taking phenytoin. A possible explanation for the inconsistent effect of phenobarbitone on plasma phenytoin levels is mentioned above.

Drugs which are transformed to phenobarbitone in the body (e.g. methylphenobarbitone and primidone) might be expected to have similar effects to phenobarbitone. Lander, Eadie and Tyrer (1975) found no evidence of effects of methylphenobarbitone or primidone on plasma phenytoin levels. Sherwin, Loynd, Bock and Sokolowski (1974) also found that primidone had no effect, whereas Windorfer and Sauer (1977) found that primidone therapy tended to reduce plasma phenytoin levels.

Carbamazepine. Hansen, Siersboek-Nielsen and Skovsted (1971) found that carbamazepine caused a fall in plasma phenytoin concentration in 3 of 7 patients. Molholm, Siersback-Nielsen and Skovsted (1971), Cereghino, Van Meter, Brock, Penry, Smith and White (1973) and Windorfer and Sauer (1977) described similar findings. However, Cereghino, Brock, Van Meter, Penry, Smith and White (1975) and Richens and Houghton (1975) found no definite effect of carbamazepine on plasma phenytoin levels. Hooper, Dubetz, Eadie and Tyrer (1974) showed that plasma phenytoin levels fell in 7 of 8 subjects as carbamazepine dose was increased (Fig. 6.24). They found that the regression for the relation between plasma phenytoin level and phenytoin dose differed for 62 persons taking phenytoin

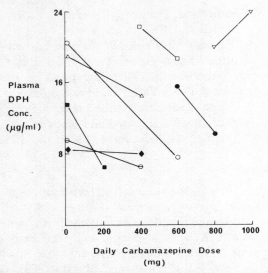

Fig. 6.24 Plasma phenytoin (DPH) levels tended to fall as carbamazepine doses were increased in 8 subjects (Hooper, Dubetz, Eadie and Tyrer, 1974).

alone, and for 59 persons taking phenytoin with carbamazepine (Fig. 6.25). In a subsequent study on an extended group of patients using multivariate linear regression analysis, Lander, Eadie and Tyrer (1975) found that carbamazepine had a tendency to raise rather than lower plasma phenytoin levels. The effect was almost statistically significant, but the magnitude of the rise would have been negligible clinically. This apparent conflict in findings from different workers may perhaps be explained by the data of Fig. 6.25. As the mean phenytoin dose in a

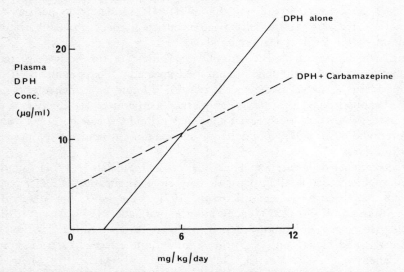

Fig. 6.25 Regression for steady-state plasma phenytoin (DPH) level on phenytoin dose in 62 patients taking phenytoin alone, and in 59 patients taking phenytoin with carbamazepine (Hooper, Dubetz, Eadie and Tyrer, 1974).

group of patients exceeded 6 mg/kg/day (just above the usual adult dose) one was more likely to see lowered plasma phenytoin levels in patients also taking carbamazepine. As illustrated in Fig. 6.26, increasing the carbamazepine dose in a particular individual may consistently cause a reduction in plasma phenytoin level.

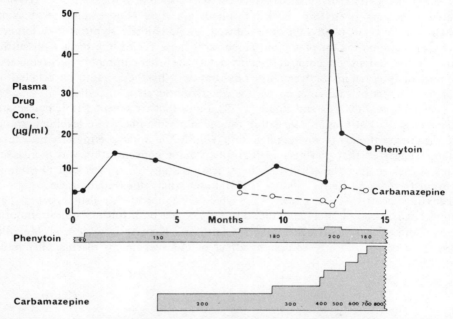

Fig. 6.26 Time-courses of plasma phenytoin and carbamazepine concentrations in a patient given different phenytoin and carbamazepine doses at different times in the endeavour to control epilepsy. On three occasions increases in carbamazepine dose, without alteration in phenytoin dose, were associated with a fall in plasma phenytoin level (Lander, Eadie and Tyrer, 1975).

Sulthiame. Several authors have noted that use of sulthiame led to raised plasma phenytoin levels in patients taking the latter drug. Hansen, Kristensen and Skovsted (1968) detected this effect in 4 cases out of 4, Hoglmeier and Wenzel (1969) in a single case, Olesen and Jensen (1969) in 7 cases out of 7, and Richens and Houghton (1973) in 6 cases out of 7. Houghton and Richens (1974a) showed that withdrawal of sulthiame caused a fall in plasma phenytoin level in all cases studied, while commencement of sulthiame therapy raised plasma phenytoin levels in 4 cases out of 4. Houghton and Richens (1974b) described shortened phenytoin half-lives in 2 cases after sulthiame was withdrawn from the therapeutic regime. However plasma phenytoin levels fell in these circumstances and, as explained earlier, phenytoin half-life is concentration dependent. Therefore the reduced half-lives do not necessarily mean that sulthiame withdrawal itself directly increases the rate of phenytoin elimination. Richens and Houghton (1975), using radio-labelled phenytoin, showed that sulthiame increased the half-life of phenytoin, and decreased the plasma concentration ratio of p-hydroxyphenytoin to phenytoin. Earlier Morselli, Rizzo and Garattini (1970) had shown that, in rats, brain phenytoin levels were higher relative to phenytoin dose when sulthiame was given concurrently, though blood phenytoin levels were not altered.

Despite this evidence of a consistent effect of sulthiame on plasma phenytoin concentrations, the present authors have failed to find an example of this interaction in their own material (Lander, Eadie and Tyrer, 1975). A multiple variable linear regression analysis of plasma phenytoin level data in 400 patients detected no statistically significant effect of sulthiame dosage on the relation between plasma phenytoin level and phenytoin dose. Regressions for plasma phenytoin level on phenytoin dose showed no statistically significant difference between patients taking phenytoin alone, and those taking the drug with sulthiame. These statistical techniques readily detect the other commonly-occurring and consistent interactions between anticonvulsants. Why they should have failed to detect an effect of sulthiame on plasma phenytoin levels is uncertain.

Clonazepam. Edwards and Eadie (1973) found that treatment with clonazepam caused a statistically significant fall in the mean plasma phenytoin level in a group of 17 patients already receiving phenytoin (Fig. 6.27). Some preliminary measurements suggested that plasma p-HPPH-glucuronide concentration was increased. This suggested that the effect may be at least partly due to increased phenytoin biotransformation. Eeg Olofsson (1973) noted that clonazepam raised plasma phenytoin levels in some cases. Windorfer and Sauer (1977) also reported that clonazepam raised plasma phenytoin levels. However both Johanessen, Strandjord and Munthe-Kaas (1977) and Nanda, Johnson, Keogh, Lambie and Melville (1977) failed to find any consistent effect of clonazepam on plasma phenytoin

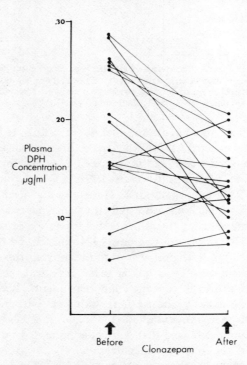

Fig. 6.27 Plasma phenytoin (DPH) levels before and after the addition of clonazepam to phenytoin therapy in 17 patients. Phenytoin doses were unchanged. The mean plasma phenytoin level fell from $18 \cdot 3 \, \mu$g/ml to $13 \cdot 5 \, \mu$g/ml, a statistically significant difference ($p < 0 \cdot 025$).

levels. Possibly the effect of clonazepam on plasma phenytoin levels is the result of a bidirectional interaction, as was discussed above in relation to the effect of phenobarbitone on phenytoin.

Diazepam. Vajda, Prineas and Lovell (1971) and Rogers, Haslam, Longstreth and Lietman (1977) found that addition of diazepam to phenytoin therapy caused raised plasma phenytoin levels. In two subjects the latter authors showed that K_m values for phenytoin were considerably reduced when diazepam was added to therapy, though changes in V_{max} were relatively small. In rat liver homogenate, Kutt and Verebely (1970) showed that diazepam inhibited phenytoin metabolism. However, Richens and Houghton (1975) found that diazepam therapy decreased plasma phenytoin levels. Perhaps the effects of diazepam on plasma phenytoin levels are also bidirectional.

Ethosuximide. Frantzen, Hansen, Hansen and Kristensen (1967) found that ethosuximide therapy caused raised plasma phenytoin levels in patients taking phenytoin. Richens and Houghton (1975) failed to find evidence of this interaction. An example of the interaction is shown in Fig. 6.28.

Valproate. Windorfer and Sauer (1977) stated that valproate therapy caused a short term increase in plasma phenytoin level, but a longer-term decrease. Vajda, Morris, Drummer and Bladin (1975) also noted a rise in plasma phenytoin level when valproate was added to phenytoin therapy. The opposite effect (i.e. a fall in plasma phenytoin level when valproate is added to therapy) is illustrated in Fig.

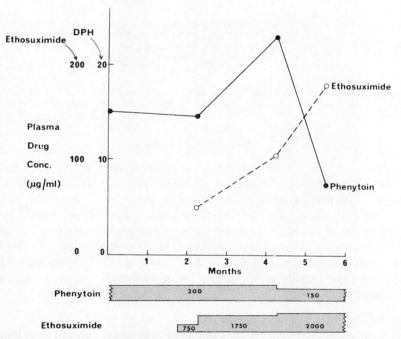

Fig. 6.28 In the subject illustrated plasma phenytoin level rose from 14·5 μg/ml to 23·0 μg/ml when ethosuximide was added to phenytoin therapy, taken in constant dosages to that time (Lander, Eadie and Tyrer, 1975).

6.29. This effect of valproate in reducing plasma phenytoin levels has also been reported by Adams, Luders and Pippenger (1978).

Troxidone. This drug is said to raise plasma phenytoin levels (Roseman, 1961).

Methoin. Roseman (1961) claimed that methoin raised plasma phenytoin levels.

Phenylacetylurea. Huisman, Van Heycop ten Ham and Van Zijl (1970) showed that this drug raised plasma phenytoin levels in 7 cases out of 7.

Pheneturide. Richens and Houghton (1975) found that pheneturide caused raised plasma phenytoin concentrations.

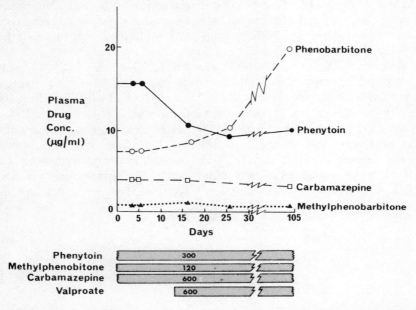

Fig. 6.29 Despite constant daily dosage of phenytoin, methylphenobarbitone and carbamazepine, plasma phenytoin levels fell and plasma phenobarbitone levels rose, when valproate was added to this patient's therapy.

Anticoagulants

Dicumarol therapy was associated with raised plasma phenytoin levels in 6 out of 6 cases studied by Hansen, Kristensen, Skovsted and Christensen (1966), though Skovsted, Kristensen, Hansen and Siersbaek-Nielsen (1976) found that dicumarol did not alter phenytoin half-life, nor raise plasma phenytoin levels. The latter authors also found that warfarin did not alter plasma phenytoin levels, though both bishydroxycoumarin and phenprocoumon did. Earlier Rothermich (1966) had reported that warfarin did raise plasma phenytoin levels. Thus there are conflicting reports in the literature regarding the effects of different anticoagulants on plasma phenytoin levels.

Sulphonamides

A number of sulphonamides slow the elimination of phenytoin and raise its plasma levels. The drugs involved include sulphaphenazole, sulphadiazine, sulphamethiazole and co-trimoxazole (Hansen, Kristensen, Skovsted and Christensen, 1966; Skovsted, Hansen, Kristensen and Christensen, 1974; Lumholtz, Siersbaek-Nielsen, Skovsted, Kampmann and Hansen, 1975; Molholm Hansen, Siersbaek-Nielsen, Skovsted, Kampmann and Lumholtz, 1975).

Folates
Olesen and Jensen (1970), Baylis, Crowley, Preece, Sylvester and Marks (1971), Glazko (1973) and Mattson, Gallagher, Reynolds and Glass (1973) all reported that plasma phenytoin levels fell when folic acid was given to folate-deficient epileptics taking phenytoin. This effect is illustrated in Fig. 6.30. However, Buch Andreasen, Hansen, Skovsted and Siersbaek-Nielsen (1971) reported that folic

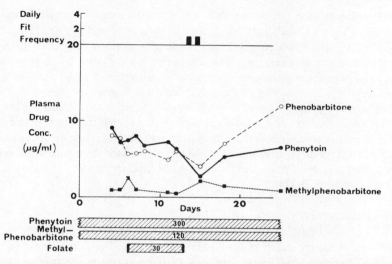

Fig. 6.30 Therapy with folic acid (30 mg per day) has been associated with a fall in plasma phenytoin and phenobarbitone levels and relapse of epilepsy in the patient illustrated. Plasma anticonvulsant levels rose again when folate therapy was ceased (Eadie, Lander and Tyrer, 1977).

acid therapy did not alter the half-life of phenytoin in man. The mechanism of the interaction therefore remains uncertain.

Ethyl alcohol
According to Kutt and Louis (1972) ethanol, like phenobarbitone, has a two-way effect on phenytoin metabolism: it may reduce plasma phenytoin levels by inducing the liver drug-metabolizing mixed oxidase enzymes, but it also inhibits these enzymes. Kater, Roggin, Tobon, Zieve and Iber (1969) found that the plasma half-life of phenytoin was shorter in chronic alcoholics than in controls. However, as mentioned earlier (see page 81), mild or moderate alcohol consumption does not appear to alter the relation between steady-state plasma phenytoin level and drug dose.

Methylphenidate
Garrettson, Perel and Dayton (1969) and Kutt and Louis (1972) reported raised

plasma phenytoin levels when methylphenidate was given, but Mirkin and Wright (1971) and Kupferberg, Jeffrey and Hunninghake (1972) could not confirm this interaction.

Isoniazid
Isoniazid has been found to raise plasma phenytoin levels in 10 per cent of patients taking phenytoin (Kutt, Winters and McDowell, 1966). Brennan, Dehija, Kutt, Verebely and McDowell (1970) observed that plasma phenytoin levels tended to rise particularly in patients who were slow inactivators of isoniazid.

Calcium sulphate
In 1968 an interaction which reduced the bioavailability of phenytoin occurred in Australasia (Tyrer, Eadie, Sutherland and Hooper, 1970; Bochner, Hooper, Tyrer and Eadie, 1972). A widely-used phenytoin preparation contained calcium sulphate dihydrate as an excipient. The excipient was replaced by lactose and many instances of phenytoin intoxication followed in patients who had been stabilized on the former preparation. The calcium sulphate had apparently interacted with the phenytoin in the preparation to convert about 25 per cent of the drug into a form insoluble in chloroform and unlikely to absorb from the gut. When all the drug was available for absorption after calcium sulphate was no longer included in the excipient, the increased phenytoin bioavailability caused drug intoxication in many patients who had been previously stabilized on the preparation that was no longer marketed (see Fig. 6.31).

Tricyclic antidepressants
Perucca and Richens (1977) reported two cases in whom imipramine therapy appeared to cause increased plasma phenytoin levels. Pond, Graham, Birkett and Wade (1975) showed that the elimination half-life of phenytoin was not altered by chronic intake of amitripytline or nortriptyline.

Disulfiram
Kiorboe (1966) and Olesen (1966, 1967) reported that disulfiram therapy caused raised plasma phenytoin levels. More recently Svendsen, Kristensen, Hansen and Skovsted (1976) showed that after 4 days of therapy with disulfiram, phenytoin half-life rose from $11 \cdot 0 \pm 1 \cdot 2$ hours to $19 \cdot 0 \pm 3 \cdot 3$ hours, and phenytoin clearance fell from $51 \cdot 2 \pm 17 \cdot 2$ ml/minute to $33 \cdot 9 \pm 12 \cdot 0$ ml/minute in 10 volunteers.

Certain other interactions have been reported in which plasma phenytoin levels were raised following the administration of certain drugs. These include the following:

calcium carbimide	Olesen (1967)
chloramphenicol	Christensen and Skovsted (1969); Ballek, Reidenberg and Orr (1973); Skovsted, Hansen, Kristensen and Christensen (1974)
chlordiazepoxide	Kutt and McDowell (1968); Vajda, Prineas and Lovell (1971)
chlorpheniramine	Pugh, Geddes and Yeoman (1975)
chlorpromazine	Kutt and McDowell (1968)

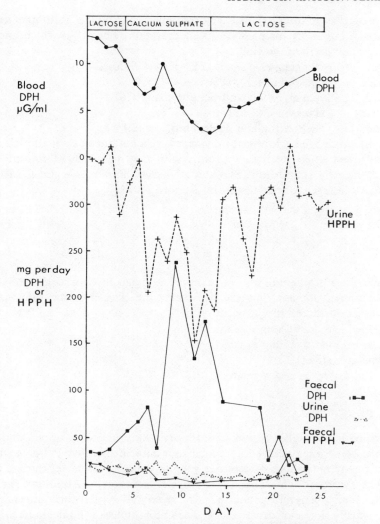

Fig. 6.31 The effect of a change in excipient from lactose to calcium sulphate, and then back to lactose, in a subject taking a constant daily phenytoin dose (400 mg). Blood phenytoin (DPH) levels and 24 hour urinary and faecal excretions of phenytoin and 5-(p-hydroxyphenyl)-5-phenylhydantoin (HPPH) were followed for 25 days (Bochner, Hooper, Tyrer and Eadie, 1972-b).

clofibrate   Skovsted, Hansen, Kristensen and Christensen (1974)
frusemide   Personal unpublished data; [Ahman, Clarke, Hewett and Richens (1976) found no effect of frusemide on plasma phenytoin level.]
halothane   Karlin and Kutt (1970)
phenylbutazone   Hansen, Kristensen, Skovsted and Christensen (1974)
phenyramidol   Solomon and Schrogie (1967)
prochlorperazine   Kutt and McDowell (1968)
propoxyphene   Kutt (1971)
propranolol   personal unpublished data

A lesser number of interactions have been reported in which addition of a second drug caused a fall in plasma phenytoin concentration. The drugs which interacted in this way include the following:

antacids   Pippenger (1973)—cited by Kutt (1975)
diazoxide   Roe, Podosin and Blaskovics (1975)
oxacillin   Fincham, Wiley and Schottelius (1976)
pyridoxine   Hansson and Sillanpaa (1976)
tolbutamide   Wesseling and Mols-Thurkow (1975)

In the literature a few additional substances are mentioned as not altering plasma phenytoin levels when given concurrently with that drug. These non-interacting substances include allopurinol (Skovsted, Hansen, Kristensen and Christensen, 1974) and vitamin D (Christiansen and Rodbro, 1974a).

TOXICITY

The toxic effects of phenytoin were reviewed in detail by Sparberg (1963). Much additional information has appeared since that time. The unwanted effects may be conveniently considered in 4 groups:

1. local effects at site of administration
2. dose-determined systemic effects
3. idiosyncratic effects
4. effects on the fetus and neonate

LOCAL EFFECTS

In a few patients orally administered phenytoin produces upper abdominal discomfort, sometimes relieved by concurrent antacid therapy. Patients who bite into their phenytoin tablets or capsules generally dislike the taste, though a more attractively flavoured chewable tablet is also marketed. Although parenteral preparations of phenytoin are at a strongly alkaline pH their intramuscular injection usually does not cause undue discomfort unless the injections are given repeatedly (Dam and Olsen, 1966). There is a possibility that phenytoin injected into intravenous solutions may partly precipitate out at physiological pH, but there is little reported evidence of adverse effects as a result of this. However, the solvent in parenteral phenytoin preparations (propylene glycol) may produce hypotension when given intravenously (Wallis, Kutt and McDowell, 1968).

DOSE-DETERMINED SYSTEMIC EFFECTS

Neurotoxicity

As Kutt, Winters, Kokenge and McDowell (1964) pointed out, once enough phenytoin has been given to raise the plasma phenytoin level above 20 μg/ml, first degree horizontal nystagmus tends to appear. However, sometimes nystagmus is absent even at much higher plasma phenytoin levels (Perlo and Schwab, 1969). If phenytoin dosage is increased and plasma levels rise further, side-effects such as ataxia of gait, double vision, nausea, vomiting and drowsiness usually occur. The correlations between plasma phenytoin level and such clinical effects were considered in detail earlier. The EEG of the over-dosed patient often shows slowing of the alpha rhythm and the appearance of bilaterally symmetrical 4–7 Hz activity and occasional slower components. Sometimes control of epilepsy lessens when plasma phenytoin levels become too high (Levy and Fenichel, 1965; Perlo and Schwab, 1969; Lascelles, Kocen and Reynolds, 1970; Troupin and Ojemann, 1976). Less typical neurotoxic features of phenytoin overdosage (e.g. mental changes, incontinence, a raised CSF protein) may sometimes occur (Logan and Freeman, 1969). There has been a report of total external ophthalmoplegia due to the drug (Spector, Davidoff and Schwartzman, 1976), and an instance of widespread fasciculation which recovered when phenytoin was ceased (Direkze and Fernando, 1977). Some patients merely feel vaguely unwell or depressed when overdosed with the drug. Others experience no neurological ill-effects even with plasma phenytoin levels up to 35 μg/ml. However, the overall incidence of neurological disturbances increases as plasma phenytoin levels rise.

There have also been several reports that phenytoin overdosage may lead to reversible dyskinesia, rather than the more usual pattern of neurological disturbance viz. nystagmus, ataxia of gait and diplopia. The dyskinetic movements have usually been choreic or choreo-athetoid in pattern, but there have occasionally been oro-facial dyskinesias, myoclonus, dystonia and asterixis (Kooiker and Sumi, 1974; McLellan and Swash, 1974; Murphy and Goldstein, 1974; Ahmad, Laidlaw, Houghton and Richens, 1975; Chadwick, Reynolds and Marsden, 1976; Chalhub, Devivo and Volpe, 1976; Luhdorf and Lund, 1977; Rasmussen and Kristensen, 1977). The occurrence of such involuntary movements may be due to phenytoin being a dopamine antagonist (Mendel, Cotzias, Mena and Papavasiliou, 1975).

There have been reports that sustained phenytoin overdosage may lead to permanent cerebellar damage in man with, in particular, loss of Purkinje cells (Hofmann, 1958; Kokenge, Kutt and McDowell, 1965; Hoglmeier and Wenzel, 1969). Dam (1972) carried out a series of studies on this matter, published in a small monograph. He was unable to demonstrate permanent histological changes in the cerebellum of animals chronically overdosed with phenytoin. He therefore favoured the view that the cerebellar changes in man allegedly due to chronic phenytoin intoxication were really due to hypoxia during epileptic seizures. The vulnerability of Purkinje cells to hypoxia is well known (Scholz, 1953; Eadie, Tyrer and Kukums, 1971) and it has also been observed that the cerebellum of the epileptic may show Purkinje cell loss (Meyer, 1958). Further instances of cerebellar atrophy in epileptic patients taking phenytoin continue to be reported (Ghatak, Santoso and McKinney, 1976; Iivanainen, Viukari and Helle, 1977). In such instances there has not been proof that the phenytoin intake was causally related to the cerebellar atrophy.

A number of authors found that chronic phenytoin therapy was associated with slowing of motor conduction in peripheral nerves without clinical peripheral neuropathy (Lovelace and Horowitz, 1968; Birket-Smith and Krogh, 1971; Chokroverty and Rubino, 1973; Eisen, Woods and Sherwin, 1974; Encinoza, 1974; Chokroverty and Sayeed, 1975). Slowed motor conduction in peripheral nerves occurs frequently in patients taking phenytoin. Encinoza (1974) found that the phenomenon in 52 per cent of 300 patients who had taken the drug for between $2\frac{1}{2}$ and 9 years. The frequency of the finding was increased in persons older than 20 years, in persons who had taken the drug for more than 4 years, and in those who took the drug in doses over 4·5 mg/kg/day. Sensory conduction as well as motor conduction was sometimes slowed. Dobkin (1977) reported a single instance of clinically apparent sensorimotor peripheral polyneuropathy seemingly due to phenytoin intake.

Brumlik and Jacobs (1974) described an instance of myasthenia which appeared causally related to phenytoin therapy.

Gum changes
Gingival hypertrophy is a characteristic side effect of chronic phenytoin therapy (Kimball, 1939). It probably occurs to a slight degree in a majority of patients taking the drug (Angelopoulos and Goaz, 1972) but often begins to become prominent about the time overdosage manifestations appear. Gum hypertrophy tends to be less severe in edentulous areas. It is made worse by poor dental hygiene and tends to be more severe in children than in adults. It disappears within a few months of ceasing phenytoin (Livingston and Livingston, 1969).

Merritt (1958) and Kutt and McDowell (1968) stated that gum hypertrophy was unrelated to plasma phenytoin level. However, Kapur, Girgis, Little and Masotti (1973), Conard, Jeffay, Boshes and Steinberg (1974) and Little, Girgis and Masotti (1975) all found that gum hypertrophy was related to plasma phenytoin concentrations. Aarli (1976) raised the possibility that lowered salivary levels of IgA in patients taking phenytoin (see page 86) might contribute to gum hypertrophy.

Altered hair growth
Overgrowth of hair on the trunk and limbs occurs in about 5 per cent of patients taking phenytoin (Livingston, 1972). Young females in particular may regard the change as cosmetically undesirable. It tends to persist after phenytoin intake is ceased (Merritt, 1958).

Connective tissue alterations
Apart from the occurrence of gingival hypertrophy, there are a number of observations suggesting that phenytoin alters collagen synthesis. Thus Bazin and Delaunay (1972) found that phenytoin accelerated the maturation of collagen both in normal skin and in granulomas in rats. The drug promoted the formation of stable intermolecular bonds derived from aldehyde groups on proteins. Blumenkrantz and Asboe-Hansen (1974) found that phenytoin inhibited collagen biosynthesis in the 10 day old chick embryo. Lefebvre, Haining and Labbé (1972) and Falconer and Davidson (1974) noted a coarsening of the facial features in patients taking phenytoin, though the drug was used with other anticonvulsants. Kattan (1975) noted that the incidence of thickening of the heel pad increased with duration of phenytoin therapy. After 10 years of therapy heel pad thickening was present in 7 of 12 subjects. Altered collagen in pulmonary alveolar walls may have contributed to the finding that almost 50 per cent of a group of 40 patients who had taken phenytoin for over two years had a decreased pulmonary gaseous diffusion capacity (Hazlett, Ward and Madison, 1974).

Hypocalcaemia and osteomalacia

Low serum calcium levels have been reported in patients taking phenytoin (Kruse, 1968; Richens and Rowe, 1970; Hunter, Maxwell, Stewart, Parsons and Williams, 1971; Hahn, Hendin, Scarp and Haddad, 1972; Christiansen, Rodbro and Lund, 1973; Lifshitz and Maclaren, 1973; Rodbro, Christiansen and Lund, 1974). Several of these authors, and also Kazamatsuri (1970), noted raised serum alkaline phosphatase levels in such patients. Hypocalcaemia occurred in about 30 per cent of the cases of Richens and Rowe (1970) and of Hunter, Maxwell, Stewart, Parsons and Williams (1971), and in about 19 per cent of those of Hahn, Hendin, Scharp and Haddad (1972). It tended to become more frequent as total anticonvulsant dose became higher. In the majority of patients with such hypocalcaemia so far described multiple anticonvulsants were being taken. Therefore phenytoin intake may not necessarily have been responsible for the abnormalities. However, low serum calcium levels have occurred in patients taking phenytoin alone (Hahn, Hendin, Scharp and Haddad, 1972; Varkey, Raman, Bhaktaviziam, and Taori, 1973). Christiansen, Nielsen and Rodbro (1974) reported mildly reduced serum magnesium levels in patients taking anticonvulsants. Serum levels of magnesium did not correlate with serum calcium levels. Katz, Gerstman, Lautenbacher and Hediger (1976) and Stewart (1976) failed to confirm the finding of reduced serum magnesium levels in patients taking anticonvulsants.

Dent, Richens, Rowe and Stamp (1970) found four instances of osteomalacia in patients taking phenytoin together with barbiturates. Stoegman (1971) noted disturbed ossification in 22 per cent of 81 epileptic children who had taken phenytoin or primidone for more than 3 years. There have been a number of further reports of biochemically and/or radiologically diagnosed osteomalacia in patients receiving long term anticonvulsant therapy (Christiansen, Rodbro and Lund, 1973; Ganapathy, Krishana Rao and Gouri Devi, 1973; Lifshitz and Maclaren, 1973; Rodbro, Christiansen and Lund, 1974; Mosekilde and Melsen, 1976). The bone disorder seems to appear after some months of anticonvulsant therapy. Rarely, secondary hyperparathyroidism has occurred (Campbell, Tam and Sheppard, 1977). Marsden, Reynolds, Parsons, Harris and Duchen (1973) reported a single instance of myopathy associated with osteomalacia in a patient taking phenytoin with phenobarbitone. The myopathy recovered when vitamin D was given. Lefebvre, Haining and Labbe (1972) described a syndrome of 'coarse facies, calvarial thickening and hyperphosphatasia associated with long-term anticonvulsant therapy'.

Dent, Richens, Rowe and Stamp (1970), Hunter, Maxwell, Stewart, Parsons and Williams (1971) and Hahn (1976) all suggested that anticonvulsants may induce the liver enzymes which metabolize these drugs and also vitamin D. This increased biotransformation may lead to a relative deficiency of biologically active vitamin D, because of increased formation of inactive metabolites of the vitamin (Stamp, 1974). In keeping with these suggestions Hahn, Hendin, Scarp and Haddad (1972) showed that serum 25-hydroxy-cholecalciferol levels were reduced by 33 per cent in their chronic epileptic patients receiving both phenytoin and phenobarbitone. Despite this, plasma levels of the hormonal form of vitamin D (1,25-dihydroxycholecalciferol) were not reduced (Jubiz, Haussler, McCain and Tolman, 1977). Vitamin D therapy reversed some, but not all, of the serum and bone biochemical abnormalities of anticonvulsant osteomalacia (Christiansen and Rodbro, 1974b; 1976). However, Christiansen, Rodbro, Munch and Munch (1975) argued that rather more than mere diversion of vitamin D to inactive metabolites is involved in the pathogenesis of anticonvulsant osteomalacia. These workers found that calciferol (vitamin D_2) did not fully correct the abnormalities of this osteomalacia (bone mineral content was restored, but serum calcium levels did not rise). On the other hand cholecalciferol (vitamin D_3) and its hepatic metabolite 25-hydroxy-cholecalciferol restored serum calcium levels but not the bone mineral content in cases of anticonvulsant osteomalacia. The exact pathophysiology of anticonvulsant osteomalacia is not yet fully known.

Another factor possibly involved in the anticonvulsant-induced disturbance of mineral metabolism may have been detected by Koch, Kraft, Von Herrath and Schaefer (1972). These workers showed that phenytoin, but not phenobarbitone, decreased calcium absorption from the intestine of vitamin D deficient rats. Caspary (1972) obtained a similar result. Harris, Jenkins and Willis (1974) showed that phenytoin, at a concentration of 15 μg/ml, inhibited effect of parathormone in promoting calcium resorption from bone. This action would interfere with a mechanism which might tend to restore calcium levels to normal.

Mosenkilde and Melsen (1976) defined the risk factors in anticonvulsant osteomalacia as including (1) a low dietary vitamin D intake, (2) a low exposure to sunlight, (3) a high hepatic clearance of phenytoin, (4) therapy with anticonvulsant combinations, and (5) being male. Practising in an affluent society (in the U.S.A.) may have been the reason that Livingston, Berman and Pauli (1973) found no osteomalacia or metabolic disorders in 5500 epileptics despite the comparatively high incidence of the disorder reported from northern Europe and the United Kingdom. The present writers also practise in an affluent society in a sunny sub-tropical climate. They have seen virtually no anticonvulsant osteomalacia. Where diet is suboptimal and where exposure to sunlight is below average, there may be a case for the routine use of vitamin D in patients, particularly children, taking high doses of anticonvulsants. However, such prophylaxis does not appear necessary in every patient given anticonvulsants. Rodbro, Christiansen and Lund (1975) noted that vitamin D therapy did not relieve symptoms such as back pain, tiredness and irritability, which might conceivably have been related to vitamin D deficiency in patients on chronic anticonvulsant therapy.

Folate deficiency

Some reference to this matter has been made both in Chapter 4, and earlier in the present Chapter, in relation to the role of folate deficiency in producing an anti-epileptic effect. The possible mechanisms whereby phenytoin may cause folate deficiency were considered earlier in the present Chapter.

For 20 years it has been known that phenytoin therapy occasionally caused megaloblastic anaemia (Stokes and Fortune, 1958) which responded to folic acid therapy. When serum folate measurements became readily available, reports appeared that anticonvulsant therapy was associated with low serum folate levels (Klipstein, 1964; Malpas, Spray and Witts, 1966) and low CSF folate levels (Reynolds, Preece and Chanarin, 1969; Mauguiere and Karlin, 1975). However there have been contrary findings (Wickman and Lehtovarra, 1968). In a series of papers Reynolds (e.g. 1958) proposed the view that anticonvulsant-induced folic acid deficiency led to impaired mental functioning and personality change in epileptics. Further he suggested that the anti-epileptic action of anticonvulsants might be inseparable from the production of folic acid deficiency. He found (Reynolds, 1967) that folic acid therapy improved the mental state of 22 of 26 epileptics, but worsened the control of seizures of 13 of 26. Neubauer (1970) used combined folic acid and vitamin B_{12} therapy and found an improved mental condition in some of his epileptics without deterioration in the control of their epilepsy. In such studies many, but not all, patients had received phenytoin, though it was often used in conjunction with other anticonvulsants. Therapy with phenytoin alone may cause folate deficiency (Davis and Woodliff, 1971). However there is no close correlation between serum phenytoin and serum folate levels (Korczyn, Elian, Don and Bornstein, 1974). There have been several careful studies showing that folic acid therapy does not alter the behaviour, personality or epilepsy control of folate-deficient epileptics (Grant and Stores, 1970; Jensen and Olesen, 1970; Ralston, Snaith and Hinley, 1970; Norris and Pratt, 1974). Thus it seems that phenytoin may at times cause reduced serum folate levels, and that these rarely lead to megaloblastic anaemia. However, it is uncertain if this folate deficiency has any deleterious effect on nervous system function in patients with epilepsy.

Immunological abnormalities
Immunological abnormalities were found by Sorrell, Forbes, Burness and Rischbieth (1971) in an appreciable proportion of patients taking phenytoin. There were low levels of immunoglobulin A in 21 per cent, failure of antibody response to Salmonella typhi antigen in 9 per cent, absence of delayed hypersensitivity to three common skin test antigens in 22 per cent, and depression of *in vitro* lymphocyte transformation by phytohaemagglutinin in 27 per cent. The pictures of the cellular and humoral immunological suppression associated with phenytoin intake were regarded as similar to those found in Hodgkin's disease and malignant lymphoma. Grob and Herold (1972) also noted immunological abnormalities associated with hydantoin intake. Beernink and Miller (1973) found an increased incidence of antinuclear antibodies in children taking phenytoin, while Shakir, Behan, Dick and Lambie (1978) noted decreased cell function in 23 per cent of a series of patients receiving the drug.

As was discussed above, there have been several recent reports that phenytoin intake is associated with decreased levels of various immunoglobulins in blood, saliva and CSF (see page 86).

Altered insulin secretion
Goldberg and Sanbar (1969) reported two cases of nonketotic hyperglycaemic coma following the intravenous administration of phenytoin. Knopp, Sheinin and Freinkel (1972) encounted an instance in which the diagnosis of insulinoma was obscured by phenytoin therapy. The drug had decreased the insulin secretion from the tumor. Other workers have also shown that phenytoin decreased insulin release from the apparently normal pancreas (Malherbe, Burrill, Levin, Karam and Forsham, 1972; Toyka, Janka and Janka, 1975) even when plasma phenytoin

levels were in the therapeutic range (Mohd Amin Arnaout and Salti, 1967). However, Cummings, Rosenbloom, Kohler and Wilder (1973) and Madsen, Hansen and Deckert (1974) found that phenytoin, in non-toxic doses, had little effect on glucose-stimulated insulin release in man. Castleden and Richens (1973) found a lower incidence of diabetes mellitus in the members of an epileptic colony than in the general population. Thus continued exposure to phenytoin did not increase the risk of diabetes, despite the action of the drug in decreasing the secretion of insulin.

IDIOSYNCRATIC EFFECTS

Skin
In a small percentage of patients phenytoin may produce skin rashes. These are often morbilliform and generally occur within 1 to 2 weeks of the onset of therapy. Rarely the skin changes are more severe, leading to exfoliative dermatitis (Stein and Pembrook, 1965) or erythema multiforme exudativum (Watts, 1962). It would appear prudent not to use phenytoin again in a given patient if a skin rash occurs. Sometimes lymphadenopathy, fever and eosinophilia may be associated with the skin rashes. The combination of erythema multiforme exudativum and lupus erythematosus has occurred in patients taking phenytoin (Rallinson, Carlisle, Lee, Vernier and Good, 1961).

Blood
Instances of toxic damage to bone marrow elements have been described, causing leucopenia (Kurtzke, 1961), and erythroid aphasia (Brittingham, Lutcher and Murphy, 1964; Jeong, Jung and River, 1974). It has sometimes been uncertain whether phenytoin or a concurrently administered drug has been responsible. On one occasion panmyeloid hypoplasia appeared to be dose-dependent (Parker and Gumnit, 1974).

The present authors have encountered occasional patients who complain of symptoms compatible with a blood coagulation defect (e.g. easy bruising, menorrhagia) which appear soon after phenytoin therapy is commenced. Investigation has not shown any alteration in coagulation but the symptoms have ceased once the phenytoin was replaced by another anticonvulsant. This observation may be relevant in view of the occurrence of definite coagulation defects in some neonates who have been exposed to anticonvulsants *in utero* (see page 106).

Lymphoid tissue
The most potentially serious idiosyncratic side-effect of phenytoin is a pseudo-lymphoma syndrome. Knowledge of this pseudo-lymphoma syndrome was reviewed by Saltzstein and Ackerman (1959). The syndrome often appears within 4 weeks of the commencement of therapy, and comprises painless generalized lymphadenopathy, sometimes associated with skin rashes and other signs of a systemic reaction. Histologically the enlarged nodes show changes in the cellular architecture with reticulum-cell hyperplasia, eosinophil and plasma cell infiltration and focal necroses. The changes do not extend into the capsule of the node and there are no Reed-Sternberg giant cells. The lymphadenopathy disappears within a

few weeks of ceasing phenytoin therapy, but may recur if the drug is resumed.

It has also been suggested that phenytoin therapy may be associated with malignant lymphoma. In patients taking phenytoin Hyman and Sommers (1966) found possible instances of malignant lymphoma which had not developed from the progression of a pseudo-lymphoma reaction. Other authors (e.g. Rausing and Trell, 1971) have reported single cases of malignant lymphoma. Indirect evidence for an association between phenytoin and malignant lymphoma was obtained by Charlton and Lunsford (1971). These authors studied 300 consecutively biopsied persons with malignant lymphoma at the Columbia Presbyterian Medical Centre, New York. Among these patients there were some 5 times as many persons who took phenytoin as would have been expected on purely random grounds. Endtz, Leeksma, Kerkhofs, Mulder, Mosmans and Meinardi (1973) found that a disproportionately high number of their cases of acute leukaemia were taking phenytoin. However Clemmesen, Fugslang-Frederiksen and Plum (1974) found no evidence of an association between anticonvulsant intake (not specifically phenytoin intake) and neoplasia in a statistical study of 9136 patients with epilepsy.

Miscellaneous effects

Several instances of hepatitis following phenytoin intake have been reported (Gropper, 1956; Crawford and Jones, 1962; Martin and Rickers, 1972; Dhar, Ahamed, Pierach and Howard, 1974; Weedon, 1975). The syndrome may be associated with a rubella-like rash, or an illness resembling infectious mononucleosis. Kuiper (1969) found that the drug might occasionally produce thyroiditis. Agarwal, Cabebe and Hoffman (1977) reported an instance of reversible renal failure following exposure to phenytoin.

EFFECTS ON THE FETUS AND NEONATE

Dysmorphogenesis

In some infra-human species (e.g. rats and mice) exposure to phenytoin between the 10th and 14th day of gestation may lead to an increased incidence of fetal resorption, cleft lip and cleft plate, ectrodactyly, hydronephrosis, hydrocephalus, peritoneal and renal haemorrhage and decreased growth of the long bones of the appendicular skeleton (Harbison and Becker, 1969; 1972; Mercier-Parot and Tuchmann-Duplessis, 1974). Meadow (1970) reported an increased incidence of hare lip and cleft palate in the offspring of women taking anticonvulsants. However, there was no control group and not all of the subjects he studied had received phenytoin. Speidel and Meadow (1972) found major congenital abnormalities (congenital heart disease, cleft lip with or without cleft palate, and microcephaly) at least twice as often in the 427 offspring of 186 epileptic mothers as in the offspring of non-epileptic mothers (also see Table 6.1). In the offspring of the epileptic mothers there was an increased perinatal mortality due either to the malformation or to spontaneous haemorrhages. Phenytoin, alone or in combination, was taken by the mothers of only 9 of the 17 babies with malformations. Phenobarbitone was taken by mothers of 10, and some mothers also took other anticonvulsants. No malformations occurred in the 62 offspring of 27 epileptic mothers taking no anticonvulsants. The reason for these latter epileptic mothers being untreated was not discussed. Possibly they had less severe epilepsy than the mothers who took anticonvulsants. The paper of Speidel and Meadow (1972) was followed by a spate of reports of the incidence of possible anticonvulsant related dysmorphogenesis (summarized in Table 6.1). Often the anticonvulsants involved were not clearly indicated. The available literature was reviewed by Annegers, Elveback, Hauser and Kurland (1974). There have also been reports of instances of phenytoin-associated dysmorphogensis which have not contained incidence figures (Loughnan, Gold and Vance, 1973).

The original reports of anticonvulsant dysmorphogenesis drew attention to the occurrence of cleft palate and hare lip. Subsequently an association was found between these drugs and heart, gastro-intestinal and central nervous system malformations (Speidel and Meadow, 1974). Danks, Barry and Sheffield (1974) and Barr, Poznanski and Schmickel (1974) pointed out the frequent occurrence of digital hypoplasia in the offspring of women taking phenytoin and other anticonvulsants during pregnancy.

There appears to be strong evidence that maternal phenytoin intake is associated with a doubled or trebled risk of dysmorphogenesis. However there is no rigid proof that phenytoin itself causes dysmorphogenesis in humans. The association between phenobarbitone intake during pregnancy and dysmorphogenesis is nearly as close as that which applies for phenytoin. However, Shapiro, Hartz, Siskind, Mitchell, Slone, Rosenberg, Monson, Heinonen, Idanpaan-Heikkila, Haro and Saxén (1976) found no increased incidence of dysmorphogenesis in the offspring of non-epileptic women who had taken phenobarbitone during pregnancy. This finding raises the possibility that dysmorphogenesis is more closely related to having epilepsy than to taking anticonvulsant drugs. If this is the case one might also expect an increased incidence of malformations in the offspring of epileptic males and non-epileptic females. Meyer (1973) obtained evidence that this was so, whereas Annegers, Elveback, Hanser and Kurland (1974) did not. It should be pointed out that if certain anticonvulsants (including phenytoin) were teratogens by virtue of a mutagenic effect, there would also be an increased incidence of malformation in the offspring of treated fathers and non-treated mothers. The difficulty of obtaining control series of untreated pregnant epileptics matched for type and severity of epilepsy with treated pregnant epileptics, has made it virtually impossible so far to settle the question of whether phenytoin produces serious dysmorphogenesis in humans.

In the present state of knowledge most authors (e.g. Janz, 1975) agree that the risks for the fetus of continuing anticonvulsant therapy during pregnancy are less than the maternal and fetal risks if treatment is ceased.

Coagulation and other haematological effects
Mountain, Hirsch and Gallus (1970) pointed out that anticonvulsant therapy in the mother (often involving barbiturate anticonvulsants as well as phenytoin) could lead in the newborn to deficiency of vitamin K-dependent blood clotting factors (factor II—prothrombin, and factor VII—convertin). These workers encountered this sequel in 8 of 16 infants born of mothers taking anticonvulsants. Solomon, Hilgartner and Kutt (1972) traced reports of 26 affected infants in the literature, though Bleyer and Skinner (1976) in a more recent report did not find as many

Table 6.1 Malformation rates in offspring of epileptic mothers (per 1000 live births)

Author	Live births to epileptic mothers Total	All malformations	Cleft lip/palate	CHD	Live births in control population Total	All malformations	Cleft lip/palate	CHD
Janz and Fuchs (1964)	225±	22	13	4	—	—	—	—
	133*	0	0	0				
Elshove and van Eck (1971)	65±	154	77	30	12051	19	2·7	0
Watson and Spellacy (1971)	51±	59	0	20	50	0	0	0
South (1972)	23±	90	90	0	7675	24·2	1·8	—
	9*	0	0	0				
Speidel and Meadow (1972)	329±	51	9	18	448	16	2	2
	59*	0	0	0				
Bjerkedal and Bahna (1973)	371	45	18	—	112328	22	1·6	—
Fredrick (1973)	217±	138	4·6	9	649	56	0	8
Koppe et al. (1973)	125±	88	8	32	123000	35	1·7	0
Kuenssberg and Knox (1973)	48±	100	0		14668	34	6	
Lowe (1973)	134±	56	7·5	7·5	31877	28	1·6	
	111*	27	0	0				
Meyer (1973)	199±	185	25	25	394†	124	0	2·5
Millar and Nevin (1973)	110±	64	18	0	32227	38	2·2	—
Monson et al. (1973)	306	46	3	10	50897	25		—
Niswander and Wertelecki (1973)	413	41	7·3	12	347087	27	1·5	4·1
Annegers et al. (1974)	141±	71	21	43	—	—	1·9	5·7
	56*	18	0	0				
Barry and Danks (1974)	62±	161			—	—	—	—

CHD: Congenital heart disease; ±: all treated with anticonvulsants; *: not receiving anticonvulsants; †: included offspring of untreated epileptics.

instances. The mothers of the affected infants did not have coagulation defects, and the children tended to bleed on their first post-natal day, earlier than the time of bleeding in haemorrhagic disease of the new born. Possibly this effect of anticonvulsant therapy is a consequence of liver enzyme induction which accelerates the metabolic breakdown of coagulation factors. However Solomon, Hilgartner and Kutt (1972) suggested that phenytoin may be a competitive inhibitor of vitamin K. These observations on neonatal coagulation defects suggest the wisdom of giving vitamin K at term to women taking phenytoin or other anticonvulsants.

Massimo, Pantarotto and Vianello (1974) reported that of 15 babies born to women taking phenytoin during pregnancy, 9 had bone marrow hypoplasia or aplasia. There was also some evidence of depressed immunological function in the babies. There do not appear to have been reports corroborating these findings.

PREPARATIONS AVAILABLE

Phenytoin sodium

Capsules: 30 mg; 100 mg
Tablets: 100 mg

Phenytoin
   Tablets (chewable): 50 mg
   Suspension (for oral use): 30 mg per 5 ml; 100 mg per 5 ml
   Amploules (for injection): 250 mg per 5 ml

OTHER HYDANTOINS

At the present time the other hydantoin anticonvulsants are little used. They are either more toxic and/or less effective than phenytoin, and have been subject of little study by modern clinical pharmacological methods.

METHOIN (MEPHENYTOIN)

The structural resemblance between the molecules of methoin (5-ethyl-5-phenyl-3-methyl-hydantoin) and that of phenytoin is shown above. As compared with phenytoin, methoin has a methyl group added at the 3 position on the hydantoin ring, and has an ethyl group substituted for one of the benzene rings at the 5 position. Butler (1953) showed that methoin was N-demethylated in the body to form 5-ethyl-5-phenylhydantoin. This latter substance is the drug 'Nirvanol', an anticonvulsant notorious for its capacity to cause bone marrow aplasia (Jones and Jacobs, 1932). This desmethylated derivative of methoin undergoes subsequent aromatic hydroxylation, to be excreted in urine as 5-ethyl-5(p-hydroxyphenyl) hydantoin (Butler, 1956).

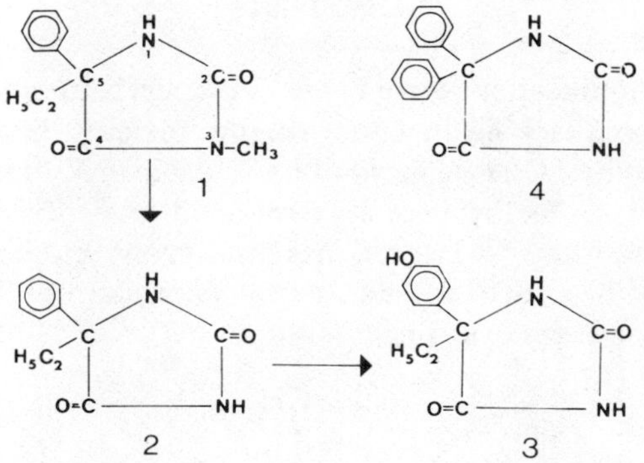

Fig. 6.32 Methoin (Mephenytoin)
1. 5-ethyl-5-phenyl-3-methylhydantoin (Methoin)
2. 5-ethyl-5-phenylhydantoin (Nirvanol)
3. 5-ethyl-5-(p-hydroxyphenyl) hydantoin
4. 5,5^1-diphenylhydantoin (Phenytoin), shown for comparison

In mice, the maximum electroshock test shows 'Nirvanol' to be a better anticonvulsant than methoin on a molar basis (Kupferberg and Yonekawa, 1975). In these animals, after a single methoin dose, brain methoin: 'Nirvanol' ratios were approximately 2·5:1 after 30 minutes, but 1:3 after 24 hours, suggesting that the metabolite was more slowly eliminated than the parent drug.

Troupin, Ojemann and Dodrill (1976) recently reinvestigated methoin as an anticonvulsant in 93 epileptic patients. Epilepsy control was improved in 72 per cent, but there was one death from aplastic anaemia. These authors found that presumed steady-state plasma methoin concentrations were 7·7 per cent ± 4·55 per cent of combined methoin-'Nirvanol' concentrations. This result would correlate with the possibility that methoin is more rapidly eliminated than 'Nirvanol'. In two cases Troupin, Ojemann and Dodrill (1976) found the half-lives of 'Nirvanol' were 74 and 144 hours respectively, while in one case the half-life of methoin was 32 hours. Combined levels of methoin plus 'Nirvanol' in CSF were 64 per cent (range 50–76 per cent) and in saliva 62 per cent (range 49–79 per cent) of the simultaneous levels of these two substances in plasma. Coradello (1973) claimed he could not detect methoin in the milk of patients taking this drug.

The anticonvulsant effect of methoin in man is said to correlate equally well with plasma concentrations of methoin, or 'Nirvanol', or of both combined (Troupin, Ojemann and Dodrill, 1976). The latter authors proposed a provisional therapeutic range of plasma concentration of the two substances (measured together) of 25–40 μg/ml.

In apparently similar circumstances, methoin sometimes proves a more effective anticonvulsant than phenytoin (Lennox and Lennox, 1960). It is less likely to cause cerebellar disturbance, gum hypertrophy and hair overgrowth. Yet all these advantages are more than offset by the relatively frequent occurrence of skin rashes, and the appreciable incidence of fatal aplastic anaemia (Robins, 1962).

DELTOIN

Various chemical modifications were made to the methoin molecule in the hope of achieving a substance lacking in bone marrow toxicity, but retaining adequate anticonvulsant activity. One such product, deltoin ('Methetoin'), differs from methoin in that it is methylated at position 1 on the hydantoin ring, and demethylated at position 3. Deltoin has undergone clinical trials (Selby and Lorenz, 1966), but has not come into any widespread use, probably because it lacks sufficient advantages over phenytoin.

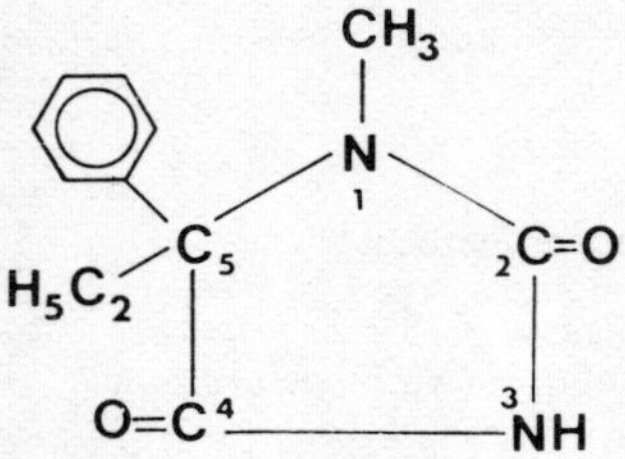

Fig. 6.33 Deltoin

ETHOTOIN

Ethotoin (3-ethyl-5-phenylhydantoin) has been available for about 20 years, but has never achieved any large scale use as an anticonvulsant, largely because of its lack of potency relative to phenytoin. The biotransformation of the drug in dogs was investigated by Dudley, Bius and Butler (1970). The drug undergoes N-dealkylation at position 3, or aromatic parahydroxylation, followed by glucuronide conjugation. In man little of the drug is excreted unchanged in urine (Sjo, Hvidberg, Larsen, Lund and Naestoft, 1975). As in the case of phenytoin, steady-state plasma levels increase disproportionately with dose increments, raising the possibility of dose-dependent elimination kinetics. CSF levels of the drug are $11 \cdot 6 \pm 11 \cdot 4$ per cent of its plasma levels (Miyamoto, Seino and Ikeda, 1975), suggesting that ethotoin undergoes substantial binding to plasma protein.

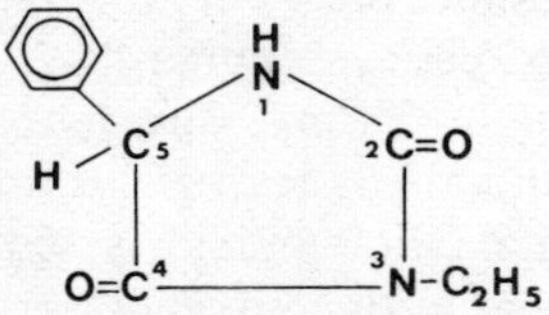

Fig. 6.34 Ethotoin

ALBUTOIN

Albutoin (3-allyl-5-isobutyl-2-thiohydantoin) was investigated as an anticonvulsant in the USA (Millichap and Ortiz, 1967). The drug was moderately potent, but tended to produce drowsiness. It does not seem to have achieved any general popularity of use. Cereghino, Brock, van Meter, Penry, Smith, Fisher and Ellenberg (1974) considered it less effective than phenytoin or phenobarbitone.

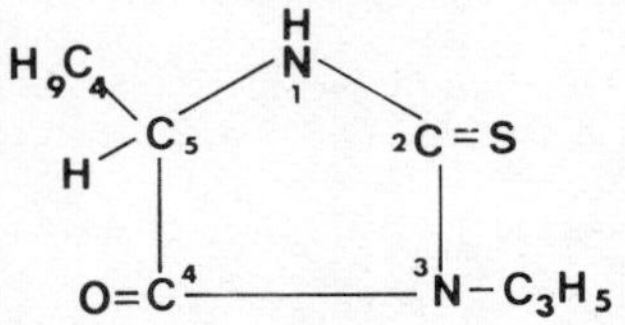

Fig. 6.35 Albutoin.

REFERENCES

Aarli, J. A. (1976) Phenytoin-induced depression of salivary IgA and gingival hyperplasia. *Epilepsia* (Amst.), **17**, 283–291.

Aarli, J. A. & Tonder, O. (1975) Effect of antiepileptic drugs on serum and salivary IgA. *Scand. J. Immunol.*, **4**, 391–396.

Abe, Y., Tamagawa, K. & Eguchi, M. (1973) Liver functions in children during antiepileptic drug therapy: serum γ-glutamyl transpeptidase activity. *Brain Develop.*, **5**, 274–280.

Adler, D. S., Martin, E., Gamertoglio, J. G., Tozer, T. N. & Spire, J. P. (1975) Hemodialysis of phenytoin in a uremic patient. *Clin. Pharmacol. Therap.*, **18**, 65–69.

Agarwal, B. N., Cabebe, F. G. & Hoffman, B. I. (1977) Diphenylhydantoin induced acute renal failure. *Nephron*, **18**, 249–251.

Agarwal, S. P. & Blake, M. I. (1968) Determination of the pK_a value for 5,5-diphenylhydantoin. *J. Pharm. Sci.*, **57**, 1434–1435.

Agnew, D. C. & Goldberg, V. C. (1976) A brief trial of phenytoin therapy for thalamic pain. *Bull. Los Angeles Neurol. Soc.*, **41**, 9–11.

Ahmad, S., Laidlaw, J., Houghton, G. W. & Richens, A. (1975) Involuntary movements caused by phenytoin intoxication in epileptic patients. *J. Neurol. Neurosurg. Psychiat.*, **38**, 225–231.

Albert, K. S., Hallmark, M. R., Sakmar, E., Weidler, D. J. & Wagner, J. G. (1974) Plasma concentrations of diphenylhydantoin, its para-hydroxylated metabolite, and corresponding glucuronide in man. *Res. Commun. Chem. Path. Pharmacol.*, **9**, 463–469.

Albert, K. S., Sakmar, E., Hallmark, M. R., Weidler, D. J. & Wagner, J. G. (1974) Bioavailability of diphenylhydantoin. *Clin. Pharmacol. Therap.*, **16**, 727–735.

Angelopoulos, A. P. & Goaz, P. W. (1972) Incidence of diphenylhydantoin gingival hyperplasia. *Oral Surg.*, **34**, 898–906.

Annegers, J. F., Elveback, L. R., Hauser, W. A. & Kurland, L. T. (1974) Do anticonvulsants have a teratogenic effect. *Arch. Neurol.* (Chic.), **31**, 364–373.

Arakawa, T., Honda, Y. & Narisawa, K. (1973) Decreased hepatic histidase activity induced by diphenylhdantoin administration as a cause of decrease in urinary formininoglutamic acid in rats. *Tohuku. J. Exp. Med.* **110**, 49–57.

Arnold, K. & Gerber, N. (1970) The rate of decline of diphenylhydantoin in human plasma. *Clin. Pharmacol. Therap.* **11**, 121–134.

Arnold, K., Gerber, N. & Levy, G. (1970) Absorption and dissolution studies on sodium diphenylhydantoin capsules. *Canad. J. Pharm. Sci.*, **5**, 89–92.

Ashley, J. J. & Levy, G. (1972) Inhibition of diphenylhydantoin elimination by its major metabolite. *Res. Commun. Chem. Pathol. Pharmacol.* **4**, 297–306.

Ashley, J. J. & Levy, G. (1973) Kinetics of diphenylhydantoin elimination in rats. *J. Pharmacokinet. Biopharmaceutics*, **1**, 99–102.

Askari, A. (editor) (1974) Properties and functions of (Na^+, K^+)-activated adenosinetriphophatase. *Ann. N.Y. Acad. Sci.*, **242**, 1–741.

Atkinson, A. J. Jr., MacGee, J., Strong, J., Garteiz, D. & Gaffney, T. E. (1970) Identification of 5-meta-hydroxyphenyl-5-phenylhydantoin as a metabolite of diphenylhydantoin. *Biochem. Pharmacol.* **19**, 2483–2491.

Atkinson, A. J. & Shaw, J. M. (1973) Pharmacokinetic study of a patient with diphenylhydantoin toxicity. *Clin. Pharmacol. Therap.* **14**, 521–528.

Ayala, G. F., Lin, S. & Johnston, D. (1977) The mechanism of action of diphenylhydantoin on invertebrate neurons. I. Effects on basic membrane properties. *Brain. Res.* (Amst.) **121**, 245–258.

Ayala, G. F. & Johnston, D. (1977) 'The influence of phenytoin on the fundamental electrical properties of simple neural systems. *Epilepsia* (Amst.), **18**, 299–307.

Azzaro, A. J., Gutrecht, J. A. & Smith, D. J. (1973) Effect of diphenylhydantoin on the uptake and catabolism of L-(^{3}H)norepinephrine *in vitro* in rat cerebral cortical tissue. *Biochem. Pharmacol.*, **22**, 2719–2729.

Baeyer, A. (1861) Ann. **119**, 126–128, cited by Ware, E. (1950) *loc. cit.*

Ballek, R. E., Reidenberg, M. M. & Orr, L. (1973) Inhibition of diphenylhydantoin metabolism by chloramphenicol. *Lancet*, **1**, 150.

Barlow, C. F., Firemark, H. & Roth, L. J. (1962) Drug-plasma binding measured by Sephadex. *J. Pharm. Pharmacol.*, **14**, 550–555.

Barr, M. Jr., Poznanski, A. K. & Schmickel, R. D. (1974) 'Digital hypoplasia and anticonvulsants during gestation: a teratogenic syndrome? *J. Pediat.* **84**, 254–256.

Barry, J. E. & Danks, D. (1974) Anticonvulsants and congenital abnormalities. *Lancet*, ii, 48–49.

Barth, N., Alvan, G., Borga, O. & Sjoqvist, F. (1976) Two fold interindividual variation in plasma protein binding of phenytoin in patients with epilepsy. *Clin. Pharmacokinetics*, **1**, 444–452.

Batt, A. M., Ziegler, J. M. & Siest, G. (1975) Competitive inhibition of glucuronidation by p-hydroxyphenyl hydantoin. *Biochem. Pharmacol.*, **24**, 152–154.

Baugh, C. M. & Krumdieck, C. L. (1969) Effects of phenytoin of folic acid conjugases in man. *Lancet*, **2**, 519–521.

Bazin, S. & Delaunay, A. (1972) Action exercée par la diphenylhydantoine sur la muturation du collagene dans la peau normale et un tissu granulomateux. *C. R. Acad. Sci. Ser, D.* (Paris), **275**, 509–511.

Beernink, D. H. & Miller, J. J. III (1973) Anticonvulsant induced antinuclear antibodies and lupus like disease in children. *J. Pediat.*, **82**, 113–117.

Berlet, H. (1975) Serum levels of phenytoin in children, in *Clinical pharmacology of antiepileptic drugs* ed. Schneider, H., Janz, D., Gardner-Thorpe, C., Meinardi, H. & Sherwin, A. L. Berlin: Springer, 63–69.

Bianchi, C., Beani, L. & Bertelli, A. (1975) Effects of some antiepileptic drugs on brain acetylcholine. *Neuropharmacology*, **14**, 327–332.

Bigger, J. T. Jr., Schmidt, D. H. & Kutt, H. (1968) Relationship between the plasma level of diphenylhydantoin sodium and its cardiac antiarrhythmic effect. *Circulation*, **38**, 363–374.

Blitz, H. (1908) Uber die Konstitution der Einwirkungsbrodukte von substituierten Harnstoffen auf Benzil und uber einige neue Methoden zur Darstellung der 5,5-Diphenylhydantoine. *Berischte der Deutschen Chemischen Gesellschaft*, **41**, 1379–1393.

Birket-Smith, E. & Krogh, E. (1971) Motor nerve conduction velocity during diphenylhydantoin intoxication. *Acta Neurol. Scandinav.* **47**, 265–271.

Bjerkedal, T. & Bahna, S. L. (1973) The course and outcome of pregnancy in women with epilepsy. *Acta. Obstet. Gynaecol. Scand.*, **52**, 245–248.

Blaschke, T. F., Meffin, P. J., Melmon, K. L. & Rowland, M. (1975) Influence of acute viral hepatitis on pheytoin kinetics and protein binding. *Clin. Pharmacol. Therap.*, **17**, 685–691.

Bleyer, W. A. & Skinner, A. L. (1976) Fatal neonatal hemorrhage after maternal anticonvulsant therapy. *J. Amer. Med. Ass.*, **235**, 626–627.

Blum, J. E., Haefely, W., Jalfre, M., Polc, P. & Schärer, K. (1973) Pharmakologie und Toxicologie des Antiepileptikums Clonazepam. *Arzheim. Forsch.* **23**, 377–389.

Blum, M. R., Riegelman, S. & Becker, C. E. (1972) Altered protein binding of diphenylhydantoin in uraemic plasma. *New Eng. J. Med.* **286**, 109.

Blumenkrantz, N. & Asboe-Hansen, G. (1974) Effect of diphenylhydantoin on connective tissue. *Acta. Neurol. Scandinav.* **50**, 302–306.

Bochner, F., Hooper, W. D., Eadie, M. J. & Tyrer, J. H. (1975) Decreased capacity to metabolize diphenylhydantoin in a patient with hypersensitivity to warfarin. *Aust. N.Z. J. Med.*, **5**, 462–466.

Bochner, F., Hooper, W. D., Sutherland, J. M., Eadie, M. J. & Tyrer, J. H. (1973) The renal handling of diphenylhydantoin and 5-(p-hydroxyphenyl)-5-phenylhydantoin. *Clin. Pharmacol. Therap.* **14**, 791–796.

Bochner, F., Hooper, W. D., Sutherland, J. M., Eadie, M. J. & Tyrer, J. H. (1974) Diphenylhydantoin concentrations in saliva. *Arch. Neurol.* (Chic.), **31**, 57–59.

Bochner, F., Hooper, W. D., Tyrer, J. H. & Eadie, M. J. (1972a) The effect of dosage increments on blood phenytoin concentrations. *J. Neurol. Neurosurg. Psychiat.*, **35**, 873–876.

Bochner, F., Hooper, W. D., Tyrer, J. H. & Eadie, M. J. (1972b) Factors involved in an outbreak of phenytoin intoxication. *J. Neurol. Sci.* **16**, 481–487.

Bochner, F., Hooper, W. D., Tyrer, J. H. & Eadie, M. J. (1972c) The effect of a delayed action phenytoin preparation on blood phenytoin concentration. *J. Neurol. Neurosurg. Psychiat.*, **35**, 682–684.

Bochner, F., Hooper, W., Tyrer, J. & Eadie, M. (1973) Clinical implications of certain aspects of diphenylhydantoin metabolism. *Proc. Aust. Assoc. Neurol.*, **9**, 171–178.

Bogoch, S. & Dreyfus, J. (1970) The broad range of use of diphenylhydantoin. Dreyfus Medical Foundation.

Bonnycastle, D. D., Giarman, N. J. & Paasonen, M. K. (1957) Anticonvulsant compounds and 5-hydroxytryptamine in rat brain. *Brit. J. Pharmacol.*, **12**, 228–231.

Bonnycastle, D. D., Paasonen, M. K. & Giarman, N. J. (1956) Diphenylhydantoin and brain levels of 5-hydroxytryptamine. *Nature*, **178**, 990–991.

Booker, H. E. (1975) Idiosyncratic reactions to the antiepileptic drugs. *Epilepsia* (Aust.), **16**, 171–181.

Booker, H. E. & Darcey, B. (1973) Serum concentrations of free diphenylhydantoin and their relationship to clinical intoxication. *Epilepsia* (Amst.), **14**, 177–184.

Booker, H. E., Tormey, A. & Toussaint, J. (1971) Concurrent administration of phenobarbital and diphenylhydantoin: Lack of an interference effect. *Neurology* (Minneap.), **21**, 383–385.

Borga, O., Azarnoff, D. L., Forshell, G. P. & Sjöqvist, F. (1969) Plasma protein binding of tricyclic antidepressants in man. *Biochem. Pharmacol.* **18**, 2135–2143.

Borga, O., Garle, M. & Gutova, M. (1972) Identification of 5(3,4-dihydroxyphenyl)-5-phenylhydantoin as metabolite of 5,5-diphenylhydantoin (phenytoin) in rats and man. *Pharmacology* (Basel), **7**, 129–137.

Borofsky, L. G., Louis, S. & Kutt, H. (1973) Diphenylhydantoin in children. Pharmacology and efficacy. *Neurology* (Minneap.), **23**, 967–972.

Borofsky, L. G., Louis, S., Kutt, H. & Roginsky, M. (1972) Diphenylhydantoin: efficacy, toxicity and dose serum level relationship in children. *J. Pediat.* **81**, 995–1002.

Borondy, P., Chang, T. & Glazko, A. J. (1972) Inhibition of diphenylhydantoin (DPH) hydroxylation by 5-(p-hydroxyphenyl)-5-phenylhydantoin (p-HPPH). *Fed. Proc.* **31**, 582.

Borondy, P., Dill, W. A., Chang, T., Buchanan, R. A. & Glazko, A. J. (1973) Effect of protein binding on the distribution of 5,5-diphenylyhdantoin between plasma and red cells. *Ann. N.Y. Acad. Sci.*, **226**, 82–87.

Braithwaite, R. A., Flanagan, R. J. & Richens, A. (1975) Steady state plasma nortriptyline concentrations in epileptic patients. *Brit. J. Clin. Pharmacol.*, **2**, 469–471.

Brennan, R. W., Dehejia, H., Kutt, H., Verebely, K. & McDowell, F. (1970) Diphenylhydantoin intoxication attendant to slow inactivation of isoniazid. *Neurology* (Minneap.), **30**, 687–693.

Brittingham, T. E., Lutcher, C. L. & Murphy, D. L. (1964) Reversible erythyroid aplasia induced by diphenylhydantoin. *Arch. Intern. Med.*, **113**, 764–768.

Brumlik, J. & Jacobs, R. S. (1974) Myasthenia gravis associated with diphenylhydantoin therapy for epilepsy. *Canad. J. Neurol. Sci.*, **1**, 127–129.

Buchanan, R. A. & Allen, R. J. (1971) Diphenylhydantoin (Dilantin) and phenobarbital blood levels in epileptic children. *Neurology* (Minneap.), **21**, 866–871.

Buchanan, R. A., Kinkel, A. W., Goulet, J. R. & Smith, T. C. (1972) The metabolism of diphenylhydantoin (Dilantin) following once-daily administration. *Neurology* (Minneap.), **22**, 126–130.

Buchanan, R. A., Turner, J. L. & Heffelfinger, J. C. (1973) Single daily dose of diphenylhdantoin in children. *I. Pediat.* **83**, 479–483.

Buch Andreasen, P., Hansen, M. J., Skovsted, L., & Siersbaek-Nielsen, K. (1971) Folic acid and the half-life of diphenylhydantoin in man. *Acta Neurol. Scandinav.* **47**, 117–119.

Buchthal, F. & Lennox-Buchthal, M. A. (1972) Phenobarbital. Relation of serum concentration to control of seizures, in *Antiepileptic drugs* ed. Woodbury, D. M., Penry, J. K., Schmidt, R. P. New York: Raven Press, pp. 335–343.

Buchthal, F. & Svensmark, O. (1959) Aspects of the pharmacology of phenytoin (Dilantin) and phenobarbital relevant to their dosage in the treatment of epilepsy. *Epilepsia* (Amst.) **1**, 373–384.

Buchthal, F., Svensmark, O. & Schiller, P. J. (1960) Clinical and electroencephalographic correlations with serum levels of diphenylhydantoin. *Arch. Neurol.* (Chic.), **2**, 624–630.

Butler, T. C. (1953) Quantitation studies of the physiological disposition of 3-methyl-5-ethyl-5-phenylhydantoin (Mesantoin) and 5-ethyl-5-phenylhydantoin (Nirvanol). *J. Pharmacol. exp. Therap.*, **109**, 340–345.

Butler, T. C. (1956) The metabolic conversion of 3-methyl-5-ethyl-5-phenylhydantoin (mesantoin) and of 5-ethyl-5-phenylhydantoin (nirvanol) to 5-ethyl-5-(p-hydroxyphenyl)hydantoin. *J. Pharmacol. exp. Therap.*, **117**, 160–165.

Butler, T. C. (1957) The metabolic conversion of 5,5-diphenylhydantoin to 5-(p-hydroxyphenyl)-5-phenylhydantoin. *J. Pharmacol. exp. Therap.* **119**, 1–11.

Butler, T. C., Dudley, K. C., Johnson, D. & Roberts, S. B. (1976) 'Studies of the metabolism of 5,5-diphenylhydantoin relating principally to the stereoselectivity of the hydroxylation reaction in man and the dog. *J. Pharmacol. exp. Therap.*, **199**, 82–92.

Cantor, F. K. (1972) Phenytoin treatment of thalamic pain. *Brit. Med. J.* **4**, 590.

Cantu, R. C. & Schwab, R. S. (1966) Ceruloplasmin rise and PBI fall in serúm due to diphenylhydantoin. *Arch. Neurol.* (Chic.), **15**, 393–396.

Cantu, R. C., Schwab, R. S. & Timberlake, W. H. (1968) Comparison of blood levels with oral and intramuscular diphenylhydantoin. *Neurology* (Minneap.), **18**, 782–784.

Carnay, L. & Grundfest, S. (1974) Excitable membrane stabilization by diphenylhydantoin and calcium. *Neuropharmacology* **13**, 1097–1108.

Caspary, W. F., (1972) Inhibition of intestinal calcium transport by diphenylhydantoin in rat duodenum. *Nauyn-Schmeideberg's Arch. exp. Path. Pharmak.* **274**, 146–153.

Castleden, C. M. & Richens, A. (1973) Chronic phenytoin therapy and carbohydrate tolerance. *Lancet* **2**, 966–967.

Cereghino, J. J., Brock, J. T., van Meter, J. C., Penry, J. K., Smith, L. D., Fisher, P. & Ellenberg, J. (1974) Evaluation of albutoin as an antiepileptic drug. *Clin. Pharmacol. Therap.* **15**, 406–416.

Cereghino, J. J., Brock, J. T., van Meter, J. C., Penry, J. K., Smith, L. D. & White, B. G. (1975) The efficacy of carbamazepine combinations in epilepsy. *Clin. Pharmacol. Therap.* **18**, 733–741.

Chadwick, D., Reynolds, E. H. & Marsden, C. D. (1976) Anticonvulsant-induced dyskinesias: a comparison with dyskinesias induced by neuroleptics. *J. Neurol. Neurosurg. Psychiat.* **39**, 1210–1218.

Chalhub, E. G., Devivo, D. C. & Volpe, J. J. (1976) Phenytoin induced dystonia and choreoathetosis in two retarded epileptic children. *Neurology* (Minneap.) **26**, 494–498.

Chang, T., Okerholm, R. A. & Glazko, A. J. (1972a) Identification of 5-(3,4-dihydroxyphenyl)-5-phenylhydantoin: a metabolite of 5,5-diphenylhydantoin (Dilantin) in rat urine. *Anal. Letters* **5**, 195–202.

Chang, T., Okerholm, R. A. & Glazko, A. J. (1972b) A 3-0-methylated catechol metabolite of diphenylhydantoin (Dilantin) in rat urine. *Res. Commun. Chem. Path. and Pharmacol.*, **4**, 13–23.

Chang, T., Savory, A. & Glazko, A. J. (1970) A new metabolite of 5,5-diphenylhydantoin (Dilantin). *Biochem. Biophys. Res. Com.* **38**, 444–449.

Charlton, M. H. & Lunsford, D. (1971) *Minerva Med.*, **62**, 43. Cited by *Lancet* leading article (1971), **2**, 1071–1072.

Chase, T. N., Katz, R. J. & Kopin, I. J. (1969) Effect of anticonvulsants on brain serotonin. *Trans. Amer. Neurol. Ass.*, **94**, 236–238.

Choi, Y., Thrasher, K., Werk, E. E. Jr., Sholiton, L. J. & Olinger, C. (1971) Effect of diphenylhydantoin on cortisol kinetics in humans. *J. Pharmacol. exp. Therap.*, **176**, 27–34.

Chokroverty, S. & Rubino, F. A. (1973) Motor nerve conduction study in patients on long term diphenylhydantoin therapy: correlation with clinical states and serum levels of diphenylhydantoin, folate and cyanocobalamin. *Electromyography Clin. Neurophysiol.*, **13**, 139–140.

Chokroverty, S. & Sayed, Z. A. (1975) Motor nerve conduction study in patients on diphenylhydantoin therapy. *J. Neurol. Neurosurg. Psychiat.* **38**, 1235–1239.

Christensen, L. K. & Skovsted, L. (1969) Inhibition of drug metabolism by chloramphenicol. *Lancet*, **2**, 1397–1399.

Christiansen, C., Nielsen, S. P. & Rodbro, P. (1974) Anticonvulsant hypomagnesaemia. *Brit. Med. J.* **1**, 198–199.

Christiansen, C. & Rødbro, P. (1974a) Effect of vitamin D$_2$ on serum phenytoin. A controlled therapeutic trial. *Acta Neurol. Scandinav.*, **50**, 661–664.

Christiansen, C. & Rødbro, P. (1974b) Initial and maintenance doses of vitamin D$_2$ in the treatment of anticonvulsant osteomalacia. *Acta. Neurol. Scandinav.*, **50**, 631–641.

Christiansen, C. & Rødbro, P. (1976) Treatment of anticonvulsant osteomalacia with vitamin D. *Calcified Tissue Res.* (Berl.), **21**, suppl. 252–259.

Christiansen, C., Rødbro, P. & Lund, M. (1973) Incidence of anticonvulsant osteomalacia and the effect of vitamin D: controlled therapeutic trial. *Brit. Med. J.* **4**, 695–701.

Christiansen, C., Rødbro, P., Munck, O. & Munck, O. (1975) Actions of vitamins D$_2$ and D$_3$ and 25-OH D$_3$ in anticonvulsant osteomalacia. *Brit. Med. J.*, **2**, 363–365.

Christiansen, J. & Dam, M. (1973) Influence of phenobarbital and diphenylhydantoin on plasma carbamazepine levels in patients with epilepsy. *Acta Neurol. Scandinav.* **49**, 543–540.

Clemminsen, J., Fuglsang Frederiksen, V. & Plum, C. M. (1974) Are anticonvulsant oncogenic? *Lancet*, **i**, 705–707.

Cocks, D. A., Critchley, E. M. R., Hayward, H. W., Owen, V., Mawer, G. E. & Woodcock, B. G. (1975) Control of epilepsy with a single daily dose of phenytoin sodium. *Brit. J. clin. Pharmacol.* **2**, 449–453.

Conard, G. J., Haavik, C. O. & Finger, K. F. (1971) Binding of 5,5-diphenylhydantoin and its major metabolite to human and rat plasma proteins. *J. Pharm. Sci.*, **60**, 1642–1646.

Conard, G. J., Jeffay, H., Boshes, L. & Steinberg, A. D. (1974) Levels of 5,5-diphenylhydantoin and its major metabolite in human serum, saliva and hyperplastic gingiva. *J. Dent. Res.*, **53**, 1323–1329.

HYDANTOIN ANTICONVULSANTS 115

Conney, A. H. (1967) Pharmacological implications of microsomal enzyme induction. *Pharmacol. Rev.*, **19**, 317–366.
Cook, C. E., Amerson, E., Poole, W. K., Lesser, P. & O'Tauma, U. (1975) Phenytoin and phenobarbital concentrations in saliva and plasma measured by radioimmuneassay. *Clin. Pharmacol. Therap.*, **18**, 742–747.
Coradello, H. (1973) Ueber die Ausscheidung von Antiepileptika in die Muttermilch. *Wein. Klin. Wschr.*, **85**, 695–697.
Cowger, M. L. & Labbe, R. F. (1967) The inhibition of terminal oxidation by porphyrinogenic drugs. *Biochem. Pharmacol.*, **16**, 2189–2199.
Cranford, R. E., Leppik, I. E., Patrick, B., Anderson, C. B. & Kostick, B. (1977) Intravenous phenytoin: clinical and pharmacokinetic aspects. *Neurology* (Minneap.), **27**, 376.
Crawford, S. E. & Jones, C. K. (1962) Fatal liver necrosis and diphenylhydantoin sensitivity. *Pediatrics*, **30**, 595–600.
Cucinell, S. A., Conney, A. H., Sansur, M. & Burns, J. J. (1965) Drug interactions in man. 1. Lowering effect of phenobarbital on plasma levels of bishydroxycoumarin (Dicumarol) and diphenylhydantoin (Dilantin). *Clin. Pharmacol. Therap.*, **6**, 420–429.
Cudworth, A. G. & Cunningham, J. L. (1974) The effect of diphenylhydantoin on insulin response. *Clin. Sci. Mol. Med.*, **46**, 131–136.
Cummings, N. P., Rosenbloom, A. L., Kohler, W. C. & Wilder, B. J. (1973) Plasma glucose and insulin responses to oral glucose with chronic diphenylhydantoin therapy. *Pediatrics* **51**, 1091–1093.
Dam, M. (1972) The density and ultrastructure of the Purkinje cells following diphenylhydantoin treatment in animals and man. *Acta Neurol. Scand. Suppl.*, **49**, 1–65.
Dam, M., Mygind, K. I. & Christiansen, J. (1976) Antiepileptic drugs, plasma clearance during pregnancy. In *Epileptology* ed. Janz, D., Stuttgart. Thieme 179–183.
Dam, M. & Olsen, V. (1966) Intramuscular administration of phenytoin. *Neurology* (Minneap.), **16**, 288–292.
Danks, D. M., Barry, J. E. & Sheffield, L. J., (1974) Digital hypoplasia and anticonvulsants during pregnancy. *J. Pediatrics.*, **85**, 877.
Davies, J. E., Edmundson, W. F., Carter, C. H. & Barquet, A. (1969) Effect of anticonvulsant drugs on dicophane (DDT) residues in man. *Lancet*, **2**, 7–9.
Davis, R. E. & Woodliffe, H. J. (1971) Folic acid deficiency in patients receiving anticonvulsant drugs. *M.J. Australia*, **2**, 1070–1072.
Dayton, P. G., Cucinell, S. A., Weiss, M. & Perel, J. M. (1967) Dose dependence of drug plasma level decline in dogs. *J. Pharmacol. exp. Therap.*, **158**, 305–316.
Dayton, P. G. & Perel, J. M. (1971) Physiological and physicochemical bases of drug interactions in man. *Ann. N.Y. Acad. Sci.*, **179**, 67–87.
Deitrick, R. A. & Erwin, G. V. (1975) Involvement of biogenic amine metabolism in ethanol addiction. *Fed. Proc.*, **34**, 1962–1968.
de Leacy, E. A., McLeay, C. D., Eadie, M. J. & Tyrer, J. H. (1979) Effects of subjects' sex and intake of tobacco, alcohol and oral contraceptives on plasma phenytoin levels. *Brit. J. Clin. Pharmacol* (in press).
de Lorenzo, R. J., Eample, G. P. & Glaser, G. H. (1977) Regulation of the level of endogenous phosphorylation of specific brain proteins by diphenylhydantoin. *J. Neurochem.*, **28**, 21–30.
de Lorenzo, R. J. & Freedman, S. D. (1977) Possible role of calcium-dependant protein phosphorylation in mediating neurotransmitter release and anticonvulsant action. *Epilepsia* (Amst.), **18**, 357–365.
Dent, C. E., Richens, A., Rowe, D. J. F. & Stamp, T. C. B. (1970) Osteomalacia with long-term anticonvulsant therapy in epilepsy. *Brit. Med. J.*, **4**, 69–72.
Deupree, J. D. (1976) Evidence that diphenylhydantoin does not affect adenosine triphosphatases from brain. *Neuropharmacology*, **15**, 187–195.
Deupree, J. D. (1977) The role or non-role of ATPase activation by phenytoin in the stabilization of excitable membranes. *Epilepsia* (Aust.), **18**, 308–315.
Dhar, G. J., Ahamed, P. N., Pierach, C. A. & Howard, R. B. (1974) Diphenylhydantoin induced hepatic necrosis. *Postgrad. Med.*, **56**, 128–134.
Diamond, W. D. & Buchanan, R. A. (1970) A clinical study of the effect of phenobarbital on diphenylhydantoin plasma levels. *J. Clin. Pharm.*, **10**, 306–311.
Dill, W. A., Baukema, J., Chang, T. & Glazko, A. J. (1971) Colorimetric assay of 5,5-diphenylhydantoin (Dilantin) and 5-(p-hydroxyphenyl)-5-phenylhydantoin. *Proc. Sci. Exp. Biol. Med.*, **137**, 674–679.
Dill, W. A. & Glazko, A. J. (1972) Fluorimetric assay of diphenylhydantoin in plasma or whole blood. *Clin. Chem.* **17**, 1200–1201.
Dill, W. A., Kazenko, A., Wolf, L. M. & Glazko, A. J. (1956) Studies on 5-5-diphenylhydantoin

(Dilantin) in animals and man. *J. Pharmacol. exp. Therap.*, **118**, 270–279.

Direkze, M. & Fernando, P. S. L. (1977) Transient anterior horn cell dysfunction in diphenylhydantoin therapy. *Europ. Neurol.*, **15**, 131–134.

Dobkin, B. H. (1977) Reversible subacute peripheral neuropathy induced by phenytoin. *Arch. Neurol.* (Chic.), **34**, 189–190.

Dow, R. C., Forfar, J. C. & McQueen, J. K. (1973) The effects of some anticonvulsant drugs on cobalt induced epilepsy. *Epilepsia* (Amst.), **14**, 203–212.

Dretchen, K. L., Standaert, F. G. & Raines, A. (1977) Effects of phenytoin on the cyclic nucleotide system in the motor nerve terminal. *Epilepsia* (Amst.), **18**, 337–348.

Drevon, B. & Donikian, R. (1956) Sur les protéines de la salive parotidienne humaine. *Compt. Rend. Soc. Biol.* **150**, 1206–1208.

Dudley, K. H., Bius, D. L. & Butler, T. C. (1970) Metabolic fates of 3-ethyl-5-phenylhydantoin (ethotoin, peganone),3-methyl-5-phenylhydantoin and 5-phenylhydantoin. *J. Pharmacol. exp. Therap.*, **175**, 27–37.

Eadie, M. J. (1971) Blood levels of anticonvulsants, in *Geigy symposium on epilepsy*, ed. Winton, R. R. Sydney, Australian Medical Publishing Co. p. 81–87.

Eadie, M. J. (in press) Clinical correlations of anticonvulsant drug plasma levels, in Burrows, G. & Norman, T. eds. *Plasma levels of psychotropic drugs and clinical response*. New York: Marcel Dekker.

Eadie, M. J., Lander, C. M., Hooper, W. D. & Tyrer, J. H. (1977) Factors influencing plasma phenobarbitone levels in epileptic patients. *Brit. J. clin. Pharmacol.*, **4**, 541–547.

Eadie, M. J., Lander, C. M. & Tyrer, J. H. (1977) Plasma drug level monitoring in pregnancy. *Clinical Pharmacokinetics*, **2**, 427–436.

Eadie, M. J. & Tyrer, J. H. (1977) Concentrazioni terapeutiche minimi e massime degli antiepilettici nel plasma. *Clinica Therapeutica*, **83**, 121–133.

Eadie, M. J. & Tyrer, J. H. (in press) *Neurological Clinical Pharmacology*. Auckland: Adis Press.

Eadie, M. J., Tyrer, J. H., Bochner, F. & Hooper, W. D. (1976) The elimination of phenytoin in man. *Clin. Exp. Pharmacol. Physiol.*, **3**, 217–224.

Eadie, M. J., Tyrer, J. H. & Hooper, W. D. (1970) Aspects of diphenylhydantoin metabolism. *Proc. Aust. Assocn. Neurol.*, **7**, 7–13.

Eadie, M. J., Tyrer, J. H. & Hooper, W. D. (1973) Diphenylhydantoin dosage. *Proc. Aust. Assoc. Neurol.*, **10**, 53–59.

Eadie, M. J., Tyrer, J. H. & Kukums, J. R. (1971) Selective vulnerability to ischaemia: studies in quantitative enzyme cytochemistry of single neurons and neuropil. *Brain*, **94**, 647–660.

Edmonds, H. L., Stark, L. G. & Hollinger, M. A. (1974) The effect of diphenylhydantoin, phenobarbital and diazepam on the penicillin-induced epileptogenic focus in the rat. *Exp. Neurol.*, **45**, 377–386.

Ehrnebo, M., Agurell, S., Jalling, B. & Boreus, L. O. (1971) Age differences in drug binding by plasma proteins: studies on human fetuses, neonates and adults. *Europ. J. Clin. Pharmacol.*, **3**, 189–193.

Ehrnebo, M. & Odar-Cederlöf, I. (1975) Binding of amobarbital, pentobarbital and diphenylhydantoin to blood cells and plasma proteins in healthy volunteers and uraemic patients. *Europe. J. clin. Pharmacol.*, **8**, 445–453.

Ehrnebo, M. & Odar-Cederlööf, I. (1977) Distribution of pentobarbital and diphenylhydantoin between plasma and cells in blood: effect of salicylic acid, temperature and total drug concentration. *Europ. J. Clin Pharmacol.* **11**, 37–42.

Eidelberg, E., Neer, H. M. & Miller, M. K. (1965) Anticonvulsant properties of some benzodiazepine derivatives. *Neurology* (Minneap.), **15**, 223–230.

Eisen, A. A., Woods, J. F. & Sherwin, A. L. (1974) Peripheral nerve function in long-term therapy with diphenylhydantoin. *Neurology* (Minneap.), **24**, 411–417.

Elfström, J. (1977) Plasma protein binding of phenytoin after cholecystectomy and neurosurgical operations. *Acta Neurol. Scandinav.*, **55**, 455–464.

Eling, T. E., Harbison, R. D., Becker, B. A. & Fouts, J. R. (1970) Diphenylhydantoin effect on neonatal and adult rat hepatic drug metabolism. *J. Pharmacol. exp. Therap.*, **171**, 127–134.

Elshove, K. & van Eck, J. H. M. (1971) Aangeboren misvormingen, met name gespleten lip met of zonder gespleten verhemette, bij kinderen van moeders met epilepsie. *Ned. Tijdschr Geneeskd.*, **115**, 1371–1375.

Encinoza, O. (1974) Nerve conduction velocity in patients on long-term diphenylhydantoin therapy. *Epilepsia* (Amst.), **15**, 147–154.

Endtz, J. J., Leeksma, C. H. W., Kerkhofs, H., Mulder, O. G., Mosmans, F. A. & Meinardi, H. (1973) Leucémie aiguë causée par la diphénylhydantoïne? A propos de quatre cas. *Rev. Neurol.* **129**, 296–300.

Engel, J., Cruz, M. E. & Shapiro, B. (1971) Phenytoin encephalopathy? *Lancet*, **2**, 824–825.

Escueta, A. V. & Appel, S. H. (1971) Diphenylhydantoin and potassium transport in isolated nerve

HYDANTOIN ANTICONVULSANTS 117

terminals. *J. Clin. Invest.*, **50**, 1977–1984.

Escueta, A. V. & Appel, S. H. (1972) Brain synapses. An *in vitro* model for the study of seizures. *Ann. Intern. Med.*, **129**, 333–344.

Escueta, A. V., Davidson, D., Hartwig, G. & Reilly, E. (1975) The freezing lesion. III. The effects of diphenylhydantoin on potassium transport within nerve terminals from the primary foci. *Brain Res.*, **86**, 85–96.

Esplin, D. W. (1957) Effect of diphenylhydantoin on synaptic transmission in cat spinal cord and stellate ganglion. *J. Pharmacol. exp. Therap.*, **120**, 301–323.

Falconer, M. A. & Davidson, S. (1974) Coarse features in epilepsy as a consequence of anticonvulsant therapy. *Drugs*, **7**, 394–395.

Fedrick, J. (1973) Epilepsy and pregnancy: a report from the Oxford record linkage study. *Brit. Med. J.*, **2**, 442–448.

Fehling, C., Jagerstad, M., Linstrand, K. & Westesson, A. K. (1973) The effect of anticonvulsant therapy upon the absorption of folates. *Clin. Sci.*, **44**, 595–600.

Ferrendelli, J. A. & Kinscherf, D. A. (1977) Phenytoin effects on calcium flux and cyclic nucleotides. *Epilepsia* (Amst.), **18**, 331–336.

Festoff, B. W. & Appel, S. A. (1968) Effect of diphenylhydantoin on synaptosome sodium-potassium-ATP-ase. *J. Clin. Invest.*, **47**, 2752–2758.

Fichman, M. P., Kleeman, C. R. & Bethune, J. E. (1970) Inhibition of antidiuretic hormone secretion by diphenylhydantoin. *Arch. Neurol. (Chic.)* **22**, 45–53.

Fincham, R. W., Schottelius, D. D. & Sahs, A. L. (1974) The influence of diphenylhydantoin on primidone metabolism. *Arch. Neurol.*, (Chic.), **30**, 259–262.

Fincham, R. W., Wiley, D. E. & Schottelius, D. D. (1976) Use of phenytoin serum levels in a case of status epilepticus. *Neurology* (Minneap.), **26**, 879–881.

Finucane, J. F. & Griffiths, R. S. (1976) Effect of phenytoin therapy on thyroid function. *Brit. J. clin. Pharmacol.*, **3**, 1040–1044.

Firemark, H., Barlow, C. F. & Roth, L. J. (1963) The entry accumulation and binding of diphenylhydantoin-2-C^{14} in brain. *Internat. J. Neuropharmacol.*, **2**, 25–38.

Fontana, A., Grob, P. J., Sauter, R. & Joller, H. (1976) IgA deficiency, epilepsy and hydantoin medication. *Lancet*, ii, 228–281.

Formby, B. (1970) The *in vivo* and *in vitro* effect of diphenylhydantoin and phenobarbitone on K$^+$-activated phosphorohydrolase and (Na$^+$, K$^+$)-activated ATPase in particulate membrane fractions from rat brain. *J. Pharmacy Pharmacology*, **22**, 81–85.

Fossan, G. O. (1976) Reduced CSF IgG in patients treated with phenytoin (diphenylhydantoin). *Europ. Neurol.*, **14**, 426–432.

Foster, D. B., Nagaswami, S. & Reimer, D. (1974) An inverse relationship between serum Dilantin and serum lipid levels: a preliminary report. *Epilepsia* (Amst.) **15**, 277.

Fredholm, B. B., Rane, A. & Persson, B. (1975) Diphenylhydantoin binding to proteins in plasma and its dependence on free fatty acid and bilirubin concentration in dogs and newborn infants. *Pediat. Res.* (Baltimore), **9**, 26–30.

Fujii, K., Hayashi, M. & Murata, R. (1975) Effect of diphenylhydantoin therapy on plasma 11-OHCS: interference in the effects of dexamethasone and metapirone. *Brain Develop.*, **7**, 354–360.

Ganapathy, G. R., Krishna Rao, G. V. G. & Gourie Devi, M. (1973) Bone changes after long term anticonvulsant therapy. *Neurology (Bombay)*, **31**, 159–164.

Garrettson, L. K. & Dayton, P. G. (1970) Disappearance of phenobarbital and diphenylhydantoin from serum of children. *Clin. Pharm. Therap.*, **11**, 674–679.

Garrettson, L. K. & Gomez, M. (1977) Phenytoin-primidone interaction. *Brit. J. clin. Pharmacol.*, **4**, 693–695.

Garrettson, L. K. & Jusko, W. J. (1975) Diphenylhydantoin elimination kinetics in overdosed children. *Clin. Pharmacol. Therap.*, **17**, 481–491.

Garrettson, L. K. & Kim, O. K. (1970) Apparent saturation of diphenylhydantoin metabolism in children. *Pediat. Res.*, **4**, 455.

Garrettson, L. K., Perel, J. M. & Dayton, P. G. (1969) Methylphenidate interaction with both anticonvulsants and ethyl biscoumacetate. *J. Amer. Med. Ass.*, **207**, 2053–2056.

Gauzhez, F. D., Lehr, H. J., Gauchez, G. & Von Harnack, G. A. (1973) Diphenylhydantoin bei Kindern. Klinisch pharmakologische Untersuchungen. *Dtsch. Med. Wschr.* **98**, 1391–1396.

Gerber, N., Lynn, R., Bush, M. & Oates, J. (1972) Relationship of plasma level of diphenylhydantoin (DPH) to the rate of excretion of urinary HPPH. *Clin. Pharmacol. Therap.*, **13**, 139.

Gerber, N., Lynn, R. & Oates, J. (1972) Acute intoxication with 5,5-diphenylhydantoin (Dilantin^R) associated with impairment of biotransformation. Plasma levels and urinary metabolites; and studies in healthy volunteers. *Arch. Intern. Med.*, **77**, 765–771.

Gerber, N., Seibert, R. A. & Thompson, R. M. (1973) Identification of a catechol glucuronide metabolite of 5,5-diphenylhydantoin (DPH) in rat bile by gas chromatography (GC) and mass spectrometry (MS). *Res. Commun. Chem. Path. Pharmacol.*, **6**, 499–511.

Gerber, N. & Wagner, J. G. (1972) Explanation of the dose-dependent decline of diphenylhydantoin plasma levels by fitting to the integrated form of the Michaelis-Menten equation. *Res. Com. Chem. Pathol & Pharmacol.*, **3**, 455–466.

Gerber, N., Weller, W. L., Lynn, R., Rangno, R. E., Sweetman, B. J. & Bush, M. T. (1971) Study of dose-dependent metabolism of 5,5-diphenylhydantoin in the rat using new methodology for isolation and quantitation of metabolites *in vivo* and *in vitro*. . *J. Pharmacol. exp. Therap.* **178**, 567–579.

Ghatak, N. R., Santoso, R. A. & McKinney, W. M. (1976) Cerebellar degeneration following long-term phenytoin therapy. *Neurology* (Minneap.), **26**, 818–820.

Gibberd, F. B. & Webley, M. (1975) Studies in man of phenytoin absorption and its implications. *J. Neurol. Neurosurg. Psychiat.*, **38**, 219–224.

Gilbert, J. C. & Wyllie, M. G. (1976) Effects of anticonvulsant and convulsant drugs on the ATPase activities of synaptosomes and their components. *Brit. J. Pharmacol.*, 49–57.

Glazko, A. J. (1973) Diphenylhydantoin metabolism. A prospective review. *Drug Metabolism Disposition*, **1**, 711–714.

Glazko, A. J. (1975) Antiepileptic drugs; biotransformation, metabolism and serum half-life. *Epilepsia* (Amst.), **16**, 367–391.

Glazko, A. J., Chang, T., Baukema, J., Dill, W. A., Goulet, J. R. & Buchanan, R. A. (1969) Metabolic disposition of diphenylhydantoin in normal human subjects following intravenous administration. *Clin. Pharmacol. Therap.* **10**, 498–504.

Goldberg, E. M. & Sanbar, S. S. (1969) Hyperglycemic, nonketotic coma following administration of Dilantin (diphenylhydantoin). *Diabetes*, **18**, 101–106.

Goldberg, M. A. (1977) Phenytoin, phospholipids and calcium. *Neurology* (Minneap.), **27**, 827–833.

Goldberg, M. A. & Todoroff, T. (1973) Binding of diphenylhydantoin to brain protein. *Biochem. Pharmacol.*, **22**, 2973–2980.

Goldberg, M. A. & Todoroff, T. (1976) Enhancement of diphenylhydantoin binding by lipid extraction. *J. Pharmacol. exp. Therap.*, **196**, 579–585.

Grant, R. H. E. & Stores, O. P. R. (1970) Folic acid in folate-deficient patients with epilepsy. *Brit. Med. J.*, **4**, 644–648.

Green, J. R., Halpern, L. M., Thomas, E. D. Jr. & Amick-Corkill, J. A. (1973) The effect of diphenylhydantoin on the activity of selected enzymes in chronic isolated cerebral cortex of cat. *Epilepsia* (Amst.), **14**, 223–232.

Green, A. R. & Graeme Smith, D. G. (1975) The effect of diphenylhydantoin on brain 5-hydroxytryptamine metabolism and function. *Neuropharmacology*, **14**, 107–113.

Grob, P. J. & Herold, G. E. (1972) Immunological abnormalities and hydantoins. *Brit. Med. J.*, **2**, 561–563.

Gropper, A. L. (1956) Diphenylhydantoin sensitivity. Report of fatal case with hepatitis and exfoliative dermatitis. *New Eng. J. Med.*, **254**, 522–523.

Gruhzit, O. M. (1939) Sodium diphenyl hydantoinate. Pharmacologic and histopathologic studies. *Arch. Path.*, **28**, 761–762.

Guberman, A., Gloor, P. & Sherwin, A. L. (1975) Response of generalized penicillin epilepsy in the cat to ethosuximide and diphenylhydantoin. *Neurology* (Minneap.), **25**, 758–764.

Guelen, P. J. M. (1975) in Discussion, in *Clinical pharmacology of antiepileptic drugs* ed. Schneider, H., Janz, D., Gardner-Thorpe, C., Meinardi, H. & Sherwin, A. L. Berlin: Springer. 45–46.

Gugler, R., Manion, C. V. & Azarnoff, D. L. (1976) Phenytoin: pharmacokinetics and bioavailability. *Clin. Pharmacol. Therap.*, **19**, 135–142.

Haerer, A. F. & Buchanan, R. A. (1972) Effectiveness of single daily doses of diphenylhydantoin. *Neurology* (Minneap.) **22**, 1021–1025.

Haerer, A. F. & Grace, J. B. (1969) Studies of anticonvulsant levels in epileptics. I. Serum diphenylhydantoin concentrations in a group of medically indigent outpatients. *Acta. Neurol. Scandinav.*, **45**, 18–31.

Hahn, T. J. (1976) Bone complications of anticonvulsants. *Drugs*, **12**, 201–211.

Hahn, T. J., Hendin, B. A., Scharp, C. R. & Haddad, J. G. Jr. (1972) Effect of chronic anticonvulsant therapy on serum 25-hydroxycalciferol levels in adults. *New Eng. J. Med.*, **287**, 900–904.

Hamfelt, A. & Wilmanns, W. (1965) Inhibition studies on folic acid metabolism with drugs suspected to act on the myeloproliferative system. *Clin. Chim. Acta.*, **12**, 144–152.

Handley, A. J. (1970) Phenytoin tolerance tests. *Brit. Med. J.*, **3**, 203–204.

Hansen, J. M., Kristensen, M. & Skovsted, L. (1968) Sulthiame (Ospolot) as inhibitor of diphenylhydantoin metabolism. *Epilepsia* (Amst.), **9**, 17–22.

Hansen, J. M., Kristensen, M., Skovsted, L. & Christensen, L. K. (1966) Dicoumarol-induced diphenylhydantoin intoxication. *Lancet*, ii, 265–266.

Hansen, J. M., Siersbaek-Nielsen, A., Kristensen, M., Skovsted, L. & Christensen, L. K. (1971) Effect of diphenylhydantoin on the metabolism of dicoumarol in man. *Acta Med. Scandinav.*, **189**, 15–19.

Hansen, J. M., Siersboek-Nielsen, K. & Skovsted, L. (1971) Carbamazepine-induced acceleration of diphenylhydantoin and warfarin metabolism in man. *Clin. Pharmacol. Therap.*, **12**, 539–543.

Hansotia, P. & Keran, E. (1974) Diphenylhydantoin binding by red blood cells of normal subjects. *Neurology* (Minneap.), **24**, 575–578.

Harbison, R. D. & Becker, B. A. (1969) Relation of dosage and time of administration of diphenylhydantoin to its teratogenic effect in mice. *Teratology*, **2**, 305–312.

Harbison, R. D. & Becker, B. A. (1972) Diphenylhydantoin teratogenicity in rats. *Toxicol. App. Pharmacol.*, **22**, 193–200.

Harbison, R. D., Olubadewo, J., Dwivedi, C. & Rama Sastry, B. V. (1975) Proposed role of the placental cholingeric system in the regulation of fetal growth and development, in *Basic and therapeutic aspects of perinatal pharmacology*, ed. Morselli, P. L., Garattini, S. & Sereni, F. New York: Raven Press, 107–120.

Harris, M., Jenkins, M. V. & Willis, M. R. (1974) Phenytoin inhibition of parathyroid hormone induced bone resorption *in vitro*. *Brit. J. Pharmacol.*, **50**, 405–408.

Hasbani, M., Pincus, J. H. & Lee, S. H. (1974) Diphenylhydantoin and calcium movement in lobster nerves. *Arch. Neurol.*, (Chic.) **31**, 250–254.

Hayes, M. J., Langman, M. J. S. & Short, A. H. (1975) Changes in drug metabolism with increasing age: 2. phenytoin clearance and protein binding. *Brit. J. clin. Pharmacol.*, **2**, 73–79.

Hazlett, D. R., Ward, G. W. Jr. & Madison, D. S. (1974) Pulmonary function loss in diphenylhydantoin therapy. *Chest*, **66**, 660–664.

Hitchcock, E. & Gabra-Sanders, T. (1977) Effect of diphenylhydantoin on gamma aminobutyric acid (GABA) and succinate activity in rat Purkinje cells. *J. Neurol. Neurosurg. Psychiat.*, **40**, 565–569.

Hoffbrand, A. V. & Necheles, T. F. (1968) Mechanism of folate deficiency in patients receiving phenytoin. *Lancet*, **ii**, 528–530.

Hofmann, W. W. (1958) Cerebellar lesions after parenteral Dilantin administration. *Neurology* (Minneap.) **8**, 210–214.

Hoglmeier, H. & Wenzel, U. (1969) Zerebellarer Dauerschaden durch vorübergehende Hydantoinüberdosierung. *Deutsche Med. Wochenschrift.*, **94**, 1330–1332.

Hooper, W. D., Bochner, F., Eadie, M. J. & Tyrer, J. H. (1974) Plasma protein binding of diphenylhydantoin. Effects of sex hormones, renal and liver disease. *Clin. Pharmacol. Therap.* **15**, 276–282.

Hooper, W. D., Dubetz, D. K., Eadie, M. J. & Tyrer, J. H. (1974) Preliminary observations on the clinical pharmacology of carbamazepine ('Tergretol'). *Proc. Aust. Assoc. Neurol.*, **11**. 189–198.

Hooper, W. D., Eadie, M. J. & Tyrer, J. H. (1973) Plasma diphenylhydantoin levels in Australian children. *Aust. N.Z. J. Med.*, **4**, 456–461.

Hooper, W. D., Sutherland, J. M., Bochner, F., Tyrer, J. G. & Eadie, M. J. (1973) The effect of certain drugs on the plasma protein binding of diphenylhydantoin. *Aust. N.Z. J. Med.*, **3**, 377–381.

Hoppel, C., Garle, M., Rane, A. & Sjoqvist, F. (1977) Plasma concentrations of 5-(4-hydroxyphenyl)-5 phenylhydantoin in phenytoin-treated patients. *Clin. Pharmacol. Therap.*, **21**, 294–300.

Horning, M. G., Brown, L., Nowlin, J., Letratanagkoon, K., Kellaway, P. and Zion, T. E. (1977) Use of saliva in therapeutic drug monitoring. *Clin. Chem.* **23**, 157–164.

Horning, M. G., Stratton, C., Wilson, A., Horning, E. C. & Hill, R. M. (1971) Detection of 5-(3,4-dihydroxy-1,5-cyclohexadiene-1-yl)-5-phenylhydantoin (Dilantin) in the newborn human. *Anal. Letters*, **4**, 537–545.

Houghton, G. W. & Richens, A. (1974a) Inhibition of phenytoin metabolism by sulthiame in epileptic patients. *Brit. J. clin. Pharmacol.*, **1**, 59–66.

Houghton, G. W. & Richens, A. (1974b) Phenytoin intoxication induced by sulthiame in epileptic patients. *J. Neurol. Neurosurg. Psychiat.*, **37**, 275–281.

Houghton, G. W., Richens, A. & Leighton, M. (1975) Effect of age, height, weight and sex on serum phenytoin concentration in epileptic patients. *Brit. J. clin. Pharmacol.*, **2**, 251–258.

Houghton, G. W., Richens, A., Toseland, P. A., Davidson, S. & Falconer, M. A. (1975) Brain concentrations of phenytoin phenobarbitone and primidone in epileptic patients. *Europ. J. Clin. Pharmacol.*, **9**, 73–78.

Hunter, J., Maxwell, J. D., Stewart, D. A., Parsons, V. & Williams, R. (1971) Altered calcium metabolism in epileptic children on anticonvulsants. *Brit. Med. J.*, **4**, 202–204.

Husby, J. (1963) Delayed toxicity and serum concentrations of phenytoin. *Danish Med. Bull.* **10**, 236–239.

Hvidberg, E. F. & Sjo, O. (1975) Clinical pharmacokinetic experiences with clonazepam, in *Clinical pharmacology of antiepileptic drugs*, ed. Schneider, H., Janz, D., Gardner-Thorpe, C., Meinardi, H. & Sherwin, A. L. Berlin: Springer. 242–246.

Hyman, G. A. & Sommers, S. C. (1966) The development of Hodgkin's disease and lymphoma during anticonvulsant therapy. *Blood*, **28**, 416–427.

Iivanainen, M., Viiukari, M. & Helle, E.-P. (1977) Cerebellar atrophy in phenytoin-treated mentally retarded epileptics. *Epilepsia* (Amst.), **18**, 375–386.

Izquierdo, I. & Nasello, A. G. (1973) Effects of cannabidol and of diphenylhydantoin on the hippocampus and on learning. *Psychopharmacologica* (Berl.), **31**, 167–175.

Jalling, B., Boréus, L. O., Rane, A. & Sjöqvist, F. (1970) Plasma concentrations of diphenylhydantoin in young infants. *Pharmacologica Clinica*, **2**, 200–202.

Janz, D. (1975) The teratogenic risk of antiepileptic drugs. *Epilepsia* (Amst.) **16**, 159–169.

Janz, D. & Fuchs, U. (1964) Are anti-epileptic drugs harmful when given during pregnancy? *German Medical Monthly*, **9**, 20–22.

Jensen, O. N. & Olesen, O. V. (1970) Subnormal serum folate due to anticonvulsant therapy. A double blind study of the effect of folic acid treatment in patients with drug-induced subnormal serum folates. *Arch. Neurol.* (Chic.), **22**, 181–182.

Jeong, Y. G., Jung, Y. & River, G. L. (1974) Pure RBC aplasia and diphenylhydantoin. *J. Amer. Med. Assoc.* **229**, 314–315.

Johannessen, S. I. & Strandjord, R. E. (1975) The influence of phenobarbitone and phenytoin on carbamazepine serum levels, in *Clinical pharmacology of antiepileptic drugs* ed. Schneider, H., Janz, D., Gardner-Thorpe, C., Meinardi, H. & Sherwin, A. L. Berlin: Springer. 201–205.

Jones, G. L. & Woodbury, D. M. (1976) Effects of diphenylhydantoin and phenobarbital on protein metabolism in the rat cerebral cortex. *Biochem. Pharmacol.*, **25**, 53–61.

Jones, T. D. & Jacobs, J. L. (1932) The treatment of obstinate chorea with Nirvanol with notes on its mode of action. *J. Amer. Med. Assoc.*, **99**, 18–21.

Jubiz, W., Haussler, M. R., McCain, T. A. & Tolman, K. G. (1977) Plasma 1,25-dihydroxy-vitamin D levels in patients receiving anticonvulsant drugs. *J. Clin. Endocrinol. Metab.*, **44**, 617–621.

Jubiz, W., Meikle, A. W., Levinson, R. A., Mizutani, S., West, C. D. & Tyler, F. H. (1970) Effect of phenytoin (diphenylhydantoin) on the metabolism of dexamethasone. *New Eng. J. Med.* **283**, 11–14.

Julien, R. M. (1972) Anticonvulsant action of diphenylhydantoin in mice with genetic cerebellar degeneration. *J. Pharmacol. exp. Therap.*, **180**, 239–243.

Jusko, W. J., Koup, J. R. & Alvan, G. (1976) Nonlinear assessment of phenytoin bioavailability. *J. Pharmocokinetics Biopharmaceutics*, **4**, 327–336.

Kapur, R. N., Girgis, S., Little, T. M. & Masotti, R. E. (1973) Diphenylhydantoin-induced gingival hyperplasia: its relationship to dose and serum level. *Develop. Med. Child. Neurol.*, **15**, 483–487.

Karch, F. E. & Wardell, W. M. (1977) Effect of halofenate on the serum binding of phenytoin. *Brit. J. clin. Pharmacol.*, **4**, 625–626.

Karkos, J. (1975) Effect of phenytoin on succinic dehydrogenase activity in rat cerebellum. *Bull. Pol. Med. Sci. Hist.*, **3**, 45–48.

Karlén, B., Garle, M., Rane, A., Gutova, M. & Lindborg, B. (1975) Assay of the major (4-hydroxylated) metabolites of diphenylhydantoin in human urine. *Europ. J. clin. Pharmacol.*, **8**, 359–363.

Karlin, J. M. & Kutt, H. (1970) Acute diphenylhydantoin intoxication following halothane anaesthesia. *J. Pediat.*, **76**, 941–944.

Kater, R. M. H., Roggin, G., Tobon, F., Zieve, P. & Iber, F. L. (1969) Increased rate of clearance of drugs from the circulation of alcoholics. *Amer. J. Med. Sci.*, **258**, 35–39.

Kattan, K. R. (1975) Thickening of the heel pad associated with long term Dilantin therapy. *Amer. J. Roentgenol.*, **124**, 52–56.

Katz, S. H., Gerstman, I., Lautenbacher, H. W. & Hediger, M. I. (1976) Failure to confirm anticonvulsant hypomagnesaemia. *Brit. Med. J.*, **1**, 341.

Kazamatsuri, H. (1970) Elevated serum alkaline phosphatase in epilepsy during diphenylhydantoin therapy. *New Eng. J. Med.*, **283**, 1411–1412.

Kemp, J. W. & Woodbury, D. M. (1971) Subcellular distribution of 4-^{14}C-diphenylhydantoin in rat brain. *J. Pharmacol. exp. Therap.*, **177**, 342–349.

Kimball, O. P. (1939) The treatment of epilepsy with sodium diphenyl hydantoinate. *J. Amer. med. Ass.*, **112**, 1244–1245.

Kiorboe, E. (1966) Phenytoin intoxication during treatment with antabuse (disulfiram). *Epilepsia* (Amst.), **7**, 246–249.

Klipstein, F. A. (1964) Subnormal serum folate and macrocytosis associated with anticonvulsant drug therapy. *Blood*, **23**, 68–86.

Knopp, R. H., Sheinin, J. C. & Freinkel, N. (1972) Diphenylhydantoin and an insulin secreting islet adenoma. *Arch. Intern. Med.*, **130**, 904–908.

Koch, H. U., Kraft, D., von Herrath, D. & Schaeffer, K. (1972) Influence of diphenylhydantoin and phenobarbital on intestinal calcium transport in the rat. *Epilepsia* (Amst.), **13**, 829–834.

Kokenge, R., Kutt, H. & McDowell, F. (1965) Neurological sequelae following Dilantin overdose in a patient and in experimental animals. *Neurology* (Minneap.), **15**, 823–829.

Kooiker, J. C. & Sumi, S. M. (1974) Movement disorder as a manifestation of diphenylhydantoin intoxication. *Neurology* (Minneap.), **24**, 68–71.

Koppe, J. G., Bosman, W., Oapers, V. M. *et al.* (1973) Epilepsie en aangeboren afwijkingen. *Ned. Tijdschr. Geneeskd.*, **117**, 220–224, cited by Annegers, Elveback, Hauser & Kurland (1974) *loc. cit.*

Korczyn, A. D., Elian, M., Don, R. & Bornstein, B. (1974) Phenytoin and folate deficiency: failure to show dose dependency. *J. Neurol.*, **207**, 151–153.

Korey, S. R. (1951) Effect of Dilantin and Mesantoin on the giant axon of the squid. *Proc. Soc. Exp. Biol. Med.*, **79**, 297–299.

Kostenbauder, H. B., Rapp, R. P., McGovren, J. P., Foster, T. S., Perrier, D. G., Blacker, H. M., Hulon, W. C. & Kinkel, A. W. (1975) Bioavailability and single-dose pharmacokinetics of intramuscular phenytoin. *Clin. Pharm. Therap.*, **18**, 449–456.

Kozelka, F. L. & Hine, C. H. (1943) Degradation products of Dilantin[R]. *J. Pharmacol. exp. Therap.*, **77**, 175–179.

Kristensen, M., Hansen, J. M. & Skovsted, L. (1969) The influence of phenobarbital on the half-life of diphenylhydantoin in man. *Acta Med. Scand.* **185**, 347–350.

Kruse, R. (1968) Osteopathien bei antiepileptischer Langzeittherapie (Vorlaüfige Mitteilung). *Mschr. Kinderheilk*, **116**, 378–381.

Kuenssberg, E. V. & Knox, J. D. E. (1973) Teratogenetic effects of anticonvulsants. *Lancet*, **1**, 198.

Kuiper, J. J. (1969) Lymphocytic thyroiditis possibly induced by diphenylhydantoin. *J. Amer. Med. Ass.*, **210**, 2370–2372.

Kupferberg, H. J. & Yonekawa, W. (1975) The metabolism of 3-methyl-5-ethyl-5-phenylhydantoin (mephenytoin) to 5-ethyl-5-phenylhydantoin (Nirvanol) in mice in relation to anticonvulsant activity. *Metabl. Disposition*, **3**, 26–29.

Kurata, D. & Wilkinson, G. R. (1974) Erythrocyte uptake and plasma binding of diphenylhydantoin. *Clin. Pharmacol. Therap.*, **16**, 355–362.

Kurtzke, J. F. (1961) Leukopenia with diphenylhydantoin. *J. Nerv. Ment. Dis.*, **132**, 339–343.

Kutt, H. (1971) Biochemical and genetic factors regulating Dilantin[R] metabolism in man. *Ann. N.Y. Acad. Sci.*, **179**, 704–722.

Kutt, H., Haynes, J. & McDowell, F. (1966) Some causes of ineffectiveness of diphenylhydantoin. *Arch. Neurol.* (Chic.), **14**, 489–492.

Kutt, H., Haynes, M., Verebely, K. & McDowell, F. (1969) The effect of phenobarbital on plasma diphenylhydantoin level and metabolism in man and in rat liver microsomes. *Neurology* (Minneap.), **19**, 611–616.

Kutt, H. & McDowell, F. (1968) Management of epilepsy with diphenylhydantoin sodium. *J.A.M.A.*, **203**, 969–972.

Kutt, H. & Verebely, K. (1970) Metabolism of diphenylhydantoin by rat liver microsomes—1. Characteristics of the reaction. *Biochem. Pharmacol.*, **19**, 675–686.

Kutt, H., Winters, W., Kokenge, R. & McDowell, F. (1964) Diphenylhydantoin metabolism, blood levels, and toxicity. *Arch. Neurol.* (Chic.), **11**, 642–648.

Kutt, H. (1975) Interaction of antiepileptic drugs. *Epilepsia* (Amst.), **16**, 393–402.

Kutt, H., Winters, W. & McDowell, F. H. (1966) Depression of parahydroxylation of diphenylhydantoin by antituberculosis chemotherapy. *Neurology* (Minneap.), **16**, 594–602.

Kutt, H., Wolk, M., Scherman, R. & McDowell, F. (1964) Insufficient parahydroxylation as a cause of diphenylhydantoin toxicity. *Neurology* (Minneap.), **14**, 542–548.

la Manna, J. C., Cordingley, G. & Rosenthal, M. (1977) Phenobarbital actions *in vivo*: effects on extracellular potassium activity and oxidative metabolism in cat cerebral cortex. *J. Pharmacol. exp. Therap.*, **200**, 560–569.

la Manna, J., Lothman, E., Rosenthal, M., Somjen, G. & Younts, W. (1977) Phenytoin, electrical, ionic and metabolic responses in cortex and spinal cord. *Epilepsia* (Amst.), **18**, 317–329.

Lambie, D. G., Nanda, R. D., Johnson, R. H. & Shakir, R. A. (1976) Therapeutic and pharmacokinetic effects of increasing phenytoin in chronic epileptics on multiple drug therapy. *Lancet*, **vii**, 386–389.

Lander, C. M., Eadie, M. J. & Tyrer, J. H. (1975) Interactions between anticonvulsants. *Proc. Aust. Assoc. Neurol.*, **12**, 111–116.

Lander, C. M., Eadie, M. J. & Tyrer, J. H. (1977) Factors influencing plasma carbamazepine concentrations. *Clin. Exptl. Neurol.*, **14**, 184–193.

Lander, C. M., Edwards, V. E., Eadie, M. J. & Tyrer, J. H. (1977) Plasma anticonvulsant concentrations during pregnancy. *Neurology* (Minneap.), **27**, 128–131.

Larsen, P. R., Atkinson, A. J. Jr., Wellman, H. N. & Goldsmith, R. E. (1970) The effect of diphenylhydantoin on thyroxin metabolism in man. *J. Clin. Invest.*, **49**, 1266–1279.

Lascelles, P. T., Kocen, R. S. & Reynolds, E. H. (1970) The distribution of plasma phenytoin levels in epileptic patients. *J. Neurol. Neurosurg. Psychiat.*, **33**, 501–505.

Lee, S. I. & Bass, N. H. (1970) Microassay of diphenylhydantoin. Blood and regional brain concentrations in rats during acute intoxication. *Neurology* (Minneap.), **20**, 115–124.

Lefebvre, E. B., Haining, R. G. & Labbé, R. F. (1972) Coarse facies, calvarial thickening and hyperphosphatasia associated with long-term anticonvulsant therapy. *New Engl. J. Med.*, **286**, 1301–1302.

Lennox, W. G. & Lennox, M. A. (1960) *Epilepsy and related disorders.* Vol. I. Boston, Toronto. Little, Brown & Co.

Letteri, J. M., Mellk, H., Louis, S., Kutt, H., Durante, P. & Glazko, A. (1971) Diphenylhydantoin metabolism in uraemia. *New Eng. J. Med.*, **285**, 648–652.

Levy, G. & Ashley, A. A. (1973) Effect of an inhibitor of glucuronide formation on elimination kinetics of diphenylhydantoin. *J. Pharm. Sci.*, **62**, 161–162.

Levy, L. L. & Fenichel, G. M. (1965) Diphenylhydantoin activated seizures. *Neurology* (Minneap.), **15**, 716–722.

Lewis, P. R. & Shute, C. C. D. (1967) The cholinergic limbic system: Projections to hippocampal formation, medial cortex, nuclei of the ascending cholinergic reticular system, and the subfornical organ and supraoptic crest. *Brain*, **90**, 521–540.

Leznicki, A. & Dymecki, J. (1974) The effect of certain anticonvulsants *in vivo* on enzyme activities in the rat's brain. *Neurol. Neurochir. Pol.*, **24**, 413–419.

Lifshitz, F. & Maclaren, N. K. (1973) Vitamin D dependent rickets in institutionalized, mentally retarded children receiving long term anticonvulsant therapy. 1. A survey of 288 patients. *J. Pediat.*, **83**, 612–620.

Little, T. M., Girgis, S. S. & Masotti, R. E. (1975) Diphenylhydantoin induced gingival hyperplasia: its response to changes in drug dosage. *Develop. Med. Child Neurol.*, **17**, 421–424.

Livingstone, S. (1972) *Comprehensive management of epilepsy in infancy, childhood and adolescence.* Springfield: Charles C. Thomas.

Livingstone, S. (1976) Phenytoin and serum cholesterol. *Brit. Med. J.*, **i**, 586.

Livingstone, S., Berman, W. & Pauli, L. L. (1973) Anticonvulsant drugs and vitamin D metabolism. *J. Amer. Med. Ass.*, **226**, 787.

Livingstone, S., Berman, W. & Pauli, L. L. (1975) Anticonvulsant drug blood levels. Practical applications based on 12 years' experience. *J. Amer. Med. Assoc.*, **232**, 60–62.

Livingstone, S. & Livingstone, H. L. (1969) Diphenylhydantoin gingival hyperplasia. *Amer. J. Dis. Child.*, **117**, 265–270.

Lockman, L. A., Hunninghake, D. B., Krivit, W. & Desnick, R. J. (1973) Relief of pain of Fabry's disease by diphenylhydantoin. *Neurology* (Minneap.), **23**, 871–875.

Loescher, W. & Frey, H. H. (1977) Effect of convulsant and anticonvulsant agents on level and metabolism of γ-aminobutyric acid in mouse brain. *Naunyn Schmied. Arch. Pharm.*, **296**, 263–269.

Loeser, E. W. (1961) Studies on the metabolism of diphenylhydantoin (Dilantin). *Neurology* (Minneap.), **11**, 424–429.

Logan, W. J. & Freeman, J. M. (1969) Pseudodegenerative disease due to diphenylhydantoin intoxication. *Arch. Neurol.* (Chic.), **21**, 631–637.

Loiseau, P., Brachet Liermain, A., Legroux, M. & Jogeix, M. (1977) Intérêt du dosage des anticonvulsivants dans le traitment des épilepsies. *Nouv. Presse Med.*, **6**, 813–816.

Loughnan, P. M., Gold, H. & Vance, J. C. (1973) Phenytoin teratogenicity in man. *Lancet*, **i**, 70–72.

Loughnan, P. M., Greenwald, A. & Purton, W. W. (1977) Pharmacokinetic observations of phenytoin disposition in the newborn and young infant. *Arch. Dis. Childh.* **52**, 302–309.

Louis, S., Kutt, H. & McDowell, F. (1968) Intravenous diphenylhydantoin in experimental seizures. II. Effect on penicillin-induced seizures in the cat. *Arch. Neurol.* (Chic.) **18**, 472–477.

Lovelace, R. E. & Horwitz, S. J. (1968) Peripheral neuropathy in long-term diphenylhydantoin therapy. *Arch. Neurol.* (Chic.), **18**, 69–77.

Lowe, C. R. (1973) Congenital malformations among infants born to epileptic women. *Obstet. Gynec. Surg.* **28**, 492–494.

Lühdorf, K. & Lund, M. (1977) Phenytoin-induced hyperkinesia. *Epilepsia* (Amst.), **18**, 409–415.

Lumholtz, B., Siersbaek-Nielsen, K., Skovsted, L., Kampmann, J. & Hansen, J. M. (1975) Sulfamethizole-induced inhibition of diphenylhydantoin, tolbutamide and warfarin metabolism. *Clin. Pharmacol. Therap.*, **17**, 731–734.

Lund, L. (1974) Anticonvulsant effect of diphenylhydantoin relative to plasma levels. A prospective three-year study in ambulant patients with generalized epileptic seizures. *Arch. Neurol.* (Chic.) **31**, 289–294.

Lund, L., Alvan, G., Berlin, A. & Alexanderson, B. (1974) Pharmacokinetics of single and multiple doses of phenytoin in man. *Europ. J. Clin. Pharmacol.*, **7**, 81–86.

Lund, L., Berlin, A. & Lunde, P. K. M. (1972) Plasma protein binding of diphenylhydantoin in patients with epilepsy. Agreement between the unbound fraction in plasma and the concentration in the cerebrospinal fluid. *Clin. Pharmacol. Therap.* **13**, 196–200.

Lund, L., Lunde, P. K., Rane, A., Borga, O. & Sjöqvist, F. (1971) Plasma protein binding, plasma concentrations, and effects of diphenylhydantoin in man. *Ann. N.Y. Acad. Sci.*, **179**, 723–728.

Lund, M., Jorgensen, R. S. & Kühl, V. (1964) Serum diphenylhydantoin (phenytoin) in ambulant patients with epilepsy. *Epilepsia* (Amst.), **5**, 51–58.

Lunde, P. K. M., Rane, A., Yaffe, S. J., Lund, L. & Sjöqvist, F. (1970) Plasma protein binding of diphenylhydantoin in man. Interaction with other drugs and the effect of temperature and plasma dilution. *Clin. Pharmacol. Therap.*, **11**, 846–855.

McAuliffe, J. J., Sherwin, A. L., Leppik, I. E., Fayle, S. A. & Pippenger, C. E. (1977) Salivary levels of anticonvulsants: a practical approach to drug monitoring. *Neurology* (Minneap.), **27**, 409–413.

McLellan, D. L. & Swash, M. (1974) Choreo-athetosis and encephalopathy induced by phenytoin. *Brit. Med. J.*, ii, 204–205.

Madsen, S. N., Hansen, J. M. & Deckert, T. (1974) Intravenous glucose tolerance during treatment with phenytoin. *Acta Neurol. Scandinav.*, **50**, 257–260.

Majkowski, J., Sobieszek, A., Bilinska Nigot, B. & Karlinski, A. (1976) EEG and clinical studies of the development of alumina cream epileptic focus in split brain cats. *Epilepsia* (Amst.), **17**, 257–269.

Malherbe, C., Burrill, K. C., Levin, S. R., Karram, J. H. & Forsham, P. H. (1972) Effect of diphenylhydantoin on insulin secretion in man. *New Eng. J. Med.*, **286**, 339–342.

Malpas, J. S., Spray, G. H. & Witts, L. J. (1966) Serum folic-acid and vitamin-B$_{12}$ levels in anticonvulsant therapy. *Brit. Med. J.*, i, 955–957.

Manson, J. I., Beal, S. M., Magarey, A., Pollard, A. C., O'Reilly, W. J. & Sansom, L. N. (1975) Bioavailability of phenytoin from various pharmaceutical prepations in children. *M. J. Australia*, **2**, 590–592.

Markkanen, T., Himanen, P., Pajula, R. L. & Molnar, G. (1973) Binding of folic acid to serum proteins. II. The effect of diphenylhydantoin treatment and of various diseases. *Acta Haemat.* (Basel), **50**, 284–292.

Markkanen, T., Peltola, O., Himanen, P. & Reikkinen, P. (1971) Metabolite(s) of diphenylhydantoin in human plasma inhibit(s) the pentose phosphate pathway of leucocytes. *Pharmacology* (Basel), **6**, 216–222.

Marsden, C. D., Reynolds, E. H., Parsons, V., Harris, R. & Duchen, L. (1973) Myopathy associated with anticonvulsant osteomalacia. *Brit. Med. J.*, iv, 526–527.

Martin, E., Tozer, T. N., Sheiner, L. B. & Riegelman, S. (1977) The clinical pharmacokinetics of phenytoin. *J. Pharmacokinetics Biopharmaceutics*, **5**, 579–596.

Martin, W. & Rickers, J. (1972) Cholestatische Hepatose nach Diphenylhydantoin. *Wein. Klin. Wschr.* **84**, 41–45.

Mascher, J. & Bernhardt, W. (1973), Überwachung der Langzeitmedikation mit Diphenylhydantoin. Gaschromatographische Bestimmung von Diphenylhydantoin und Hydroxy-Diphenylhydantoin. *Z. Neurol.*, **204**, 179–192.

Massimo, L., Panarotto, M. F. & Vianello, M. G. (1974) Haematological and cytogenetic effects induced in the newborn by anticonvulsant treatment of the mother during pregnancy. *Gaslini*, **6**, 166–172.

Mauguiere, F. & Karlin, R. (1975) Etude des modifications du taux de N$_5$ methyl tétrahydrofolate obsèrvés dans le LCR des epileptiques traites par les anticonvulsivants. *Rev. EEG Neurol. Physiol. Clin.*, **5**, 221–230.

Mawer, G. E., Mullen, P. W., Rodgers, M., Robins, A. J. & Lucas, S. B. (1974) Phenytoin dose adjustment in epileptic patients. *Brit. J. Clin. Pharmacol.*, **1**, 163–168.

Maynert, E. W. (1960) The metabolic fate of diphenylhydantoin in the dog, rat and man. *J. Pharmacol. exp. Therap.* **130**, 275–284.

Meadow, S. R. (1970) Congenital abnormalities and anticonvulsant drugs. *Proc. Roy. Soc. Med.*, **63**, 48–49.

Meldrum, B. S., Horton, R. W. & Toseland, P. A. (1975) A primate model for testing anticonvulsant drugs. *Arch. Neurol.* (Chic.), **32**, 287–294.

Mendel, J. S., Cotzias, G. C., Mena, I. & Papavasiliou, P. S. (1975) Diphenylhydantoin. Blocking of levodopa effects. *Arch. Neurol.* (Chic.), **32**, 44–46.

Mercier-Parot, L. & Tuchmann-Duplessis, H. (1974) The dysmorphogenic potential of phenytoin: experimental observations. *Drugs*, **8**, 340–353.

Merritt, H. H. (1958) Medical treatment in epilepsy. *Brit. Med. J.*, i, 666–669.

Merritt, H. H. & Putnam, T. J. (1938) Sodium diphenyl hydantoinate in the treatment of convulsive disorders. *J. Amer. Med. Ass.*, **111**, 1068–1073.

Meyer, A. (1958) Epilepsy, in *Neuropathology*, ed. Greenfield, J. G., Blackwood, W., McMenemey, W., Meyer, A. & & Norman, R. M. London: Edward Arnold Ltd.

Meyer, J. G. (1973) The teratological effect of anticonvulsants and the effects of pregnancy and birth. *Europ. Neurol.*, **10**, 179–190.

Midha, K. K., Hindmarsh, K. W., McGilveray, I. J. & Cooper, J. K. (1977) Identification of urinary catechol and methylated catechol metabolites of phenytoin in humans, monkeys and dogs by GLC and GLC-mass spectrometry. *J. Pharm. Sci.*, **66**, 1596–1602.

Millar, J. H. D. & Nevin, N. C. (1973) Congenital malformations and anticonvulsant drugs. *Lancet*, i, 328.

Millichap, J. G. & Ortiz, W. R. (1967) Albutoin, a new thiohydantoin derivative for grand mal epilepsies: comparison with diphenylhydantoin in a double-blind controlled study. *Neurology* (Minneap.), **17**, 162–165.

Mirkin, B. L. (1971) Diphenylhydantoin: placental transport, fetal localization, neonatal metabolism and possible teratogenic effects. *J. Pediat.* **78**, 329–337.

Mirkin, B. L. & Wright, F. (1971) Drug interactions: Effect of methylphenidate on the disposition of diphenylhydantoin in man. *Neurology* (Minneap.), **21**, 1123–1128.

Miyamoto, K., Seino, M. & Ikeda, Y. (1975) Consecutive determination of the levels of twelve antiepileptic drugs in blood and cerebrospinal fluid in *Clinical pharmacology of antiepileptic drugs*, ed. Schneider, H., Janz, D., Gardner-Thorpe, C., Meinardi, H. & Sherwin, A. L. Berlin: Springer. 323–329.

Mohd Amin Arnaout & Salti, I. (1976). Phenytoin and benign insulinoma. *Lancet*, **1**, 861.

Mølholm Hansen, J., Siersbaek-Nielsen, K., Skovsted, L., Kampmann, J. P. & Lumholtz, B. (1975) Potentiation of warfarin by Co-trimoxazole. *Brit. Med. J.*, ii, 684.

Mølholm, J., Siersbaek-Nielsen, K. & Skovsted, L. (1971) Interaktion mellan difenylhydantoin oct karbamazepin, in *Plasmakoncentrations bestämmingar av Antiepileptika: Metodologiaka och Kliniska Aspekter*. Lidingo. 48–50.

Monson, R. R., Rosenberg, L., Hartz, S., Shapiro, S., Heinonen, O. P. & Stone, D. (1973) Diphenylhydantoin and selected congenital malformations. *New Eng. J. Med.*, **289**, 1049–1052.

Mori, A. (1974) Neuropharmacologic studies on anticonvulsants. *Brain Develop.* **6**, 435–440..

Morselli, P. L., Rizzo, M. & Garattini, S. (1970) Effect of sulthiame on blood and brain levels of diphenylhydantoin in the rat. *Biochem. Pharmacol.*, **19**, 1846–1847.

Morselli, P. L., Rizzo, M. & Garattini, S. (1971) Interaction between phenobarbital and diphenylhydantoin in animals and in epileptic patients. *Proc. N.Y. Acad. Sci.*, **179**, 88–107.

Mosekilde, L. & Melsen, F. (1976) Anticonvulsant osteomalacia determined by quantitative analysis of bone changes: population study and possible risk factors. *Acta Med. Scand.*, **199**, 349–355.

Mountain, K. R., Hirsch, J. & Gallus, A. S. (1970) Neonatal coagulation defect due to anticonvulsant drug treatment in pregnancy. *Lancet*, i, 265–268.

Munsat, T. L. (1967) Therapy of myotonia. A double-blind evaluation of diphenylhydantoin, procainamide, and placebo. *Neurology* (Minneap.), **17**, 359–367.

Murphy, M. J. & Goldstein, M. N. (1974) Diphenylhydantoin induced asterixis. A clinical study. *J. Amer. Med. Ass.*, **229**, 538–540.

Musgrave, F. S. & Purpura, D. P. (1963) Effect of dilantin on focal epileptogenic activity of cat neocortex. *Electroenceph. clin. Neurophysiol.*, **15**, 923.

Mygind, K. I., Dam, M. & Christiansen, J. (1976) Phenytoin and phenobarbitone plasma clearance during pregnancy. *Acta Neurol. Scandinav.*, **54**, 160–166.

Narisawa, K., Honda, Y., Yoshida, T. & Arakawa, T. (1972) *In vitro* inhibition study of diphenylhydantoin upon rat liver enzymes concerned in folic acid metabolism. *Tohoku J. Exp. Med.*, **106**, 249–251.

Neubauer, C. (1970) Mental deterioration in epilepsy due to folate deficiency. *Brit. Med. J.*, ii, 759–761.

Neuvonen, P. J., Pentikainen, P. J. & Elfving, S. M. (1977) Factors affecting the bioavailability of phenytoin. *Int. J. Clin. Pharmacol. Biopharm.* **15**, 84–89.

Neuvonen, P. J., Penttila, O., Lehtovarra, R. & Aho, K. (1975) Effect of antiepileptic drugs on the elimination of various tetracycline derivatives. *Europ. J. clin. Pharmacol.*, **9**, 147–154.

Nielsen, T. & Cotman, C. (1971) The binding of diphenylhydantoin to brain and subcellular fractions. *Europ. J. Pharmacol.*, **14**, 344–350.

Niswander, J. D. & Wertelecki, W. (1973) Congenital malformations among offspring of epileptic women. *Lancet*, i, 1062.

Noach, E. L., Woodbury, D. M. & Goodman, L. S. (1958) Studies on the absorption, distribution, fate and excretion of 4-C^{14}-labelled diphenylhydantoin. *J. Pharmacol. exp. Therap.*, **122**, 301–314.

Nolte, R. & Brugmann, G. (1975) Problems in controlled anti-epileptic treatment with phenytoin in children. I., in *Clinical pharmacology of antiepileptic drugs*, ed. Schneider, H., Janz, D., Gardner-Thorpe, C., Meinardi, H. & Sherwin, A. L. Berlin: Springer. 70–77.

Norell, E., Lilienberg, G. & Gamstorp, I. (1975) Systematic determination of the serum phenytoin level as an aid in the management of children with epilepsy. *Europ. Neurol.*, **13**, 232–244.

Norris, J. W. & Pratt, R. F. (1974) Folic acid deficiency and epilepsy *Drugs*, **8**, 366–385.

Odar-Cederlöf, I. & Borgå, O. (1974) Kinetics of diphenylhydantoin in uraemic patients: consequences of decreased plasma protein binding. *Europ. J. clin. Pharmacol.*, **7**, 31–37.

Odar-Cederlöf, I. & Borgå, O. (1976) Lack of relationship between serum free fatty acids and impaired plasma protein binding of diphenylhydantoin in chronic renal failure. *Europe. J. clin. Pharmacol.*, **10**, 403–405.

Odar-Cederlöf, I., Lunde, P. & Sjoqvist, F. (1970) Abnormal pharmacokinetics of phenytoin in a patient with uraemia. *Lancet*, **ii**, 831–832.

Olesen, O. V. (1966) Disulfiramum (Antabuse) as inhibitor of phenytoin metabolism. *Acta Pharmacol. et Toxicol.*, **24**, 317–322.

Olesen, O. V. (1967) The influence of disulfiram and calcium carbimide on the serum diphenylhydantoin. Excretion of HPPH in the urine. *Arch. Neurol.* (Chic.), **16**, 642–644.

Olesen, O. V. & Jensen, O. N. (1969) Drug-interaction between sulthiame (Ospolot[R]) and phenytoin in the treatment of epilepsy. *Danish Med. Bull.*, **16**, 154–158.

Olesen, O. V. & Jensen, O. N. (1970) The influence of folic acid on phenytoin (DPH) metabolism and the 24-hour fluctuation in urinary output of 5-(p-hydroxyphenyl)-5-phenyl-hydantoin (HPPH). *Acta pharmacol. et toxicol.*, **28**, 265–269.

Olsen, G. D., Bennet, W. M. & Porter, G. A. (1975) Morphine and phenytoin binding to plasma proteins in renal and hepatic failure. *Clin. Pharmacol. Therap.*, **17**, 677–684.

Olsen, R. W., Lamar, E. E. & Bayless, J. D. (1977) Calcium-induced release of γ-aminobutyric acid from synaptosomes: effects of tranquilliser drugs. *J. Neurochem.*, **28**, 299–305.

O'Malley, W. E., Denckla, M. B. & O'Doherty, D. S. (1969) Oral absorption of diphenylhydantoin as measured by gas liquid chromatography. *Trans. Amer. Neurol. Assocn.*, **94**, 318–319.

Painter, M. J., Pippinger, C., Carter, G. & Pitlick, W. (1977) Metabolism of phenobarbital and phenytoin by neonates with seizures. *Neurology* (Minneap.), **27**, 370.

Parker, W. A. & Gumnit, R. J. (1974) Diphenylhydantoin toxicity: dose dependent blood dyscrasia. *Neurology* (Minneap.), **24**, 1178–1180.

Patsalos, P. M. & Lascelles, P. T. (1977) *In vitro* hydroxylation of diphenylhydantoin and its inhibition by other commonly used anticonvulsant drugs. *Biochem. Pharmacol.*, **26**, 1929–1933.

Paxton, J. W., Rowell, F. J., Ratcliffe, J. G., Lambie, D. G., Nanda, R., Melville, I. D. & Johnson, R. H. (1977) Salivary phenytoin radioimmunoassay. A simple method for the assessment of non-protein bound drug concentrations. *Europ. J. clin. Pharmacol.*, **11**, 71–74.

Pelkonen, R., Fogelholm, R. & Nikkilä, E. A. (1975) Increase in serum cholesterol during phenytoin treatment. *Brit. Med. J.*, **iv**, 85.

Penfield, W. & Jasper, H. (1954) *Epilepsy and the functional anatomy of the human brain*. Boston: Little, Brown & Co.

Pennybacker, J. (1961) Some observations on trigeminal neuralgia, in Garland, H. *Scientific Aspects of Neurology*. Edinburgh: Livingstone. 153–167.

Pentikainen, P. J., Neuvonen, P. J. & Elfving, S. M. (1975) Bioavailability of four brands of phenytoin tablets. *Europ. J. clin. Pharmacol.*, **9**, 213–218.

Penttila, O., Neuvonen, P. J., Aho, K. & Lehtovarra, R. (1974) Interaction between doxycycline and some antiepileptic drugs. *Brit. Med. J.*, **ii**, 470–472.

Perlo, V. P. & Schwab, R. S. (1969) Unrecognised dilantin intoxication, in *Modern Neurology*, ed. Locke, S. Boston. Little, Brown and Co. pp. 589–597.

Perucca, E. & Richens, A. (1977) Interaction between phenytoin and imipramine. *Brit. J. clin. Pharmacol.*, **4**, 485–486.

Petereit, L. B. & Meikle, A. W. (1977) Effectiveness of prednisolone during phenytoin therapy. *Clin. Pharmacol. Therap.*, **22**, 912–916.

Peterson, D. I. & Zweig, R. W. (1974) Absorption of anticonvulsants after jejunoileal bypass. *Bull. Los Angeles Neurol. Soc.* **39**, 51–55.

Petruch, F., Schüppel, R. V. A. & Steinhilber, G. (1974) Effect of diphenylhydantoin on hepatic drug hydroxylation. *Europ. J. clin. Pharmacol.*, **7**, 281–285.

Pieri, L. & Haefely, W. (1959) Cerebellar Purkinje cells discharge rate after diphenylhydantoin or diazepam. *Experientia* (Basel), **31**, 731.

Pieri, L. & Haefely, W. (1976) The effect of diphenylhydantoin, diazepam and clonazepam on the activity of Purkinje cells in the rat cerebellum. *Nauyn-Schmied. Arch. Pharm.*, **296**, 1–4.

Pincus, J. H. (1972) Diphenylhydantoin and ion flux in lobser nerve. *Arch. Neurol.* (Chic), **26**, 4–10.

Pincus, J. H. & Gairman, N. J. (1967) The effect of diphenylhydantoin on sodium, potassium, magnesium stimulated adenosine triphosphatase activity of rat brain. *Biochem. Pharmacol.*, **16**, 600–603.

Pincus, J. H., Grove, I., Marino, B. B. & Glaser, G. E. (1970) Studies on the mechanism of action of diphenylhydantoin. *Arch. Neurol.* (Chic.), **22**, 566–571.

Pincus, J. H. & Lee, S. H. (1973) Diphenylhydantoin and calcium. Relation to norepinephrine release from brain slices. *Arch. Neurol.* (Chic.), **29**, 239–244.

Pincus, J. H. & Rawson, M. D. (1969) Diphenylhydantoin and intracellular sodium concentration. *Neurology* (Minneap.), **19**, 419–422.

Plaa, G. L. & Hine, C. C. (1960) Hydantoin and barbiturate blood levels observed in epileptics. *Arch. int. Pharmacodyn*, **128**, 375–382.

Pond, S. M., Graham, G. G., Birkett, D. J. & Wade, D. N. (1975) Effects of tricyclic antidepressants on drug metabolism. *Clin. Pharmacol. Therap.*, **18**, 191–199.

Porter, R. J. & Layzer, R. B. (1975) Plasma albumin concentration and diphenylhydantoin binding in man. *Arch. Neurol.* (Chic.), **32**, 298–303.

Pruitt, A. W., Zwiren, G. T., Patterson, J. H., Dayton, P. G., Cook, C. E. & Wall, M. E. (1975) A complex pattern of disposition of phenytoin in severe intoxication. *Clin. Pharmacol. Therap.*, **18**, 112–120.

Pugh, R. N. H., Geddes, A. M. & Yeoman, W. B. (1975) Interaction of phenytoin with chlorpheniramine. *Brit. J. Clin. Pharmacol.*, **2**, 173–175.

Racine, R. J., Livingstone, K. & Joaquin, A. (1975) Effects of procaine HCl, diazepam, and diphenylhydantoin on cortical and subcortical structures in rats. *Electroenceph. Clin. Neurophysiol.*, **38**, 355–365.

Rallison, M. L., Carlisle, J. W., Lee, R. E., Vernier, R. L. & Good, R. A. (1961) Lupus erythematosus and Stevens-Johnson syndrome. *Amer. J. Dis. Child.*, **101**, 725–738.

Ralston, A. J., Snaith, R. P. & Hindley, J. B. (1970) Effects of folic acid on fit frequency and behaviour in epileptics on anticonvulsants. *Lancet*, **i**, 867–868.

Ramsay, R. E., Strauss, R. G., Wilder, B. J. & Willmore, L. J. (1978) Status epilepticus in pregnancy: Effect of phenytoin malabsorption on seizure control. *Neurology* (Minneap.), **28**, 85–89.

Rane, A., Garle, M., Borga, O. & Sjöqvist, F. (1974) Plasma disappearance of transplacentally transferred diphenylhydantoin in the newborn studied by mass fragmentography. *Clin. Pharmacol. Therap.*, **15**, 39–45.

Rane, A., Lunde, P. K. M., Jalling, B., Yaffe, S. J. & Sjöqvist, F. (1971) Plasma protein binding of diphenylhydantoin in normal and hyperbilirubinemic infants. *J. Pediat.*, **78**, 877–882.

Rasmussen, S. & Kristensen, M. (1977) Choreoathetosis during phenytoin treatment. *Acta Med. Scand.* **201**, 239–241.

Rausing, A. & Trell, E. (1971) Malignant lymphogranulomatosis and anticonvulsant therapy. *Acta Med. Scand.*, **189**, 131–136.

Reidenberg, M. M., Odar-Cederlöf, I., von Bahr, C., Borga, A. & Sjöqvist, F. (1971) Protein binding of diphenylhydantoin and desmethylimipramine in plasma from patients with poor renal function. *New Eng. J. Med.* **285**, 264–267.

Reinken, L. (1973) Die Wirkung von Hydantoin und Succinimid auf den Vitamin B$_6$ Stoffwechsel. *Clin. Chim. Acta*, **48**, 435–436.

Remmer, H., Hirschmann, J. & Greiner, J. (1969) Die Bedeutung von Kumulation und Elimination fur die Dosierung von Phenytoin (Diphenylhydantoin). *Deutsche Medizinesche Wochen.*, **94**, 1265–1272.

Reynolds, E. H. (1967) Effects of folic acid on the mental state and fit-frequency of drug-treated epileptic patients. *Lancet*, **i**, 1086–1088.

Reynolds, E. H. (1968) Mental effects of anticonvulsants, and folic acid metabolism. *Brain*, **91**, 197–214.

Reynolds, E. H. (1976) Folate and epilepsy, in Bradford, H. B. & Marsden, C. D. *Biochemistry and Neurology*. London: Academic Press, 247–252.

Reynolds, E. H., Chadwick, D. & Galbraith, A. W. (1976) One drug (phenytoin) in the treatment of epilepsy. *Lancet* **i**, 923–926.

Reynolds, E. H., Fenton, G., Fenwick, P., Johnson, A. L. & Laundy, M. (1975) Interaction of phenytoin and primidone. *Brit. Med. J.*, **ii**, 594–595.

Reynolds, E. H., Preece, J. & Chanarin, J. (1969) Folic acid and anticonvulsants. *Lancet*, **i**, 1264–5.

Reynolds, E. H. & Travers, R. D. (1974) Serum anticonvulsant concentration in epileptic patients with mental symptoms. A preliminary report. *Brit. J. Psychiat.*, **124**, 440–445.

Reynolds, F., Ziroyanis, P. N., Jones, N. F. & Smith, S. E. (1976) Salivary phenytoin concentrations in epilepsy and in chronic renal failure. *Lancet*, **vii**, 384–386.

Reynolds, J. W. & Mirkin, B. L. (1973) Urinary corticosteroid and diphenylhydantoin metabolite patterns in neonates exposed to anticonvulsant drugs in utero. *Clin. Pharmacol. Therap.*, **14**, 891–897.

Richens, A. (1974) Drug estimation in the treatment of epilepsy. *Proc. Roy. Soc. Med.* **67**, 1227–1229.
Richens, A. (1975) Discussion, in *Clinical pharmacology of antiepileptic drugs*, ed. Schneider, H., Janz, D., Gardner-Thorpe, C., Meinardi, H. & Sherwin, A. L. Berlin: Springer. 46–47.
Richens, A. & Dunlop, A. (1975) Serum-phenytoin levels in management of epilepsy. *Lancet*, ii, 247–248 and *Lancet*, ii, 1305–1306.
Richens, A. & Houghton, G. W. (1973) Phenytoin intoxication caused by sulthiame. *Lancet*, ii, 1442–1443.
Richens, A. & Houghton, G. W. (1975) Effect of drug therapy on the metabolism of phenytoin, in *Clinical pharmacology of anti-epileptic drugs* ed. Schneider, H., Janz, D., Gardner-Thorpe, C., Meinardi, H. & Sherwin, A. L. Berlin: Springer. 87–95.
Richens, A. & Rowe, D. J. F. (1970) Disturbance of calcium metabolism by anticonvulsant drugs. *Brit. Med. J.*, iv, 73–76.
Riker, W. K., Downes, H., Olsen, G. D. & Smith, B. (1978) Conjugate lateral gaze nystagmus and free phenytoin concentrations in plasma: lack of correlation. *Epilepsia (Amst.)* **19**, 93–98.
Rizzo, M., Morselli, P. L. & Garattini, S. (1972) Further observations on the interactions between phenobarbital and diphenylhydantoin during chronic treatment in the rat. *Biochem. Pharmacol.*, **21**, 449–454.
Robins, M. M. (1962) Aplastic anaemia secondary to anticonvulsants. *Amer. J. Dis. Child.*, **104**, 614–624.
Rødbro, P., Christiansen, C. & Lund, M. (1974) Development of anticonvulsant osteomalacia in epileptic patients on phenytoin treatment. *Acta Neurol. Scandinav.*, **50**, 527–532.
Rødbro, P. Christiansen, C. & Lund, M. (1975) Subjective symptoms in epileptic patients on anticonvulsant drugs. A controlled therapeutic trial on the effect of vitamin D. *Acta Neurol. Scandinav.*, **52**, 87–93.
Roe, T. F., Podosin, R. L. & Blaskovics, M. E. (1975) Drug interaction: diazoxide and diphenylhydantoin. *J. Pediat.* **87**, 480–484.
Rose, J. Q., Choi, H. K. & Schentag, J. J. (1977) Intoxication caused by interaction of chloramphenicol and phenytoin. *J. Amer. Med. Assoc.*, **237**, 2630–2631.
Roseman, E. (1961) Dilantin toxicity. A clinical and electroencephalographic study. *Neurology* (Minneap.), **11**, 912–921.
Rosenberg, I. H., Godwin, H. A., Streiff, R. R. & Castle, W. B. (1968) Impairment of intestinal deconjugation of dietary folate. A possible explanation of myeloblastic anaemia associated with phenytoin therapy. *Lancet*, ii, 530–532.
Rothermich, N. O. (1966) Diphenylhydantoin intoxication. *Lancet*, ii, 640.
Rowan, A. J., Pippenger, C. E., McGregor, P. A. & French, J. H. (1975) Seizure activity and anticonvulsant drug concentration. *Arch. Neurol.* (Chic.) **32**, 281–288.
Rudman, D., Bixler, T. J. II & Del Rio, A. E. (1971) Effect of free fatty acids on binding of drugs by bovine serum albumin, by human serum albumin and by rabbit serum. *J. Pharmacol. exp. Therap.*, **176**, 261–272.
Saad, S. F., El Masry, A. M. & Scott, P. M. (1972) Influence of certain anticonvulsants on the concentration of γ aminobutyric acid in the cerebral hemispheres of mice. *Europ. J. Pharmacol.* **17**, 386–392.
Saltzstein, S. L. & Ackerman, L. V. (1959) Lymphadenopathy induced by anticonvulsant drugs and mimicking clinically and pathologically malignant lymphomas. *Cancer*, **12**, 164–182.
Sansom, L. B., O'Reilly, W. J., Wiseman, C. W., Stern, L. M. & Derham, J. (1975) Plasma phenytoin levels produced by various phenytoin preparations. *M. J. Australia*, **2**, 593–595.
Savariaryan, F. & Dixey, G. M. (1959) Syncope following uterosigmoidostomy. *J. Urol.* **101**, 844–845.
Sawaya, M. C. B., Horton, R. W. & Meldrum, B. S. (1975) Effects of anticonvulsant drugs on the cerebral enzymes metabolizing GABA. *Epilepsia (Amst.)*, **16**, 649–655.
Schallek, W. & Kuehn, A. (1963) Effects of trimethadione, diphenylhydantoin and chlordiazepoxide on after-discharges in brain of cat. *Proc. Soc. exp. Biol. NY.*, **112**, 813–817.
Schmidt, D. (1975) The effect of phenytoin and ethosuximide on primidone metabolism in patients with epilepsy. *J. Neurol.*, **209**, 115–123.
Schmidt, D. & Kupferberg, H. J. (1975) Diphenylhydantoin, phenobarbital and primidone in saliva, plasma and cerebrospinal fluid. *Epilepsia (Amst.)*, **16**, 735–741.
Schneider, H. (1975) Carbamazepine: the influence of other anti-epileptic drugs on its serum level, in *Clinical pharmacology of anti-epileptic drugs* ed. Schneider, H., Janz, D., Gardner-Thorpe, C., Meinardi, H. & Sherwin, A. L. Berlin: Springer. 189–195.
Scholz, W. (1953) Selective neuronal necrosis and its topistic patterns in hypoxemia and oligemia. *J. Neuropath. exp. Neurol.*, **12**, 249–261.
Schuppel, R., Petruch, F. & Steinhilber, E. (1973) Hepatic drug hydroxylation in epileptic patients: effect of diphenylhydantoin (DPH) therapy. *Naunyn. Schmied. Arch. Pharm.*, **279**, R48.

Schussler, G. C. (1971) Diazepam competes for thyroxine binding sites. *J. Pharmacol. exp. Therap.* **178**, 204–209.

Schwartz, P. A., Rhodes, C. T. & Cooper, J. W. Jr. (1977) Solubility and ionization characteristics of phenytoin. *J. Pharm. Sci.*, **66**, 994–997.

Seager, J., Wilson, J., Jamison, D. L., Hayward, A. R. & Soothill, J. F. (1975) IgA deficiency, epilepsy and phenytoin treatment. *Lancet*, ii, 632–635.

Selby, G. & Lorentz, I. T. (1966) Methetoin (N_3): a trial of a new anticonvulsant drug. *M. J. Australia*, **2**, 940–942.

Selzer, M. E. (1978) The action of phenytoin on a composite electrical-chemical synapse in the lamprey spinal cord. *Ann. Neurol.*, **3**, 202–206.

Serrano, E. E., Roye, D. B., Hammer, R. H. & Wilder, B. J. (1973) Plasma diphenylhydantoin values after oral and intramuscular administration of diphenylhydantoin. *Neurology* (Minneap.), **23**, 311–317.

Serrano, E. E. & Wilder, B. J. (1974) Intramuscular administration of diphenylhydantoin. Histologic follow-up study. *Arch. Neurol.* (Chic.), **31**, 276–278.

Shakir, R. A., Behan, P. O., Dick, H. & Lambie, D. G. (1978) Metabolism of immunoglobulin A, lymphocyte function, and histocompatibility antigens in patients on anticonvulsants. *J. Neurol. Neurosurg. Psychiat.*, **41**, 307–311.

Shanes, A. M. (1958) Electrochemical aspects of physiological and pharmacological action in excitable cells. *Pharmacol. Rev.*, **10**, 59–273.

Shapiro, S., Hartz, S. C., Siskind, V., Mitchell, A. C., Slone, D., Rosenberg, L., Monson, R. R., Heinonen, O. P., Idanpaan-Heikkila, J., Haro, S. & Saxén, L. (1976) Anticonvulsants and parental epilepsy in the development of birth defects. *Lancet*, i, 272–275.

Sherwin, A. L., Eisen, A. A. & Sokolowski, C. D. (1973) Anticonvulsant drugs in human epilpetogenic brain. *Arch. Neurol.* (Chic.), **29**, 73–77.

Sherwin, A. L., Harvey, C. D., Leppik, I. E. & Gonda, A. (1976) Correlation between red cell and free plasma phenytoin levels in renal disease. *Neurology* (Minneap.), **26**, 874–878.

Sherwin, A. L., Loynd, J. S., Bock, G. W. & Sokolowski, C. D. (1974) Effect of age, sex, obesity and pregnancy on plasma diphenylhydantoin levels. *Epilepsia* (Amst.), **15**, 507–521.

Sherwin, I. (1973) Suppressant effect of diphenylhydantoin on the cortical epileptogenic focus. *Neurology* (Minneap.), **23**, 274–281.

Shoeman, D. W. & Azarnoff, D. L. (1972) The alteration of plasma proteins in uremia as reflected in their ability to bind digitoxin and diphenylhydantoin. *Pharmacology*, **7**, 169–177.

Shoeman, D. W., Benjamin, D. M. & Azarnoff, D. L. (1973) The alteration of plasma proteins in uraemia as reflected in the ability to bind diphenylhydantoin. *Ann. N.Y. Acad. Sci.*, **226**, 127–130.

Shute, C. C. D. & Lewis, P. R. (1967) The ascending cholinergic reticular system: Neocortical, olfactory and subcortical projections. *Brain*, **90**, 497–520.

Siegel, G. J. & Goodwin, B. B. (1972) Sodium-potassium activated adenosine triphosphatase of brain microsomes: modification of sodium inhibition by diphenylhydantoin. *J. Clin. Invest.*, **51**, 1164–1169.

Siersbaek-Nielsen, K., Skovsted, L., Hansen, J. M. & Kristensen, M. (1971) Phenytoin tolerance tests. *Brit. Med. J.*, **1**, 231.

Sjo, O., Hvidberg, E. F., Larsen, N. E., Lund, M. & Naestoft, J. (1975) Dose dependent kinetics of ethotoin in man. *Clin. Exp. Pharmacol. Physiol.*, **2**, 185–192.

Skou, J. C. (1965) Enzymatic basis for active transport of Na^+ and K^+ across cell membrane. *Physiol. Rev.*, **45**, 596–617.

Skovsted, L., Kristensen, M., Hansen, J. M. & Siersbaek-Nielson, K. (1976) The effect of different oral anticoagulants on diphenylhydantoin (DPH) and tolbutamide metabolism. *Acta Med. Scandinav.*, **199**, 513–515.

Skovsted, L., Hansen, J. M., Kristensen, M. & Christensen, L. K. (1974) Inhibition of drug metabolism in man, in Morselli, P. L., Garattini, S. & Cohen, S. N. *Drug interactions.* New York: Raven Press. 81–90.

Smith, R. G., Davies, G. D., Lynn, R. K. & Gerber, N. (1977) Hydantoin ring glucuronidation: characterization of a new metabolite of 5,5-diphenylhydantoin in man and the rat. *Biomed. Mass. Spectrometry*, **4**, 275–279.

Smith, R. L. & Williams, R. T. (1966) Implication of the conjugation of drugs and other exogenous compounds, in *Glucuronic acid, free and combined*. Ed. Dutton, G. J. New York and London: Academic Press. 457–491.

Snider, S. R. & Snider, R. S. (1977) Phenytoin and cerebellar lesions. Similar effects of cerebral catecholamine metabolism. *Arch. Neurol.* (Chic.), **34**, 162–167.

Sohn, R. S. & Ferrendelli, J. A. (1976) Anticonvulsant drug mechanisms. Phenytoin, phenobarbital, and ethosuximide and calcium flux in isolated presynaptic endings. *Arch. Neurol.* (Chic.), **33**, 626–629.

Solomon, G. E., Hilgartner, M. W. & Kutt, H. (1972) Coagulation defects caused by diphenylhydantoin. *Neurology* (Minneap.), **22**, 1165–1171.

Solomon, H. M., Reich, S., Spirt, N. & Abrams, W. B. (1971) Interactions between digitoxin and other drugs *in vitro* and *in vivo*. *Ann. N. Y. Acad. Sci.*, **79**, 362–369.

Solomon, H. M. & Schrogie, J. J. (1976) The effect of phenyramidol on the metabolism of diphenylhydantoin. *Clin. Pharm. Therap.*, **8**, 554–556.

Sorrell, T. C., Forbes, I. J., Burness, F. R. & Rischbieth, R. H. C. (1971), Depression of immunological function in patients treated with phenytoin sodium (sodium diphenylhydantoin). *Lancet*, **ii**, 1233–1235.

South, J. (1972) Teratogenic effect of anticonvulsants. *Lancet*, **ii**, 1154.

Sotaniemi, E., Arvela, P., Hakkarainen, H. & Huhti, E. (1970) Serum levels of antiepileptic drugs during chronic treatment. *Scand. J. Clin. Lab. Invest.*, **25**, 90.

Sparberg, M. (1963) Diagnostically confusing complications of diphenylhydantoin therapy. *Ann. Intern. Med.*, **59**, 914–930.

Spector, R. G. (1972) The influence of anticonvulsant drugs on formyl tetrahydrofolic acid stimulation of rat brain respiration *in vitro*. *Biochem. Pharmacol.*, **21**, 3198–3201.

Spector, R. H., Davidoff, R. A. & Schwartzman, R. J. (1976) Phenytoin-induced opthalmoplegia. *Neurology* (Minneap.), **26**, 1031–1034.

Speidel, B. D. & Meadow, S. R. (1972) Maternal epilepsy and abnormalities of the fetus and newborn. *Lancet*, **ii**, 839–843.

Stamp, T. C. B. (1974) Effects of long-term anticonvulsant therapy on calcium and vitamin D metabolism. *Proc. roy. Soc. Med.*, **67**, 64–68.

Stein, S. & Pembrook, R. C. (1965) Cross-sensitivity to Dilantin (Diphenylhydantoin) and Celontin (methosuximide). *J. Pediat.*, **66**, 799–801.

Stewart, M. J. (1976) Failure to confirm anticonvulsant hypomagnesaemia. *Brit. Med. J.*, **i**, 649.

Stewart, M. J. Ballinger, B. R., Devlin, E. J., Miller, A. Y. & Ramsay, A. C. (1975) Bioavailability of phenytoin. A comparison of two preparations. *Europ. J. clin. Pharmacol.*, **9**, 209–212.

Stoegmann, W. (1971) Ossifikationsstoerungen bei antikonvulsiver Langzeitbehandlung. *Paediat. Paedol.*, **6**, 280–286.

Stokes, J. B. & Fortune, C. (1958) Megaloblastic anaemia associated with anticonvulsant drug therapy. *Aust. Ann. Med.*, **7**, 118–125.

Strandjord, R. E. & Johannessen, S. I. (1972) One daily dose of diphenylhydantoin (DPH) to patients with epilepsy. *Acta Neurol. Scandinav.*, Suppl. 51. Vol. **48**, 499–500.

Strandjord, R. E. & Johannessen, S. I. (1974) One daily dose of diphenylhydantoin for patients with epilepsy. *Epilepsia* (Amst.), **15**, 317–327.

Steinberg, M. S. & Doctor, B. P. (1976) Studies on the effect of 5,5-diphenylhydantoin on *in vitro* protein synthesis in rat brain. *J. Pharmacol. exp. Therap.*, **198**, 648–654.

Stensrud, P. A. & Palmer, H. (1964) Serum phenytoin determinations in epileptics. *Epilepsia* (Amst), **5**, 364–370.

Suzkui, I., Saitoh, Y. & Nishihara, K. (1970) Kinetics of diphenylhydantoin disposition in man. *Chem. Pharm. Bull.* **18**, 405–411.

Svendsen, T. L., Kristensen, M. B., Hansen, J. M. & Skovsted, L. (1976) The influence of disulfiram on the half-life and metabolic clearance rate of diphenylhydantoin and tolbutamide in man. *Europ. J. clin. Pharmacol.*, **9**, 439–441.

Svensmark, O. & Buchthal, F. (1964) Diphenylhydantoin and phenobarbital. Serum levels in children. *Amer. J. Dis. Child.*, **108**, 82–87.

Svensmark, O., Schiller, P. J. & Buchthal, F. (1960) 5,5-diphenylhydantoin (Dilantin^R) blood levels after oral or intravenous dosage in man. *Acta Pharmacol. et Toxicol.*, **16**, 331–346.

Takeda, A., Goto, H., Amano, Y. & Kukino, K. (1976) A study on serum and cerebrospinal fluid levels of sodium valproate (DPA), a new antiepileptic drug. *Brain Develop.*, **8**, 401–408.

Tammisto, P., Kauro, K. & Viukari, M. (1976) Bioavailability of phenytoin. *Lancet*, **i**, 254–255.

Tappaz, M. & Pacheco, H. (1973) Effets de convulsivants et d'anticonvulsivants sur le capture de GABA. *J. Pharmacol.* (Paris), **4**, 295–306.

Taylor, J. D., Krahn, P. M. & Higgins, T. N. (1974) Serum copper levels and diphenylhydantoin. *Amer. J. Clin. Path.*, **61**, 577–578.

Thompson, R. M., Beghin, J., Fife, W. K. & Gerber, N. (1976) 5,5-bis (4-hydroxyphenyl) hydantoin, a minor metabolite of diphenylhydantoin (Dilantin) in the rat and human. *Drug. Metab. Disposition.* **4**, 349–356.

Tokya, K. V., Janka, G. E. & Janka, H. U. (1975) Effect of intravenous diphenylhydantoin on glucose tolerance and insulin response in children. *Neuropadiatrie*, **6**, 176–183.

Travers, R: D., Reynolds, E. H. & Gallagher, B. B. (1972) Variation in response to anticonvulsants in a group of epileptic patients. *Arch. Neurol.* (Chic.) **27**, 29–33.

Triedman, H. M., Fisman, R. A. & Yahr, M. D. (1960) Determination of plasma and cerebrospinal fluid levels of Dilantin in the human. *Trans. Amer. Neurol. Assocn.*, **85**, 166–170.

Troupin, A. S. & Friel, P. (1975) Anticonvulsant levels in saliva, serum, and cerebrospinal fluid. *Epilepsia* (Amst.), **16**, 223–227.

Troupin, A. S. & Ojemann, L. M. (1976) Paradoxical intoxication—a complication of anticonvulsant intoxication. *Epilepsia* (Amst.), **16**, 753–758.

Troupin, A. S., Ojemann, L. M. & Dodrill, C. B. (1976) Mephenytoin: a reappraisal. *Epilepsia* (Amst.), **17**, 403–414.

Tyrer, J. H., Eadie, M. J., Sutherland, J. M. & Hooper, W. D. (1970) An outbreak of anticonvulsant intoxication in an Australian city. *Brit. Med. J.*, iv., 271–273.

Vajda, F. J. E., Merory, J. & Bladin, P. F. (1975) Fluctuation of plasma phenytoin levels on single dose and twice daily dosage regimes. *Proc. Aust. Assoc. Neurol.*, **12**, 61–64.

Vajda, F., Williams, F. M., Davidson, S., Falconer, M. A. & Breckenridge, A. (1974) Human brain, cerebrospinal fluid, and plasma concentrations of diphenylhydantoin and phenobarbital. *Clin. Pharmacol. Therap.* **15**, 597–603.

Van der Kleijn, E., Guelen, P. J. M., van Wijk, C. & Baars, I. (1975) Clinical pharmacokinetics in monitoring chronic medication with anti-epileptic drugs, in *Clinical pharmacology of antiepileptic drugs*, ed. Schneider, H., Janz, D., Gardner-Thorpe, C., Meinardi, H. & Sherwin, A. L. Berlin: Springer, 11–33.

Van Meter, J. C., Buckmaster, H. S. & Shelley, L. L. (1970) Concurrent assay of phenobarbital and diphenylhydantoin in plasma by vapour-phase chromatography. *Clin. Chem.* **16**, 135–138.

Vapaatalo, H. & Lehtinen, L. (1971) Variations of serum diphenylhydantoin concentrations in epileptic out-patients. *Europ. Neurol.*, **5**, 303–310.

Varkey, K., Raman, P. T., Bhaktaviziam, A. & Taori, G. M. (1973) Osteomalacia due to phenytoin sodium. A case report with reviews of literature. *J. Neurol. Sci.*, **19**, 287–295.

Vasiliades, J. & Shawawneh, T. (1975) Effect of diphenylhydantoin on serum copper, zinc and magnesium. *Clin. Chem.*, **31**, 637–638.

Vernadakis, A. & Woodbury, D. M. (1960) Effect of diphenylhydantoin and adrenocortical steroids on free glutamic acid, glutamine and gamma-aminobutyric acid concentrations of rat cerebral cortex, in *Inhibition in the nervous system and gamma-aminobutyric acid* ed. Roberts, E., Barden, C. F., van Harreveld, A., Wiersma, C. A. G., Adey, W. R. & Killam, K. F. New York: Pergamon. 242–248.

Victor, A., Lundberg, P. O. & Johansson, E. D. B. (1977) Induction of sex hormone binding globulin by phenytoin. *Brit. Med. J.* ii, 934–935.

Viukari, N. M. A. (1969) Intolerance to diphenylhydantoin in five cases of Vogt-Speilmeyer disease. *J. Ment. Defic. Res.*, **13**, 246–248.

Viukari, N. M. A. & Tammisto, P. (1969) Diphenylhydantoin as an anticonvulsant: protein binding and fluctuations of the serum and cerebrospinal fluid levels in forty mentally subnormal epileptics. *J. Ment. Defic. Res.*, **13**, 235–244.

Wada, J. A. (1977) Pharmacological prophylaxis in the kindling model of epilepsy. *Arch. Neurol.* (Chic.), **34**, 389–395.

Wallis, W., Kutt, H. & McDowell, F. (1968) Intravenous diphenylhydantoin in treatment of acute repetitive seizures. *Neurology* (Minneap.), **18**, 513–525.

Ware, E. (1950) The chemistry of the hydantoins. *Chem. Reviews*, **46**, 403–470.

Watson, J. D. & Spellacy, W. N. (1971) Neonatal effects of maternal treatment with the anticonvulsant drug diphenylhydantoin. *Obstet. Gynecol.*, **37**, 881–885.

Watts, J. C. (1962) A fatal case of erythema multiforme exudativum (Steven's-Johnson's syndrome) following therapy with Dilantin. *Pediatrics*, **30**, 592–594.

Weckman, N. & Lehtovarra, R. (1968) Serum and cerebrospinal fluid folate values in epileptics on anticonvulsant treatment. *Scand. J. Clin. Lab. Invest.* **21**, 120–121.

Weedon, A. P. (1975) Diphenylhydantoin sensitivity. A syndrome resembling infectious mononucleosis with a morbilliform rash and cholestatic hepatitis. *Aust. N.Z. J. Med.*, **5**, 561–563.

Weinberger, J., Nicklas, W. J. & Berl, S. (1976) Mechanism of action of anticonvulsants. Role of the differential effects on the active uptake of putative neurotransmitters. *Neurology* (Minneap.), **26**, 162–166.

Weiss, C. F., Heffelfinger, J. C. & Buchanan, R. A. (1969) Serial Dilantin[R] levels in mentally retarded children. *Amer. J. Mental Deficiency*, **73**, 826–830.

Wesseling, H. & Mols-Thurkow, I. (1975) Interaction of diphenylhydantoin (DPH) and tolbutamide in man. *Europ. J. clin. Pharmacol.*, **8**, 75–78.

Wilder, B. J., Buchanan, R. A. & Serrano, E. E. (1973) Correlation of acute diphenylhydantoin intoxication with plasma levels and metabolite excretion. *Neurology* (Minneap.), **23**, 1329–1322.

Wilder, B. J. & Ramsay, R. E. (1976) Oral and intramuscular phenytoin. *Clin. Pharmacol. Therap.*, **19**, 360–364.

Wilder, B. J. & Serrano, E. E. (1978) Single versus multiple daily dose diphenylhydantoin maintenance in an outpatient population. *Neurology* (Minneap.), **23**, 447.

Wilder, B. J., Serrano, E. E. & Ramsay, R. E. (1973) Plasma diphenylhydantoin levels after loading and maintenance doses. *Clin. Pharmacol. Therap.*, **14**, 797–801.

Wilder, B. J., Serrano, E. E., Ramsay, E. & Buchanan, R. A. (1974) A method of shifting from oral to intramuscular diphenylhydantoin administration. *Clin. Pharmacol. Therap.*, **16**, 507–513.

Wilder, B. J., Streiff, R. R. & Hammer, R. H. (1972) Diphenylhydantoin: absorption, distribution and excretion: clinical studies, in *Antiepileptic drugs*, ed. Woodbury, D. M., Penry, J. K. & Schmidt, R. P. New York: Raven Press. 137–148.

Wilensky, A. J. & Lowden, J. A. (1973) Inadequate serum levels after intramuscular administration of diphenylhydantoin. *Neurology* (Minneap.), **23**, 318–324.

Wilson, J. T., Hojer, B. & Rane, A. (1976) Loading and conventional dose therapy with phenytoin in children: kinetic profile of parent drug and main metabolite in plasma. *Clin. Pharmacol. Therap.*, **20**, 48–58.

Windorfer, A. Jr. & Sauer, W. (1977) Drug interactions during anticonvulsant therapy in childhood: Diphenylhydantoin, primidone, phenobarbitone, clonazepam, nitrazepam, carbamazepine and dipropylacetate. *Neuropadiatrie*, **8**, 29–41.

Winek, C. L. (1976) Tabulation of therapeutic, toxic, and lethal concentrations of drugs and chemicals in blood. *Clin. Chem.* **22**, 832–836.

Woodbury, D. M. (1955) Effect of diphenylhydantoin on electrolytes and radiosodium turnover in brain and other tissues of normal, hyponatremic and postical rats. *J. Pharmacol. exp. Therap.* **115**, 74–95.

Woodbury, D. M. (1969a) Mechanism of action of anticonvulsants, in *Basic mechanisms of the epilepsies*, ed. Jasper, H. H., Ward, A. A. & Pope, A. Boston. Little, Brown & Co. 647–681.

Woodbury, D. M. (1969b) Role of pharmacological factors in the evaluation of anticonvulsant drugs. *Epilepsia* (Amst.), **10**, 121–144.

Woodbury, D. M. & Esplin, D. W. (1959) Neuropharmacology and neurochemistry of anticonvulsant drugs. *Proc. Ass. Res. nerv. ment. Dis.*, **37**, 24–56.

Yabuki, S. & Nakaya, K. (1976) Immunoglobulin abnormalities in epileptic patients treated with diphenylhydantoin. *Folia Psychiat. Neurol. Jap.*, **30**, 93–109.

Yanagihara, T. & Hamberger, A. (1971) Distribution of diphenylhydantoin in rat organs: study with neuron-glia and subcellular fractions. *J. Pharmacol. exp. Therap.* **179**, 611–618.

Yeo, P. P. B., Bates, D., Howe, J. G., Ratcliffe, W. A., Schardt, C. W., Heath, A. & Evered, D. C. (1978) Anticonvulsants and thyroid function. *Brit. Med. J.* i, 1581–1583.

7

Carbamazepine

Common proprietary name: Tegretol

This dibenzazepine derivative, a structural congener of the antidepressant imipramine, was synthesized by Schindler in 1953 (Donaldson and Graham, 1965). The drug came into use as an anticonvulsant early in the 1960s, and soon after found its place as treatment of choice for tic douloureux (Blom, 1962). It is administered orally, and is useful in all forms of partial epilepsy and in tonic-clonic generalized seizures. It is reported to have a favourable effect on some personality disturbances (Pakesch, 1963). Carbamazepine finds an occasional use in certain pain syndromes apart from tic douloureux, and in treating diabetes insipidus (Wohlfahrth, 1972).

CHEMISTRY

Carbamazepine (5-carbamyl-5H-dibenz[b,f]azepine) is a white powder with a molecular weight of 236·3. It is soluble in the more polar organic solvents (e.g. propylene glycol, ethanol and acetone) but has a very poor solubility in water. For practical purposes the molecule is neutral and does not ionize.

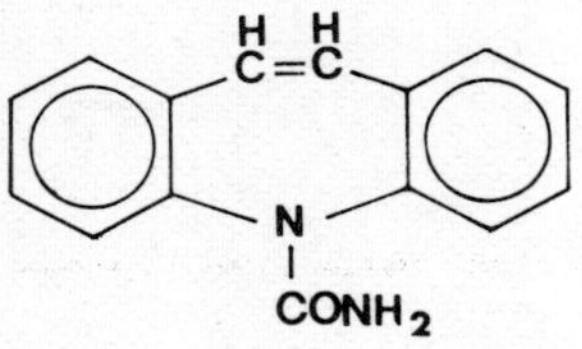

PHARMACODYNAMICS

ACTIONS IN MAN

Anticonvulsant actions

Carbamazepine appears to be effective against all varieties of partial epilepsy in man, whether or not the seizures undergo secondary generalization. The drug is also useful in those varieties of primary generalized epilepsy which present as convulsive seizures. It also exerts a degree of protective action against myoclonic seizures (Lance, 1968). Carbamazepine is of little or no use in absence seizures. Thus carbamazepine has a slightly broader spectrum of anticonvulsant action than phenytoin, but resembles this drug more than any other widely used anticonvulsant in respect to the types of epilepsy for which it is useful. In a double-blind cross-over study, carbamazepine appeared to cause fewer errors in mental tasks requiring attention and problem solving than did phenytoin (Dodrill and Troupin, 1977). In that study there was some evidence suggesting that carbamazepine treatment led to an improved emotional state.

Other actions

Carbamazepine is generally accepted as the treatment of choice for tic douloureux. It has been used with some success in other pain syndromes including glossopharyngeal neuralgia (Ekbom and Westerberg, 1966), painful crises in Fabry's disease (Shibasaki, Tabira, Inoue, Goto and Kuroiwa, 1973), tabetic lightning pains (Killian and Fromm, 1968; Ekbom, 1972) and painful diabetic peripheral neuropathy (Chakrabarti and Samantaray, 1976). It appears doubtful whether carbamazepine is effective in post-herpetic neuralgia (Killian and Fromm, 1968).

Carbamazepine may be used to treat diabetes insipidus with a reasonable success rate, though it is ineffective against the nephrogenic variety of the disorder (Wales, 1975).

ACTIONS IN ANIMALS

Models of generalized epilepsy

Carbamazepine protects against photomyclonic seizures in the baboon Papio papio, but only when given in doses that are toxic to the animals (Meldrum, Horton and Toseland, 1975). The drug is relatively ineffective against seizures induced by systemically-administered pentylenetetrazole (Theobald and Kunz, 1963). However, Julien and Hollister (1975) found that it conferred some protection against seizures produced by this agent. It also protected against seizures evoked by strychnine (Theobald and Kunz, 1963) and bicuculline (Blum, Haefely, Jalfre, Polc and Scharer, 1973). Carbamazepine protects against maximum electroshock seizures in mice (Julien and Hollister, 1975). It raises the threshold for evocation of minimum electroshock seizures (Blum, Haefely, Jalfre, Polc and Schaerer, 1973).

Models of partial epilepsy

Wada, Sato, Wake, Green and Troupin (1976) showed that carbamazepine prevented kindled focal seizures in cats. The drug did not prevent amygdala-kindled seizures in rats, even when given in doses that made the animals comatose (Wada, 1977). Carbamazepine protected against seizures arising from an alumina-induced focus in the hippocampus or sensorimotor cortex of rhesus monkeys (David and Grewal, 1976), and against seizures induced by electrical stimulation of the visual cortex of cats (Ito, Hori, Yoshida and Shimizu, 1977).

MECHANISMS OF ACTION

Neuron pools

Carbamazepine produced some diminution in paroxysmal activity at an alumina-induced cortical focus in the rhesus monkey (David and Grewal, 1976). In cats, at concentrations below 9 μg/ml, carbamazepine failed to influence spike activity at a penicillin-induced cortical focus (Julien and Hollister, 1975). At concentrations of 5–9 μg/ml, carbamazepine rather specifically suppressed activity in the antero-ventral nucleus of the thalamus in cats (Holm, Kelleter, Heinemann and Hamann, 1970). The drug limited the propagation of activity from spike foci (Julien and Hollister, 1975; David and Grewal, 1976), and increased the threshold for after-discharge instigation in limbic structures of cats (Hernandez-Peon, 1962; Kobayaski, Iwata and Mukawa, 1967), though not in the lenticular nucleus (Kobayasky, Iwata and Mukawa, 1967).

Hernandez-Peon (1965) and Fromm and Killain (1967) found that car-bamazepine decreased synaptic transmission in the spinal trigeminal nucleus of cats. In the spinal cords of rabbits (Krupp, 1969) and cats (Demieville, 1975) the drug decreased post-tetanic potentiation. However, Demieville (1975) showed that this effect occurred only in the first 20 minutes after carbamazepine administration. Later, post-tetanic potentiation became super-normal. Julien and Hollister (1975) provided further information about the effect of the drug on post-tetanic potentiation. At the therapeutic concentrations of 3·5 to 10 μg/ml carbamazepine did not alter post-tetanic potentiation, but at supratherapeutic concentrations (15–20 μg/ml) the potentiation was decreased.

Single cells
Carbamazepine decreased the membrane potential of the squid giant axon, but only when the drug was present in the supra-therapeutic concentrations of 118 to 236 μg/ml (Schauf, Davis and Marder, 1974). The low aqueous solubility of carbamazepine would make microelectrode study of the effects of the drug technically difficult.

Biochemical effects

Effects on energy production
No information is available.

Effects on inorganic ions
Schauf, Davis and Marker (1974) found that carbamazepine at supratherapeutic concentrations (0·25–1·0 m mole/litre) produced a dose-dependent fall in Na$^+$ and K$^+$ conductance in the squid giant axon.

Effects on synpatic transmitters

Acetylcholine: Consolo, Bianchi and Ladinsky (1977) found that carbamazepine increased acetylcholine concentrations in the striatum, but not in other brain regions.

Serotonin: No data are available.

Noradrenaline: At concentrations in the therapeutic range (10^{-5} M) car-bamazepine inhibited noradrenaline uptake by rabbit brain synaptosomes (Purdy, Julien, Fairhurst and Terry, 1977).

Dopamine: No data are available.

Gamma-aminobutyrate: No data are available.

Thus there appears to have been little study of the effects of carbamazepine on brain synaptic transmitters.

Effects on cyclic adenosine monophosphate (cAMP)
Lewin and Bleck (1977) found that carbamazepine inhibited the rise in rat cerebral cortex levels of cAMP induced by local ouabain application. Raised cAMP levels are associated with epileptogenesis.

Effects on folates
Carbamazepine therapy causes a fall in serum folate levels (Reizenstein and Lund, 1973).

No other data have been traced regarding the biochemical mechanisms of action of carbamazepine. The actions of the drug at a molecular level are not adequately understood.

PHARMACOKINETICS

The pharmacokinetics of carbamazepine were reviewed by Bertilsson (1978).

ABSORPTION AND BIOAVAILABILITY

Carbamazepine is given by mouth, as tablets. Levy, Pitlick, Troupin, Green and Neal (1975) found the absorption half-time of the drug from tablets averaged 1·72 hours, while Cotter, Smith, Hooper, Tyrer and Eadie (1975) obtained an average value of 7 hours for this parameter. However they found wide interindividual variation for the half-time. They also found that absorption half-time varied with carbamazepine dose (Fig. 7.1). Levy, Pitlick, Troupin, Green and Neal (1975) showed that absorption half-time was shorter if the drug was given in solution (0·29 hours) rather than as tablets (1·72 hours).

The time to achieve peak plasma level after a single oral dose of carbamazepine in tablet form has varied from study to study. Some available figures are 4–8 hours (Kauko and Tammisto, 1974), 6–24 hours (Morselli, 1975), 6–18 hours (Morselli, Gerna, De Maio, Zanda, Viani and Garattini, 1975) and 5–35 hours (Cotter, Eadie, Hooper, Lander, Smith and Tyrer, 1977). Gerardin, Abadie, Campestini and Theobald (1976) found that the T_{max} increased from a mean of 7·9 hours to a mean of 12·5 hours as carbamazepine dose increased from 100 mg to 600 mg in the same subjects. When the drug is given in solution the faster absorption may cause T_{max} to shorten (Fig. 7.2; Cotter, Smith, Hooper, Tyrer and Eadie, 1975).

Morselli (1975) stated that carbamazepine had a 58 to 85 per cent bioavailability. Morselli, Monaco, Gerna, Recchia and Riccio (1975) found no significant differences between steady state plasma carbamazepine levels produced by the drug in

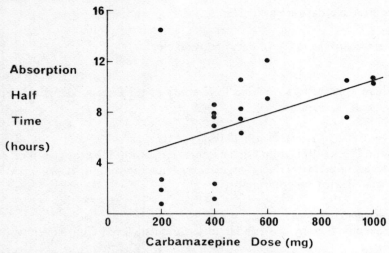

Fig. 7.1 Relation between carbamazepine absorption half-time and carbamazepine dose in 6 healthy volunteers. Carbamazepine absorption half-time showed a tendency to increase when the drug was given in increasing dosage (Cotter, Smith, Hooper, Tyrer and Eadie, 1975).

tablet and syrup form. Kauko and Tammisto (1974) found only slight differences when steady state plasma levels produced by two different brands of car-bamazepine tablets were compared. Cotter, Eadie, Hooper, Lander, Smith and Tyrer (1977) found no statistically significant differences when comparing areas under the curves for plasma carbamazepine levels in five subjects given single 400 mg doses of the drug as tablets and as a solution on different occasions. However, some of their data led them to suspect that they had studied a dose at

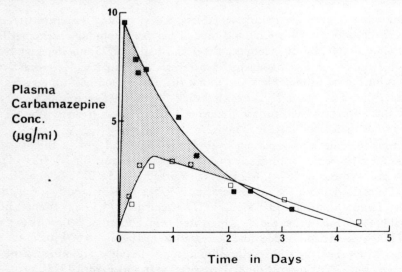

Fig. 7.2 Comparison of areas under the plasma level curves when 400 mg carbamazepine was given orally to the one subject at different times, firstly as tablets (open squares) and secondly as a specially prepared solution (solid squares). The shaded area represents a measure of increased bioavailability when the drug was given in solution (Cotter, Smith, Hooper, Tyrer and Eadie, 1975).

which plasma level-time curves had behaved in an unusual fashion as compared with plasma level-time curves at other doses. When the products of areas under the curves and k for all their data were plotted against dose, the origin did not fall within the 95 per cent confidence limits of the regression line (Fig. 7.3). This suggested that the drug in the preparation studied might be incompletely bioavailable. However, Gerardin, Abadie, Campestrini and Theobald (1976) had

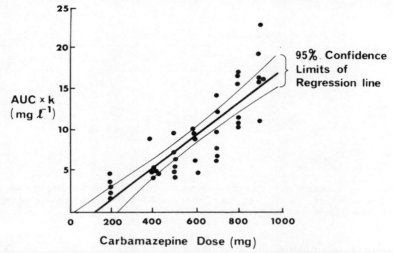

Fig. 7.3 Plot of the product of area under the plasma level curve (AUC) and elimination rate constant (k) against drug dose in 6 subjects who took single carbamazepine doses of different sizes at different times. The 95 per cent confidence limits of the regression line do not include the origin, a result consistent with carbamazepine being incompletely bioavailable (Cotter, Eadie, Hooper, Lander, Smith and Tyrer, 1977).

found that a similar plot of their data yielded a regression that did go through the origin. This discrepancy between the findings of two groups of workers may mean that they had studied carbamazepine preparations with different bioavailabilities.

The low water solubility of carbamazepine and the indications of its slow absorption in man, when given in tablet form, raise suspicion that the drug may at times be incompletely bioavailable. The studies mentioned above have not completely settled this matter. However, the drug's elimination rate constant is dose dependent and the relation between steady-state plasma levels of the drug and dosage in the individual is not linear (see pp. 141 and 150). These facts suggest that comparisons of steady-state plasma levels produced by different carbamazepine preparations may be a very insensitive way to assess the bioavailability of the drug. The observations of Faigle and Feldmann (1975) that 10–15 per cent of a carbamazepine dose is excreted unchanged in faeces also suggests that the drug may be incompletely bioavailable.

DISTRIBUTION

V_d

A number of values are available in the literature for the apparent volume of distribution of carbamazepine. No intravenous preparation of the drug has been readily available, and V_d values have been determined after oral administration of carbamazepine, with 100 per cent bioavailability being assumed. Therefore available values (Table 7.1) of V_d for carbamazepine may be overestimates of the parameter.

From the values of V_d one might anticipate that the drug is distributed throughout body water, and that it may also undergo a degree of binding to some tissue components.

Table 7.1 Values for the V_d of carbamazepine

Author	V_d(litres kg^{-1})
Cotter *et al.* (1977)	1·127 ± 0·274
	(0·825 ± 0·104)*
Eichelbaum *et al.* (1975)	1·20 ± 0·45
Morselli (1975)	0·82 – 1·30
Morselli *et al.* (1975)	0·82 – 1·04
Palmer *et al.* (1973)	1·30
Rawlins *et al.* (1975)	1·07 ± 0·22
Westenberg *et al.* (1978)	1·43 ± 0·37

*This value was determined when the drug was given in solution and may therefore represent a closer approximation to the true value of V_d than the other values shown. (Drugs in solution tend to be more bioavailable than drugs in solid dosage forms).

Plasma protein binding

Figures for the plasma protein binding of carbamazepine are 76 per cent (Di Salle, Pacifici and Morselli, 1974; Morselli, 1975), 74·2–77·5 per cent (Morselli, Gerna, De Maio, Zanda, Viani and Garrattini, 1975), 72·1 ± 1·2 per cent (Rawlins, Collste, Bertilsson and Palmer, 1975) and 73·1 ± 9·4 per cent (Hooper, DuBetz, Bochner, Cotter, Smith, Eadie and Tyrer, 1975). The percentage of carbamazepine unbound in plasma is virtually constant at drug concentrations up to 50 μg/ml (Hooper, DuBetz, Bochner, Cotter, Smith, Eadie and Tyrer, 1975—Fig. 7.4). The percentage unbound increases with temperature up to 37°C (Di Salle, Pacifici and Morselli, 1974; Hooper, DuBetz, Bochner, Cotter, Smith, Eadie and Tyrer, 1975). The main metabolite of carbamazepine so far studied, the 10,11-epoxide, is 48–53 per cent bound to plasma protein (Morselli, 1975).

The effects of other drugs, and of disease, on the plasma protein binding of carbamazepine are discussed on pages 153 and 151, respectively.

Concentrations in various body fluids

Carbamazepine is virtually non-ionized at the pH values encountered in the body. Concentrations of the drug in various body fluids, relative to stimultaneous plasma drug concentrations are likely to reflect differences in the protein contents of the respective fluids.

Blood

Hooper, DuBetz, Bochner, Cotter, Smith, Eadie and Tyrer (1975) showed that red blood cell carbamazepine concentration was 38·3 ± 17·9 per cent of the simultaneous plasma concentration of the drug. One might therefore expect that whole blood

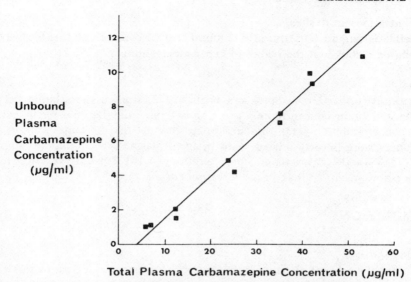

Fig. 7.4 The linear relation between unbound and total plasma carbamazepine concentrations (Hooper, Dubetz, Bochner, Cotter, Smith, Eadie and Tyrer, 1975).

carbamazepine concentrations would be about 75 per cent of plasma concentration. Carbamazepine-epoxide is said not to enter red cells (Pynnonen and Yrjana, 1977).

Cerebrospinal fluid

CSF carbamazepine concentrations average 20 per cent of plasma drug concentrations (Eichelbaum, Bertilsson, Lund, Palmer and Sjoqvist, 1976), 21 per cent (Johannessen and Strandjord, 1972), 22 per cent (Johannessen and Strandjord, 1973), 19–25 per cent (Morselli, 1975), 19–30 per cent (Johannessen, Gerna, Bakke, Strandjord and Morselli, 1976) or 33 per cent (Pynnonen, Silaanpaa, Frey and Iisalo, 1977). Thus for practical purposes the CSF carbamazepine concentration is similar to the drug concentration simultaneously present in plasma water.

CSF carbamazepine-epoxide levels are 34–71 per cent of the plasma levels of this metabolite (Johannessen, Gerna, Bakke, Strandjord and Morselli, 1976) or 41 per cent (Pynnonen, Silaanpaa, Frey and Iisalo, 1977).

Saliva

Salivary carbamazepine concentrations average $26 \pm 2 \cdot 4$ per cent of simultaneous whole plasma levels of the drug (McAuliffe, Sherwin, Leppik, Fayle and Pippenger, 1977) or 26 ± 1 per cent (Westenberg, van der Kleijn, Oei and de Zeeuw, 1978). Troupin and Friel (1975) and Rylance, Butcher and Moreland (1977) also showed that salivary and plasma water carbamazepine levels were similar.

Milk

Carbamazepine levels in human milk are 60 per cent and carbamazepine-epoxide 93 per cent of those in maternal plasma (Pynnonen and Silaanpaa, 1975).

Concentrations in tissues

Morselli, Gerna and Garattini (1971) found that carbamazepine was fairly evenly distributed throughout the bodies of experimental animals.

Brain

Morselli, Baruzzi, Gerna, Bossi and Porta (1977) studied the relation between plasma and brain concentrations of carbamazepine and its epoxide in patients undergoing craniotomy for tumour. Brain and plasma concentrations of both substances were linearly related, with brain to plasma carbamazepine rations of $1 \cdot 1 \pm 0 \cdot 1 : 1 \cdot 0$ and carbamazepine-epoxide ratios of $1 \cdot 1 – 1 \cdot 2 : 1 \cdot 0$. Levels were higher in the parieto-occipital than in the temporal cortex.

ELIMINATION

Elimination rate

A number of workers have studied the kinetics of carbamazepine after a single dose of the drug was given. In these circumstances the elimination in man appears to be monoexponential. Values for the half-life were $35 \cdot 6 \pm 15 \cdot 3$ hours (Eichelbaum, Ekbom, Bertilsson, Ringberger and Rane, 1975), $37 \cdot 7 \pm 5 \cdot 7$ hours (Gerardin, Abadie, Campestrini and Theobald, 1976), 31–35 hours (Levy, Pitlick, Troupin, Green and Neal, 1975), 25–65 hours (Morselli, 1975), 31–55 hours (Morselli, Gerna, De Maio, Zanda and Garattini, 1975), $35 \cdot 9 \pm 8 \cdot 3$ hours (Rawlins, Collste, Bertilsson and Palmer, 1975) and $37 \cdot 5 \pm 13 \cdot 1$ hours (Cotter, Eadie, Hooper, Lander, Smith and Tyrer, 1977). Levy, Pitlick, Troupin, Green and Neal (1975) studied the kinetics of the drug after doses of 3, 6 and 9 mg per kg and found no evidence of dose-dependent elimination. However, Gerardin, Abadie, Campestrini and Theobald (1976) and Cotter, Eadie, Hooper, Lander, Smith and Tyrer (1977) found that the elimination rate constant of the drug increased with increasing drug dose (Fig. 7.5). It would also appear that the drug induces its own biotransformation. Eichelbaum, Ekbom, Bertilsson, Ringeberger and Rane (1975) found that the half-life shortened from a mean of $35 \cdot 6 \pm 15 \cdot 3$ hours after the first dose to a mean of $20 \cdot 9 \pm 5 \cdot 0$ hours after the drug had been given repeatedly. Pitlick, Levy, Troupin and Green (1976) found that the half-life decreased from $33 \cdot 9 \pm 3 \cdot 5$ hours to $19 \cdot 9 \pm 4 \cdot 0$ hours after 3 weeks of regular carbamazapine intake, while Westenberg, van der Kleijn, Oei and de Zeeuw (1978) found that the half-life was $14 \cdot 5 \pm 5 \cdot 3$ hours in 10 subjects who had been taking the drug regularly. Rane, Bertilsson and Palmer (1975) showed that the elimination rate of carbamazepine was similar in mothers and their newborn children. Continued exposure to the drug prior to the measurements had probably induced the carbamazepine biotransformation pathway in mothers and infants.

Reliable data for the elimination rate of carbamazepine-10,11-epoxide are not available.

Clearance

Values for the clearance of carbamazepine may well be overestimates, since they depend on V_d, and values for this parameter in turn have been based on the

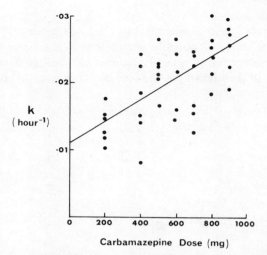

Fig. 7.5 Plot of elimination rate constant (k) against carbamazepine dose in 6 subjects who took different carbamazepine doses at different times. The rate constant tended to increase as dose was increased (Cotter, Eadie, Hooper, Lander, Smith and Tyrer, 1977).

assumption that the drug is completely bioavailable when given by mouth. As indicated above, this may not necessarily be the case. Published clearance values include the following:

1.824 ± 0.588 litres hour^{-1} (Eichelbaum, Ekbom, Bertilsson, Ringberger and Rane, 1975)

0.011–0.260 litres kg^{-1} hour^{-1} (Morselli, 1975)

1.524 ± 0.210 litres hour^{-1} (Rawlins, Collste, Bertilsson and Palmer, 1975)

0.132 ± 0.068 litres kg^{-1} hour^{-1} (Guelen, van der Kleijn and Woudstra, 1975)

0.016 ± 0.006 litres kg^{-1} hour^{-1} (Cotter, Eadie, Hooper, Lander, Smith and Tyrer, 1977)

0.076 ± 0.032 litres kg^{-1} hour^{-1} in chronically treated patients (Westenberg, van der Kleijn, Oei and de Zeeuw, 1978)

It is noticeable that the clearance values given by Guelen, van der Kleijn and Woudstra (1975) and by Westenberg, van der Kleijn, Oei and de Zeeuw (1978) are substantially higher than the values for this parameter given by other workers. However, Guelen, van der Kleijn and Woudstra (1975) and Westenberg, van der Kleijn, Oei and de Zeeuw (1978) calculated clearances when autoinduction had sufficient time to occur. All the other above mentioned authors calculated clearances after the initial dose of the drug.

Per cent excreted unchanged

Only 2 per cent of a carbamazepine dose is excreted unchanged in urine, though 28 per cent of the dose is lost in faeces, 10–15 per cent being in the form of intact carbamazepine (Faigle and Feldmann, 1975). Frigerio and Morselli (1975) also quoted the percentage excreted unchanged in urine as 2 per cent, while Morselli (1975) cited values of 0.65–1.12 per cent. It would therefore appear that most of a carbamazepine dose is eliminated by biotransformation.

Biotransformation pattern

Weist and Zicha (1967) and Goenechea and Hecke-Seibicke (1972) used thin-layer chromatography to detect 7 possible metabolites in the urine of patients taking carbamazepine. Subsequently several of these metabolites have been identified. Figure 7.6 set out of the known pathways of biotransformation of the drug and the

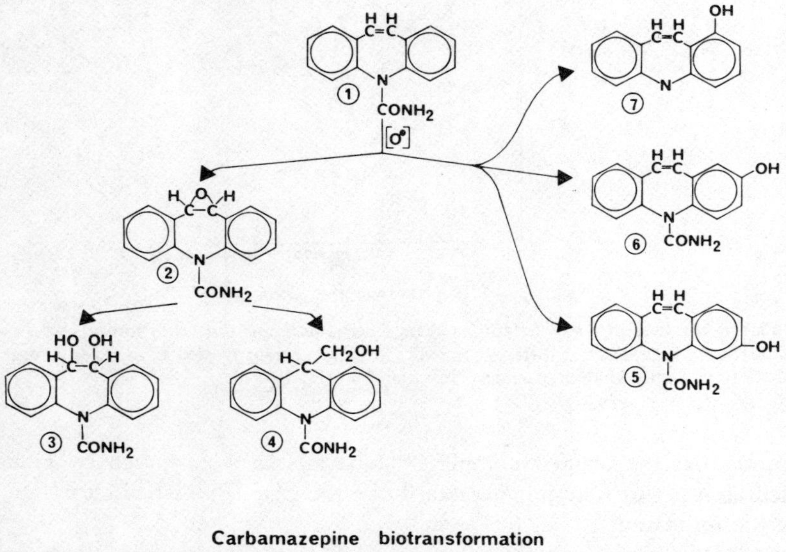

Carbamazepine biotransformation

Fig. 7.6 Biotransformation pathways for carbamazepine (with percentages of a carbamazepine dose excreted in urine as each substance)
1. Carbamazepine (0·1–2·0 per cent)
2. Carbamazepine-10,11-epoxide (0·1–2·0 per cent)
3. 10,11-dihydroxycarbamazepine (10–30 per cent)
4. 9-hydroxymethyl-10-carbamoyl acridan (<0·1 per cent)
5, 6 and 7. 3,2 and 1-hydroxycarbamazepine (each 2–10 per cent)

proportions of the dose excreted as the various metabolites (after Faigle, Brech-buhler, Feldmann and Richter, 1975). Of these metabolites, carbamazepine-10,11-epoxide is known to be an anticonvulsant (Morselli, Bossi and Gerna, 1975). The dihydroxy derivative is said to lack anticonvulsant activity (Frigerio and Morselli, 1975).

Excretion

The quantitative pattern of the renal excretion of carbamazepine and of its biotransformation products is discussed above. Information is lacking as to the renal mechanisms involved in the excretions of these various substances.

CLINICAL PHARMACOKINETICS

Time course of plasma drug levels

Single dose

A typical plot of the time course of plasma carbamazepine levels after a single oral dose of the drug, given in tablet form, is shown in Fig. 7.7. As discussed earlier, peak plasma levels occur a variable time after dosage. The T_{max} is rarely below 5 hours, and may be over 24 hours. The decline in plasma carbamazepine level is monoexponential, with a half-life of about 36 hours, after the first dose of the drug. In view of the data of Eichelbaum, Ekbom, Bertilsson, Ringberger and Rane

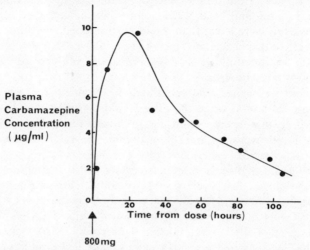

Fig. 7.7 Time course of plasma carbamazepine levels after a single oral 800 mg dose of the drug (Cotter, Eadie, Hooper, Lander, Smith and Tyrer, 1977).

(1975), the levels may decline more rapidly if measured after the drug has been given for several days, the half-life than falling to about 20 hours or less. Carbamazepine-10,11-epoxide appeared in plasma about 3 hours after the initial carbamazepine dose in a few patients studied personally, and thereafter its levels tended to parallel plasma carbamazepine levels (Fig. 7.8).

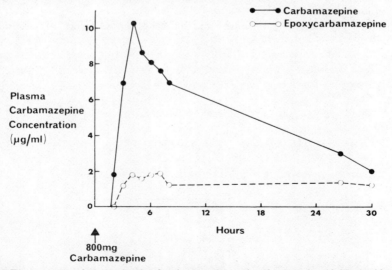

Fig. 7.8 Time courses of plasma levels of carbamazepine and carbamazepine-10,11-epoxide after an 800 mg oral dose of the drug (Eadie and Tyrer, 1977).

Repeated doses

When carbamazepine is taken regularly, one might expect that steady state plasma levels would be achieved in about 7–8 days if the half-life was 36 hours. However, if the half-life shortens with continued intake of the drug the steady state should develop more rapidly. Gerardin, Abadie, Campestrini and Theobald (1976) and Pitlick, Levy, Troupin and Neal (1976) found that the actual steady-state plasma carbamazepine levels were lower than the levels predicted from the pharmacokinetic parameters of the drug calculated after the first dose of the drug. This finding is consistent with the possibility that the elimination rate constant increases with continued exposure to the drug.

Carbamazepine is absorbed relatively slowly from tablets, and has an elimination half-life of about 24 hours, when the drug is taken in regular dosages. Therefore one might expect that there would be relatively little fluctuation in plasma carbamazepine levels over an 8 or 12 hour dosage interval, once a steady state was achieved. In the writers' experience this has been so (Figs. 7.9 and 12.3). Carbamazepine-epoxide plasma levels also show little fluctuation in the steady state. Plasma carbamazepine levels would probably fluctuate relatively little even over a 24 dosage interval. However, certain authors have stated that plasma carbamazepine levels fluctuate considerably during the day (Schneider, 1975-a; Johannessen, Gerna, Bakke, Strandjord and Morselli, 1976). Schneider (1975-a) though that the fluctuations were sufficient to make it desirable to give the drug four or five times daily. As indicated above, the present authors have not encountered such fluctuations in steady state plasma carbamazepine levels. Both on pharmacokinetic grounds and on the basis of clinical experience they consider that twice daily carbamazepine administration would keep steady-state plasma levels of the drug within acceptable limits.

Relation of plasma drug concentration and clinical effect

Anticonvulsant effects

Most authors in recent years have set the therapeutic range of plasma car-

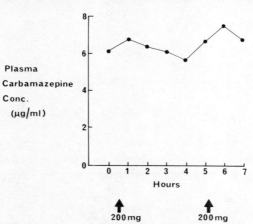

Fig. 7.9 Relative constancy of steady-state plasma carbamazepine levels over a dosage interval (Hooper, Dubetz, Eadie and Tyrer, 1974).

bamazepine levels in epilepsy at about 6 to 12 μg/ml. Thus Moller (1971) considered that plasma levels above 6 μg/ml were necessary to control epilepsy. Monaco, Riccio, Benna, Covacich, Durelli, Fantini, Furlan, Gilli, Mutani, Troni, Gerna and Morselli (1976) found that plasma carbamazepine levels of 4–10 μg/ml usually controlled epilepsy in their patients. They proposed a therapeutic range for the drug of 4–12 μg/ml. Simonsen, Olsen, Kuhl, Lund and Wendelboe (1975) set the range at 6–10 μg/ml, and Larsen, Naestoft and Hvidberg (1972) at 5–11 μg/ml, while Perchalski and Wilder (1974) stated that carbamazepine levels up to 10 μg/ml usually sufficed to control epilepsy. Schneider (1975-b) found that plasma carbamazepine levels of $4\cdot6 \pm 2\cdot2$ μg/ml were associated with 50 to 99 per cent control of complex partial seizures and levels of $5\cdot9 \pm 2\cdot7\mu$g/ml with full control. On this basis he proposed a therapeutic range of plasma levels for the drug of $6\cdot5 \pm 3\cdot0$ μg/ml.

The above correlations between plasma carbamazepine concentrations and therapeutic effect may have sometimes been established in patients who were also taking phenytoin and other anticonvulsants. As will be discussed later, Dam, Jensen and Christiansen (1975) found that concurrent phenytoin intake increased the concentration of carbamazepine-10,11-epoxide in plasma relative to the concentration of carbamazepine. If this finding is correct (the present authors' unpublished data tend to agree with it), the therapeutic range of plasma carbamazepine level may be lower in the presence of phenytoin than in its absence, since carbamazepine-epoxide is itself an anticonvulsant. A therapeutic range of plasma carbamazepine-epoxide concentrations has not yet been established.

Epilepsy may worsen when plasma carbamazepine levels exceed 20 μg/ml (Troupin and Ojemann, 1976).

Other therapeutic effects
The present authors have not seen tic douloureux controlled by plasma carbamazepine levels below 5 μg/ml. At times levels as high as 18 μg/ml have been needed to provide relief. Such levels have been tolerated without undue side-effects.

Unwanted effects
Meinardi (1972) found that nystagmus occurred in some patients taking carbamazepine once plasma levels of the drug exceeded $1\cdot5$ μg/ml. He found that, with levels in the range $8\cdot5$–$10\cdot0$ μg/ml, about 50 per cent of patients had unwanted effects such as headache, dysequilibrium and disturbed vision. Schneider (1975-b) regarded 8–9 μg/ml as the threshold for the appearance of toxic effects of the drug. He found unwanted effects in a patient with a plasma carbamazepine level as low as $5\cdot9$ μg/ml, but also found patients with levels up to $16\cdot9$ μg/ml who experienced no adverse effects. Winek (1976) considered that plasma carbamazepine levels of 8–10 μg/ml were toxic. After a single dose of carbamazepine, Levy, Pitlick, Troupin, Green and Neal (1975) could not correlate plasma drug levels with the time course of unwanted effects. However in such a study it is possible that there may not have been time for definitive steady-state equilibria to apply.

The present authors have noted that a degree of tolerance to the sedative effects of carbamazepine develops as time passes. This phenomenon may explain some of the variation in figures for the threshold values of plasma carbamazepine levels at which toxicity appears.

Plasma level—dose correlations in treated populations

A number of authors have commented on the lack of correlation between steady-state plasma carbamazepine levels and drug dose (Reynolds, 1973; Rane, Hojer and Wilson, 1976; Eichelbaum, Bertilsson, Lund, Palmer and Sjoqvist, 1976; Johannessen, Gerna, Bakke, Strandjord and Morselli, 1976; Miura, Minagawa, Yagi *et al.*, 1976; Monaco, Riccio, Benna, Covacich, Durelli, Fantini, Furlan, Gilli, Mutani, Troni, Gerna and Morselli, 1976). Hooper, DuBetz, Eadie and Tyrer (1974) studied this matter in a series of 93 patients. Although there was a wide scatter of data points about the regression line there was a statistically significant relation between plasma drug level and dose. The correlation between the two was somewhat improved by expressing dose on a body weight basis.

When the effect of concurrent phenytoin therapy in reducing plasma carbamazepine levels became known (page 153), a study of the relation between plasma carbamazepine concentration and drug dose, in patients taking carbamazepine alone, appeared desirable. It seemed possible that the poor or absent correlation between plasma carbamazepine level and drug dose referred to above might have been due to many patients being studied who were also taking phenytoin. Lander, Eadie and Tyrer (1977) therefore reinvestigated this question in a series of 217 patients, 54 of whom were taking carbamazepine alone. Again, statistically significant regressions could be fitted to the data for the whole 217 subjects, though there was a wide scatter of data points (Fig. 7.10). When the 54

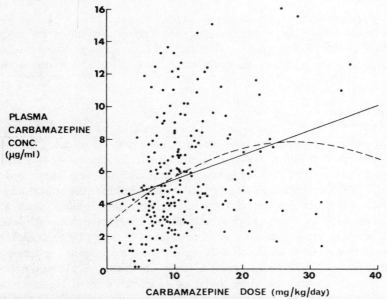

Fig. 7.10 Correlation between steady-state plasma carbamazepine concentration and drug dose in 217 subjects. The parabolic regression fits the data slightly better than the linear regression (Lander, Eadie and Tyrer, 1977).

subjects taking carbamazepine alone were considered, there was a statistically significant linear relation between plasma level and total daily dose of carbamazepine. Curiously, if the drug dose was expressed on a body weight basis, the deviations from regression increased so that it was no longer possible to fit a statistically significant linear regression to the data (Fig. 7.11).

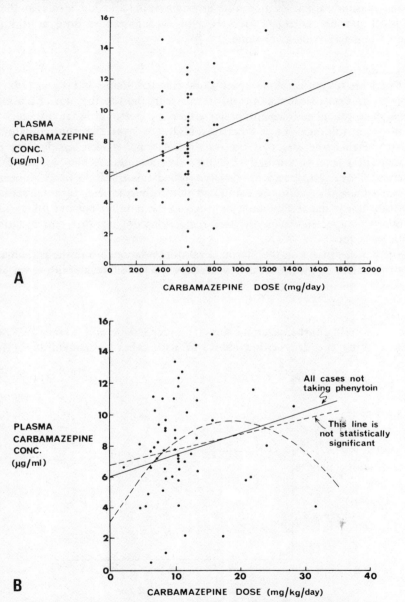

Fig. 7.11 Steady-state plasma carbamazepine concentrations plotted against drug dose in mg/day (upper half), and against drug dose per unit body weight, i.e. mg/kg/day (lower half) for 54 patients taking no other drugs. It was impossible to fit a statistically significant linear regression to the data when doses were expressed on a body weight basis (Lander, Eadie and Tyrer, 1977).

In as yet unpublished studies on 46 patients, McKauge, Eadie and Tyrer have shown that steady-state plasma carbamazepine -10,11-expoxide levels correlated better with carbamazepine dose than did plasma levels of carbamazepine itself. Plasma carbamazepine-epoxide levels showed a correlation with plasma carbamazepine levels that barely reached statistical significance. The sum of simultaneous plasma carbamazepine and carbamazepine-epoxide levels in the same individual did not correlate as well with carbamazepine dose as did plasma carbamazepine-epoxide level alone.

Effect of age
In 54 patients taking carbamazepine alone Lander, Eadie and Tyrer (1977) were unable to fit a statistically significant linear regression to the plot of plasma level against dose (on a bodyweight basis) either for persons under 14 years or for persons over this age (i.e. in persons under or over the approximate age of puberty). Hence the effect of age on the relation between steady-state plasma carbamazepine level and drug dose could not be assessed. When Hooper, DuBetz, Eadie and Tyrer (1974) had previously studied this question in 93 subjects who took carbamazepine alone, or combined with other anticonvulsants, statistically significant linear regression could be fitted to the data for persons under 13 years and over this age. However, the two regressions did not differ to a statistically significant extent (Fig. 7.12).

If age has any effect on the plasma level-dose relationship in the carbamazepine treated population, this effect is obscured by the wide interindividual variation in the data.

Effect of sex
In patients taking carbamazepine alone (Lander, Eadie and Tyrer, 1977) and in patients taking the drug either alone, or with other anticonvulsants (Hooper,

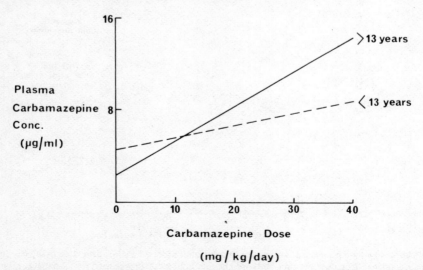

Fig. 7.12 Regressions for steady-state plasma carbamazepine levels on drug dose in persons under and over the age of 13 years (Hooper, Dubetz, Eadie and Tyrer, 1974).

Dubetz, Eadie and Tyrer, 1974), sex had no statistically significant effect on the relationship between steady-state plasma carbamazepine level and drug dose (Fig. 7.13). Frey (1971) had also noted that sex did not influence this relationship.

Effect of pregnancy
Eadie, Lander and Tyrer (1977) described a patient (Fig. 7.14) who took a constant phenytoin dose throughout pregnancy. She showed a fall in plasma carbamazepine level at the end of the second trimester despite taking a constant carbamazepine

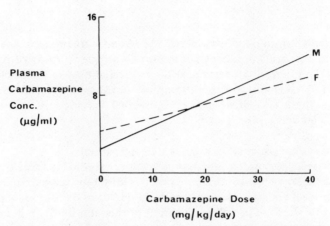

Fig. 7.13 Regressions for steady-state plasma carbamazepine levels on drug dose in males and females (Hooper, Dubetz, Eadie and Tyrer, 1974).

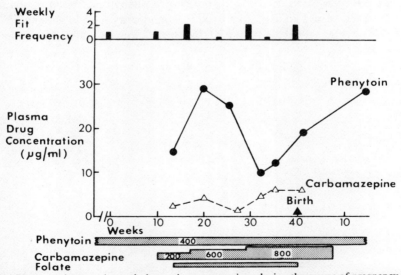

Fig. 7.14 Plasma carbamazepine and phenytoin concentrations during the course of pregnancy in one patient. Phenytoin and folate dosage were kept constant. It was necessary to increase carbamazepine dosage at the end of the second trimester in order to correct a fall in plasma carbamazepine levels (Eadie, Lander and Tyrer, 1977).

dose for approximately 3 months. In this patient there was a concurrent fall in plasma phenytoin level, and nearly always (in non-pregnant subjects) when plasma phenytoin levels fall plasma carbamazepine levels rise (page 153). Thus in this one patient pregnancy may have altered the relationship between plasma carbamazepine level and drug dose.

In other patients studied during pregnancy, carbamazepine was taken with phenytoin, and doses of this were changed. Therefore the interpretation of alterations in plasma carbamazepine levels during the course of pregnancy was uncertain in these patients.

The poor correlation between steady-state plasma carbamazepine level and drug dose in a treated population does not appear to be due to study of populations of mixed ages and sexes. Uncertain drug bioavailability and a dose-dependent elimination rate constant probably contribute to the poor correlation but it seems possible that there is a great deal of individual variation in biotransformation capacity for carbamazepine.

Plasma level—dose correlations in treated individuals

When steady-state plasma carbamazepine levels are studied in individuals given the drug as sole therapy, but in different doses at different times, the rate of rise in plasma drug level (relative to dose) tends to decrease as dose is increased in the individual (Fig. 7.15). The full explanation of this non-linearity is uncertain, but the increase in the elimination rate constant of carbamazepine with increasing dose (page 140) is likely to contribute. Incomplete and possible variable bioavailability of the drug may also play a part.

Carbamazepine is often used concurrently with phenytoin. When this is so the relation between steady-state plasma drug level and drug dose in the individual is different from that described above. In these circumstances, at lower car-

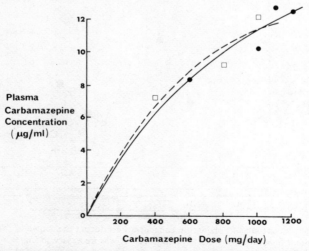

Fig. 7.15 The non-rectilinear relation between steady-state plasma carbamazepine level and drug dose in two patients (Cotter, Eadie, Hooper, Lander, Smith and Tyrer, 1977).

bamazepine doses, plasma levels usually rise less relative to dose than when the drug is used alone. However, as dose is increased further, the rate of rise in plasma drug levels increases, relative to the dose increment (Fig. 7.16). This finding may in some way depend on the phenytoin–carbamazepine interaction discussed on page 153, but the full explanation is not yet clear.

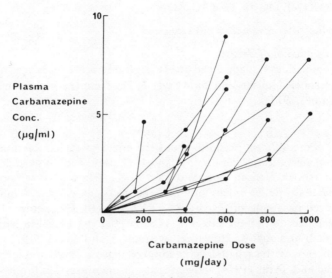

Fig. 7.16 Relation between steady-state plasma carbamazepine concentrations and drug dose in 10 patients taking carbamazepine in different doses at different times, but also taking phenytoin (Hooper, Dubetz, Eadie and Tyrer, 1974).

Effects of disease

Hooper, Dubetz, Bochner, Cotter, Smith, Eadie and Tyrer (1975) found that the plasma protein binding of carbamazepine was not altered in patients with renal disease. Binding capacity was slightly reduced in patients with hepatic disease (percentage unbound $20·5 \pm 6·0$, as compared with $18·2 \pm 5·0$ in controls). This alteration in binding capacity was not related to serum albumin or bilirubin concentrations, nor to a number of other biochemical indices of hepatic function.

We have not noticed any other descriptions of the effects of disease on the pharmacokinetics of carbamazepine.

INTERACTIONS

PHARMACODNYAMIC INTERACTIONS

As is the case for other anti-epileptic drugs, carbamazepine is sometimes given combined with a second or even a third anticonvulsant in the hope of achieving an additive or even synergistic effect against epilepsy. Thus Cereghino, Brock, van Meter, Penry, Smith and White (1975) demonstrated that the combination of carbamazepine, phenytoin and phenobarbitone was more effective than any of these drugs given singly, or in pairs. However, such a finding should not be taken as evidence of a pharmacodynamic interaction, when plasma water levels of the various drugs have not been measured to exclude the possibility of a beneficial pharmacokinetic interaction.

PHARMACOKINETIC INTERACTIONS

Carbamazepine affecting other substances

Plasma protein binding of drugs

Carbamazepine does not appear to alter the plasma protein binding of phenytoin (Hansen, Siersboek-Neilsen and Skovsted, 1971; Hooper, Sutherland, Bochner, Tyrer and Eadie, 1973).

Phenytoin

There have been conflicting reports about the effect of carbamazepine on plasma phenytoin concentration. Hansen, Siersboek-Neilsen and Skovsted (1971) and Molholm, Siersboek-Neilsen and Skovsted (1971) showed that carbamazepine decreased the half-life of phenytoin in 5 subjects. It caused a fall in plasma phenytoin level in 3 out of 7 patients. Richens and Houghton (1975) found carbamazepine had no definite effect on plasma phenytoin level in patients taking 300 mg of phenytoin daily. However, Windorfer and Sauer (1977) found that concurrent therapy with carbamazepine lowered plasma phenytoin levels. Hooper, Dubetz, Eadie and Tyrer (1974) showed that plasma phenytoin levels fell in 7 of 8 subjects taking a constant daily phenytoin dose when carbamazepine was added to therapy or when its dose was increased (Fig. 6.24). Their linear regression analysis on data from treated patients showed that steady-state plasma phenytoin levels exhibited a statistically significantly greater rate of rise, relative to phenytoin dose, when patients were taking phenytoin alone, as compared with patients who were taking the drug with carbamazepine (Fig. 6.25). However, as time has passed the present authors have encountered more instances in which an increase in carbamazepine dose has failed to cause a fall in plasma phenytoin level. They would now accept that the effect of carbamazepine on plasma phenytoin levels is inconsistent. A multiple variable linear regression analysis of plasma anticonvulsant level data was carried out in the hope of tracing interactions in a series of 400 patients (Lander, Eadie and Tyrer, 1975). It was found that carbamazepine dosage had a slight (quantitatively insignificant though nearly statistically significant) tendency to raise plasma phenytoin levels, rather than to lower them.

Primidone

Windorfer and Sauer (1977) found that carbamazepine therapy caused a fall in plasma primidone levels. Cereghino, van Meter, Brock, Penry, Smith and White (1973) noted some tentative evidence that carbamazepine might raise plasma primidone levels.

Warfarin

Hansen, Siersboek-Neilsen and Skovsted (1971) reported that carbamazepine therapy increased the metabolism of warfarin, thus decreasing its anticoagulant effect.

Tetracyclines
Carbamazepine increased the elimination of doxycycline, but not that of other tetracyclines tested (Neuvonen, Penttila, Lehtovarra and Aho, 1975).

Other substances affecting carbamazepine

Plasma protein binding
Hooper, Dubetz, Bochner, Cotter, Smith, Eadie and Tyrer (1975) were unable to demonstrate that phenytoin, phenobarbitone, ethosuximide, sulthiame, diazepam, clonazepam and aspirin altered the plasma protein binding of carbamazepine *in vitro*.

Phenytoin
With the exception of Monaco, Riccio, Benna, Covacich, Durelli, Fantini, Furlan, Gilli, Mutani, Troni, Gerna and Morselli (1976), it has been repeatedly observed that concurrent phenytoin therapy reduced plasma carbamazepine levels relative to drug dose (Christiansen and Dam, 1973; Dam and Christiansen, 1973; Hooper, Dubetz, Eadie and Tyrer, 1974; Cereghino, Brock, van Meter, Penry, Smith and White, 1975; Dam, Jensen and Christiansen, 1975; Johannessen and Strandjord, 1975; Schneider, 1975-c). The effect can be detected in treated population (Fig. 7.17) and in treated individuals (Figs. 7.18 and 6.26). Multiple linear regression analysis (Lander, Eadie and Tyrer, 1975) detected the interaction easily and indicated that, on the average, plasma carbamazepine levels fell by nearly $0.5\ \mu g/ml$ for each 1 mg/kg/day of phenytoin taken. Westenberg, van der Kleijn, Oei and de Zeeuw (1978) found a shorter carbamazepine half-life (10.6 ± 0.7 hours)

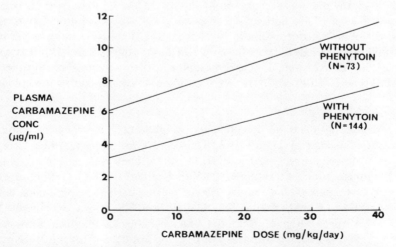

Fig. 7.17 Regressions for steady-state plasma carbamazepine level on drug dose in 144 patients taking carbamazepine with phenytoin and in 73 patients taking carbamazepine without phenytoin. For the same carbamazepine dose, plasma carbamazepine levels tend to be $2.5\ \mu g/ml$ lower when phenytoin is taken concurrently (Lander, Eadie and Tyrer, 1977).

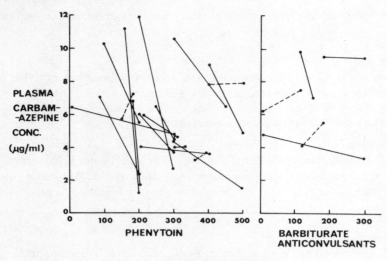

Fig. 7.18 This shows the tendency of steady-state plasma carbamazepine levels to fall in individual patients when phenytoin dose was increased, carbamazepine dose being unaltered. However, increase in the dose of various barbiturate anticonvulsants had no consistent effects on plasma carbamazepine levels (Lander, Eadie and Tyrer, 1977).

in 5 subjects taking the drug with phenytoin and/or phenobarbitone, than in 5 subjects taking carbamazepine alone (half-life $18 \cdot 3 \pm 5 \cdot 2$ hours).

This interaction between phenytoin and carbamazepine appears to be consistent, and its effects are of considerable magnitude. The mechanism is not fully worked out. Dam, Jensen and Christiansen (1975), Schneider (1975-c) and Westenberg, van der Kleijn, Oei and de Zeeuw (1978) found that the interaction was associated with a rise in plasma carbamazepine-epoxide level relative to plasma carbamazepine level. This finding is consistent with the possibility that phenytoin enhanced the biotransformation of carbamazepine. However, in an as yet unpublished study the present authors have obtained data suggesting that phenytoin may increase the conversion of carbamazepine to some metabolite other than carbamazepine-10,11-epoxide, rather than increase conversion to the epoxide.

Phenobarbitone
Phenobarbitone also has been reported to cause a fall in plasma carbamazepine levels (Christiansen and Dam, 1973; Dam and Christiansen, 1973; Cereghino, Brock, van Meter, Penry, Smith and White, 1975; Dam, Jensen and Christiansen, 1975; Johannessen and Strandjord, 1975; Schneider, 1975-c). The interaction is said to be associated with a relative rise in plasma carbamazepine-epoxide levels (Dam, Jensen and Christiansen, 1975; Schneider, 1975; Miura, Minagawa, Yagi *et al.*, 1976). Monaco, Riccio, Benna, Covacich, Durelli, Fantini, Furlan, Gilli, Murtani, Troni, Gerna and Morselli (1976) could not detect this interaction. Using multiple linear regression techniques on population data Lander, Eadie and Tyrer (1977) showed a tendency for phenobarbitone dosage to be associated with reduction in plasma carbamazepine levels. However, the effect was not statistically

significant. In individual patients, altering phenobarbitone dose had no consistent effect on plasma carbamazepine levels (Fig. 7.18). It seems possible that the interaction between phenobarbitone and carbamazepine is inconsistent, though it may be quantitatively significant in certain individuals.

Primidone

There have been reports that primidone therapy reduced plasma carbamazepine levels (Schneider, 1975; Miura, Minagawa, Yagi *et al.*, 1976). Possibly this is due to an effect of phenobarbitone produced from primidone biotransformation.

Clonazepam

Johanessen, Strandjord and Munthe-Kaas (1977) showed that clonazepam had very little effect on plasma carbamazepine levels. However, Lander, Eadie and Tyrer (1975) illustrated plasma level data from a single patient in whom stepwise withdrawal of clonazepam was associated with a decline in plasma carbamazepine levels, without any change being made in the dosage of any concurrent therapy (Fig. 7.19).

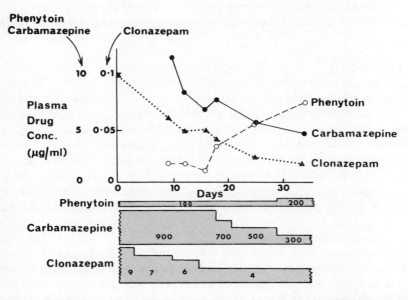

Fig. 7.19 Time courses of plasma carbamazepine, phenytoin and clonazepam levels in one patient. In the left-hand half of the Fig., phenytoin and carbamazepine doses have been kept constant. Despite this, plasma carbamazepine levels fell as clonazepam dose was reduced (Lander, Eadie and Tyrer, 1975).

Propoxyphene

Dam, Kristensen, Hansen and Christiansen (1977) found that propoxyphene caused raised plasma carbamazepine levels in 5 patients, without alteration in carbamazepine-epoxide levels.

TOXICITY

Specific aspects of carbamazepine toxicity were discussed at length by Pisciotta (1975) and Reynolds (1975).

LOCAL EFFECTS AT ADMINISTRATION SITE

In occasional patients therapeutic doses of carbamazepine may cause alimentary upset, with anorexia, nausea and vomiting.

DOSE-DETERMINED SYSTEMIC EFFECTS

Neurological

The dose-related unwanted neurological effects of carbamazepine include diplopia, nystagmus, drowsiness and fatigue, ataxia and feelings of dysequilibrium (Livingstone, Villamater, Sakata and Pauli, 1967). More recently Chadwick, Reynolds and Marsden (1976) noted that the drug could cause asterixis. Carbamazepine overdosage may make epilepsy worse (Troupin and Ojemann, 1976). Chakrabarti and Samantaray (1976) found that carbamazepine did not alter nerve conduction in cases of diabetic peripheral neuropathy, despite relieving sensory symptoms. The plasma level correlations of these effects, where known, are given on pages 144 and 145.

Non-neurological

The question of anticonvulsant-induced osteomalacia and folate deficiency were discussed in relation to phenytoin (pages 101–103). Unfortunately many authors have not distinguished the effects of the different drugs in producing these disorders when patients were taking multiple anticonvulsants. While carbamazepine intake has been associated with anticonvulsant osteomalacia one cannot be certain that other concurrently taken anticonvulsants were not responsible for the disorder. However, Reizenstein and Lund (1973) stated that carbamazepine itself could cause folate deficiency. Whether this deficiency may be responsible for symptoms in patients taking carbamazepine alone is uncertain.

Altered water and Na+ balance

Carbamazepine increases plasma antidiuretic activity (Wales, 1975) by altering hypothalamic osmoreceptor function so that there is increased release of arginine-vasopressin (Thomas, Ball, Wales and Lee, 1978). This action may make the drug useful in diabetes insipidus of extra-renal origin. Helin, Nilsson, Bjerre and Vegfors (1977) found no evidence that therapeutic doses of carbamazepine altered serum Na^+ concentration or osmolality in children. However Henry, Lawson, Reavey and Renfrew (1977) found that carbamazepine doses of more than 700 mg per day were associated with reduced serum Na^+ levels in 5 out of 16 randomly chosen patients. In 80 adult epileptics receiving carbamazepine, mean plasma osmolality was lower than in 50 epileptics receiving other anticonvulsants, though mean plasma sodium levels did not differ in the two groups (Perucca, Garratt, Hebdige and Richens, 1978). Rado (1973) reported the occurrence of water intoxication in a patient with psychogenic polydypsia who was given carbamazepine, while Stephens, Espir, Tattersall, Quinn, Gladwell, Galbraith and Reynolds (1977) reported two further instances of water intoxication related to use of the drug.

IDIOSYNCRATIC UNWANTED EFFECTS

A number of apparently idiosyncratic unwanted effects of carbamazepine have been reported. These include jaundice, aplastic anaemia (Donaldson and Graham, 1965; Dyer, Hughes and Jenkins, 1966; Fellows, 1969), purpuric rashes (Harman, 1967), generalized erythema, erythema multiforme exudativum (Stevens-Johnson syndrome), exfoliative dermatitis (Ford and Biedner, 1968) and an instance of a lupus erythematosus-like syndrome (Simpson, 1966). Livingstone, Pauli and Pruce (1978) emphasized the infrequency of serious blood disorders in patients taking carbamazepine.

EFFECTS ON THE FETUS

The role of individual anticonvulsants in relation to human dysmorphogenesis has often not been sharply differentiated. However, Starreveld-Zimmerman, Van der Kolk, Meinardi and Elshove (1973) made a rather curious observation. They found that no congenital malformations occurred in 50 offspring of mothers who took carbamazepine alone, or combined with other anticonvulsants during pregnancy, whereas there were 22 malformations in 247 live births to mothers who had taken anticonvulsants other than carbamazepine. This finding does not appear to have been confirmed by other workers. In the present authors' own experience of managing epilepsy in pregnancy, the most serious instance of dysmorphogenesis (a congenital heart lesion) occurred after maternal intake of phenytoin and carbamazepine.

PREPARATIONS AVAILABLE

Carbamazepine: 100 mg and 200 mg tablets.

REFERENCES

Bertilsson, L. (1978) Clinical pharmacokinetics of carbamazepine. *Clinical Pharmacokinetics,* **3,** 128–143.

Blom, S. (1962) Trigeminal neuralgia: its treatment with a new anticonvulsant drug (G-32883). *Lancet,* i, 839–840.

Blum, J. E., Haefely, W., Jalfre, M., Polc, P. & Schärer, K. (1973) Pharmakologie und Toxicologie des Antiepileptikums Clonazepam. *Arzneim.-Forsch.,* **23,** 377–389.

Cereghino, J. J., Brock, J. T., van Meter, J. C., Penry, J. K., Smith, L. D. & White, B. G. (1975) The efficacy of carbamazepine combinations in epilepsy. *Clin. Pharmacol. Therap.,* **18,** 733–741.

Cereghino, J. J., van Meter, J. C., Brock, J. T., Penry, J. K., Smith, L. D. & White, B. G. (1973) Preliminary observations of serum carbamazepine concentration in epileptic patients. *Neurology* (Minneap.), **23,** 357–366.

Chadwick, D., Reynolds, E. H. & Marsden, C. D. (1976) Anticonvulsant-induced dyskinesias induced by neuroleptics. *J. Neurol. Neurosurg. Psychiat.,* **39,** 140–148.

Chakrabarti, A. K. & Samantaray, S. K. (1976) Diabetic peripheral neuropathy: nerve conduction studies before, during and after carbamazepine therapy. *Aust. N.Z. J. Med.*, **6**, 565–568.

Christiansen, J. & Dam, M. (1973) Influence of phenobarbital and diphenylhydantoin on plasma carbamazepine levels in patients with epilepsy. *Acta Neurol. Scandinav.*, **49**, 543–546.

Consolo, S., Bianchi, S. & Ladinsky, H. (1976) Effect of carbamazepine on cholinergic parameters in rat brain areas. *Neuropharmacology*, **15**, 653–657.

Cotter, L. M., Eadie, M. J., Hooper, W. D., Lander, C. M., Smith, G. A. & Tyrer, J. H. (1977) The pharmacokinetics of carbamazepine. *Europ. J. clin. Pharmacol.*, **12**, 451–456.

Cotter, L. M., Smith, G. A., Hooper, W. D., Tyrer, J. H. & Eadie, M. J. (1975) The bioavailability of carbamazepine. *Proc. Aust. Assoc. Neurol.*, **12**, 123–128.

Dam, M. & Christiansen, J. (1973) Evidence of drug action on serum level of carbamazepine. *Epilepsia* (Amst.), **14**, 105–106.

Dam, M., Jensen, A. & Christiansen, J. (1975) Plasma level and effect of carbamazepine in grand mal and psychomotor epilepsy. *Acta Neurol. Scandinav. Suppl.*, **60**, 33–38.

Dam, M., Kristensen, C. B., Hansen, B. S. & Christiansen, J. (1977) Interaction between carbamazepine and propoxyphene in man. *Acta Neurol. Scandinav.*, **56**, 603–607.

David, J. & Grewal, R. S. (1976) Effect of carbamazepine (Tegretol[R]) on seizure and EEG patterns in monkeys with alumina-induced focal motor and hippocampal foci. *Epilepsia* (Amst.), **17**, 415–422.

Demieville, H. (1975) Effects of carbamazepine (Tegretol) on the monosynaptic reflex and post tetanic potentiation. *Experientia* (Basel), **31**, 727.

DiSalle, E., Pacifici, G. M. & Morselli, P. L. (1974) Studies on plasma protein binding of carbamazepine. *Pharmacol. Res. Commun.*, **6**, 193–202.

Dodrill, C. B. & Troupin, A. S. (1977) Psychotropic effects of carbamazepine in epilepsy: A double-blind comparison with phenytoin. *Neurology* (Minneap.), **27**, 1023–1028.

Donaldson, G. W. K. & Graham, J. G. (1965) Aplastic anaemia following the administration of Tegretol. *Brit. J. Clin. Practice*, **19**, 699–702.

Dyer, N. H., Hughes, D. T. D. & Jenkins, G. C. (1966) Hypoplastic anaemia following treatment with carbamazepine. *Clin. Trials*, **3**, 521–527.

Eichelbaum, M., Bertilsson, L., Lund, L., Palmér, L. & Sjöqvist, F. (1976) Plasma levels of carbamazepine and carbamazepine-10,11-epoxide during carbamazepine therapy in epileptic patients. *Europ. J. Clin. Pharmacol.*, **9**, 417–421.

Eichelbaum, M., Ekbom, K., Bertilsson, L., Ringberger, V. A. & Rane, A. (1975), Plasma kinetics of carbamazepine and its epoxide metabolite in man after single and multiple doses. *Europ. J. Clin. Pharmacol.*, **8**, 337–341.

Ekbom, K. (1972) Carbamazepine in the treatment of tabetic lightning pains. *Arch. Neurol.* (Chic.), **26**, 374–378.

Ekbom, K. A. & Westerberg, C. E. (1966) Carbamazepine in glossopharyngeal neuralgia. *Arch. Neurol.* (Chic.), **14**, 595–596.

Faigle, J. W., Brechbuhler, S., Feldmann, K. F. & Richter, W. J. (1975) The biotransformation of carbamazepine, in *International Symposium on Epileptic Seizures—Behaviour—Pain*, ed. Birkmayer, W., Berne. Huber. 127–140.

Faigle, J. W. & Feldmann, K. F. (1975) Pharmacokinetic data of carbamazepine and its major metabolites in man, in *Clinical pharmacology of antiepileptic drugs*, ed. Schneider, H., Janz, D., Gardner-Thorpe, C., Meinardi, H. and Sherwin, A. L. Berlin, Springer. 159–165.

Fellows, W. R. (1969) A case of aplastic anaemia and pancytopenia with Tegretol therapy. *Headache*, **9**, 92–95.

Ford, G. R. & Biedner, L. (1968) Exfoliative dermatitis due to carbamazepine (Tegretol), *N.Z. med. J.*, **68**, 386–387.

Frey, H. (1971) Serumkoncentrationer av Karbamazepin Los Vuxna, in *Plasmakoncentrationabestaemningar av Antiepileptika: Methodologiska och Kliniska Aspekter*, Lidingö. 68–71.

Frigerio, A. & Morselli, P. L. (1975) Carbamazepine: biotransformation, in *Advances in Neurology*, ed. Penry, J. K. & Daly, D. D. New York: Raven Press. Vol. 11. 295–308.

Fromm, G. H. & Killian, J. M. (1967) Effect of some anticonvulsant drugs on the spinal trigeminal nucleus. *Neurology* (Minneap.), **17**, 275–280.

Gerardin, A. P., Abadie, F. V., Campestrini, J. A. & Theobald, W. (1976) Pharmacokinetics of carbamazepine in normal humans after single and repeated oral doses. *J. Pharmacokinetics Biopharmaceutics*, **4**, 521–535.

Goenechea, S. & Hecke-Seibicke, E. (1972) Beitrag zum Stoffwechsel von Carbamazepin. *Z. Klin. Chem. Klin. Biochem.*, **10**, 112–113.

Guelen, P. J. M., van der Kelijn, E. & Woudstra, U. (1975) Statistical analysis of pharmacokinetic parameters in epileptic patients chronically treated with antileptic drugs, in *Clinical pharmacology of anti-epileptic drugs*, ed. Schneider, H., Janz, D., Gardner-Thorpe, C., Meinardi, H. & Sherwin, A. L. Berlin, Springer. 2–10.

Hansen, J. M., Siersboek-Nielsen, K. & Skovsted, L. (1971) Carbamazepine-induced acceleration of diphenylhydantoin and warfarin metabolism in man. *Clin. Pharm. Therap.*, **12**, 539–543.

Harman, R. R. M. (1967) Carbamazepine (Tegretol) drug eruptions. *Brit. J. Derm.*, **79**, 500.

Helin, I., Nilsson, K. O., Bjerre, I. & Vegfors, P. (1977) Serum sodium and osmolarity during carbamazepine treatment in children. *Brit. Med. J.*, ii, 558.

Henry, D. A., Lawson, D. H., Reavey, P. & Renfrew, S. (1977) Hyponatraemia during carbamazepine treatment. *Brit. med. J.*, i, 83–84.

Hernández-Péón, R. (1962), Anticonvulsive action of G32883. *Proc. Third Meet. CINP. Munich.*, 303–311.

Hernandez-Peon, R. (1965) Central actions of G32883 upon transmission of trigeminal pain impulses. *Med. Pharmacol. Exp.* (Basel.), **12**, 73–80.

Holm, E., Kelleter, R., Heinemann, H. & Hamann, K. F. (1970) Electrophysiologische Analyse der Wirkangen von Carbamazepin auf das Behirn der Katze. *Pharmakopsychiat. Neuro. Psychopharmakol.*, **3**, 187–200.

Hooper, W. D., Dubetz, D. K., Bochner, F., Cotter, L. M., Smith, G. A., Eadie, M. J. & Tyrer, J. H. (1975), Plasma protein binding of carbamazepine. *Clin. Pharmacol. Therap.*, **17**, 433–440.

Hooper, W. D., Dubetz, D. K., Eadie, M. J. & Tyrer, J. H. (1974) Preliminary observations on the clinical pharmacology of carbamazepine ('Tegretol'). *Proc. Aust. Assoc. Neurol.*, **11**, 189–198.

Hooper, W. D., Sutherland, J. M., Bochner, F., Tyrer, J. H. & Eadie, M. J. (1973) The effect of certain drugs on the plasma protein binding of diphenylhydantoin. *Aust. N.Z. J. Med.*, **3**, 377–381.

Ito, T., Hori, M., Yoshida, K. & Shimizu, M. (1977) Effect of anticonvulsants on cortical focal seizures in cats. *Epilepsia* (Amst.), **18**, 63–71.

Johannessen, S. I., Gerna, M., Bakke, J., Strandjord, R. E. & Morselli, P. L. (1976) CSF concentrations and serum protein binding of carbamazepine and carbamazepine-10,11-epoxide in epileptic patients. *Brit. J. clin. Pharmacol.*, **3**, 575–582.

Johannessen, S. I. & Stranjord, R. E. (1972) The concentration of carbamazepine (Tegretol^R) in serum and in cerebrospinal fluid in patients with epilepsy. *Acta. Neurol. Scandinav.*, **48**, Suppl. 51, 445–446.

Johannessen, S. I. & Strandjord, R. E. (1973) Concentration of carbamazepine (Tegretol^R) in serum and cerebrospinal fluid in patients with epilepsy. *Epilepsia* (Amst.) **14**, 373–379.

Johannessen, S. I. & Strandjord, R. E. (1975) The influence of phenobarbitone and phenytoin on carbamazepine serum levels, in *Clinical pharmacology of antiepileptic drugs*, ed. Schneider, H., Janz, D., Gardner-Thorpe, C., Meinardi, H. and Sherwin, A. L. Berlin: Springer. 201–205.

Johanessen, S. I., Strandjord, R. E. & Munthe-Kaas, A. W. (1977) Lack of effect on clonazepam on serum levels of diphenylhydantoin, phenobarbital and carbamazepine. *Acta Neurol. Scandinav.*, **55**, 506–512.

Julien, R. M. & Hollister, R. P. (1975) Carbamazepine: mechanism of action, in *Advances in neurology*, ed. Penry, J. K. & Daly, D. D. New York: Raven Press. Vol. 11. 263–276.

Kauko, K. & Tammisto, P. (1974) Comparison of two generically equivalent carbamazepine preparations. *Ann. Clin. Research*, **6**, (Suppl. 11) 21–25.

Killian, J. M. & Fromm, G. H. (1968) Carbamazepine in the treatment of neuralgia. *Arch. Neurol.* (Chic.), **19**, 129–136.

Kobayashi, K., Iwata, Y., & Mukawa, J. (1967) Preferential action of Tegretol (G-32883) to limbic seizures. Clinical and experimental analysis. *Brain and Nerve (Japan)*, **19**, 999–1005.

Krupp, P. (1969) The effect of Tegretol on some elementary neuronal mechanisms. *Headache*, **2**, 42–46.

Lance, J. W. (1968) Myoclonic jerks and falls: aetiology, classification and treatment. *M.J. Australia*, **1**, 113–120.

Lander, C. M., Eadie, M. J. & Tyrer, J. H. (1975) Interaction between anticonvulsants. *Proc. Aust. Assoc. Neurol.*, **12**, 111–116.

Lander, C. M., Eadie, M. J. & Tyrer, J. H. (1977) Factors influencing plasma carbamazepine concentrations. *Clin. Exptl. Neurol.*, **14**, 184–193.

Larsen, N. E., Naestoft, J. & Hvidberg, E. (1972) Rapid routine determination of some antiepileptic drugs in serum by gas chromatography. *Clin. chim. Acta*, **40**, 171–176.

Levy, R. H., Pitlick, W. H., Troupin, A. S., Green, J. R. & Neal, J. M. (1975) Pharmacokinetics of carbamazepine in normal man. *Clin. Pharmacol. Therap.*, **17**, 657–668.

Lewin, E. & Bleck, V. (1977) Cyclic AMP accumulation in cerebral cortical slices: effect of carbamazepine, phenobarbital and phenytoin. *Epilepsia* (Amst.), **18**, 237–242.

Livingstone, S., Pauli, L. L. & Pruce, I. (1978) No proven relationship of carbamazepine therapy to blood dyscrasias. *Neurology* (Minneap.), **28**, 101.

160   ANTICONVULSANT THERAPY

Livingstone, S., Villamater, C., Sakata, Y. & Pauli, L. L. (1967) Use of carbamazepine in epilepsy. Results in 87 patients. *J. Amer. Med. Ass.*, **250**, 116–120.

McAuliffe, J. J., Sherwin, A. L., Leppik, I. E., Fayle, S. A. & Pippenger, C. E. (1977) Salivary levels of anticonvulsants: a practical approach to drug monitoring. *Neurology* (Minneap.), **27**, 409–413.

Meinardi, H. (1972) Other antiepileptic drugs. Carbamazepine, in *Antiepileptic drugs*, ed. Woodbury, D. M., Penry, J. K. and Schmidt, R. P. New York: Raven Press. 487–496.

Meldrum, B. S., Horton, R. W. & Toseland, P. A. (1975) A primate model for testing anticonvulsant drugs. *Arch. Neurol.* (Chic.), **32**, 289–294.

Miura, H., Minagawa, K., Yagi, J. *et al.* (1976) Preliminary observations of plasma carbamazepine concentrations in epileptic children. *Brain Develop.*, **8**, 455–462. Translated summary in *Epilepsy Abstracts*, **10**, 342.

Mølholm, J., Siersbaek-Nielsen, K. & Skovsted, L. (1971) Interaktion mellan difenylhydantoin oct Karbamazepin, in *Plasmakoncentrationsbestämningar av Antiepileptika: Metodlogiska och Kliniska Aspekter*. Lidingo. 48–50.

Møller, J. (1971) Serumkoncentrationsbestämniar av Karbamazepin inom barnneurologin, in *Plasmakoncentrationsbestämningar av Antiepileptika: Metodologiska och Kliniska Aspekter*. Lidingö. 72–79.

Monaco, F., Riccio, A., Benna, P., Covacich, A., Durelli, L., Fantini, M., Furlan, P. M., Gilli, M., Mutani, R., Troni, W., Gerna, M. & Morselli, P. L. (1976) Further observations on carbamazepine plasma levels in epileptic patients. *Neurology* (Minneap.), **26**, 936–943.

Morselli, P. L. (1975) Carbamazepine: absorption, distribution and excretion, in *Advances in Neurology*, ed. Penry, J. K. and Daly, D. D. New York: Raven Press. Vol. 11, 279–293.

Morselli, P. L., Baruzzi, A., Gerna, M., Bossi, L. & Porta, M. (1977) Carbamazepine and carbamazepine-10,11-epoxide concentrations in human brain. *Brit. J. Clin. Pharmacol.*, **4**, 535–540.

Morselli, P. L., Bossi, L. & Gerna, M. (1975) Pharmacokinetic studies with carbamazepine in epileptic patients, in *International symposium on epileptic seizures-behaviour-pain*, ed. Birkmayer, W. Berne. Huber. 141–150.

Morselli, P. L., Gerna, M., De Maio, D., Zanda, G., Viani, F. & Garattini, S. (1975) Pharmacokinetic studies on carbamazepine in volunteers and in epileptic patients, in *Clinical pharmacology of antiepileptic drugs*, ed. Schneider, H., Janz, D., Gardner-Thorpe, C., Meinardi, H. & Sherwin, A. L. Berlin: Springer. 166–179.

Morselli, P., Gerna, M. & Garattini, S. (1971) Carbamazepine plasma and tissue levels in the rat. *Biochem. Pharmacol.*, **19**, 1846–1847.

Morselli, P. L., Monaco, F., Gerna, M., Recchia, M. & Riccio, A. (1975) Bioavailability of two carbamazepine preparations during chronic administration to epileptic patients. *Epilepsia* (Amst.), **16**, 759–764.

Neuvonen, P. J., Penttilä, O., Lehtovarra, R. & Aho, K. (1975) Effect of antiepileptic drugs on the elimination of various tetracycline derivatives. *Europ. J. clin. Pharmacol.*, **9**, 147–154.

Pakesch, E. (1963) Untersuchungen uber ein neuartiges Antiepilepticum. *Wien. med. Wschr.*, **113**, 794–796.

Palmér, L., Bertilsson, L., Collste, P. & Rawlins, M. (1973) Quantitative determination of carbamazepine in plasma by mass fragmentography. *Clin. Pharmacol. Therap.*, **14**, 827–832.

Perchalski, R. J. & Wilder, B. J. (1974) Rapid gas-liquid chromatographic determination of carbamazepine in plasma. *Clin. Chem.*, **20**, 492–493.

Perucca, E., Garratt, A., Hebdige, S. & Richens, A. (1978) Water intoxication in epileptic patients receiving carbamazepine. *J. Neurol. Neurosurg. Psychiat.*, **41**, 713–718.

Pisciotta, A. V. (1975) Hematologic toxicity of carbamazepine, in Penry, J. K. & Daly, D. D. *Advances in neurology*. Vol. 11. New York: Raven Press. 355–368.

Pitlick, W. H., Levy, R. H., Troupin, A. S. & Green, J. R. (1976) Pharmacokinetic model to describe self-induced decreases in steady-state concentrations of carbamazepine. *J. Pharm. Sci.*, **65**, 462–463.

Purdy, R. E., Julien, R. M., Fairhurst, A. S. & Terry, M. D. (1977) Effect of carbamazepine on the *in vitro* uptake and release of norepinephrine in adrenergic nerves of rabbit aorta and in whole brain synaptosomes. *Epilepsia* (Amst.), **18**, 251–257.

Pynnonen, S. & Sillanpää (1975) Carbamazepine and mother's milk. *Lancet*, **3**, 563.

Pynnonen, S., Sillanpää, M., Frey, H. & Iisalo, E. (1977) Carbamazepine and its 10,11 epoxide in children and adults with epilepsy. *Europ. J. Clin. Pharmacol.*, **11**, 129–133.

Pynnonen, S. & Yrjana, T. (1977) The significance of the simultaneous determination of carbamazepine and its 10,11 epoxide from plasma and human erythrocytes. *Int. J. Clin. Pharmacol. Biopharm.*, **15**, 222–226.

Rado, J. P. (1973) Water intoxication during carbamazepine treatment. *Brit. Med. J.*, iii, 479.

Rane, A., Bertilsson, L. & Palmér, L. (1975) Disposition of placentally transferred carbamazepine (Tegretol[R]) in the newborn. *Europ. J. Clin. Pharmacol.*, **8**, 283–284.

Rane, A., Hojer, B. & Wilson, J. T. (1976) Kinetics of carbamazepine and its 10,11-epoxide metabolite in children. *Clin. Pharmacol. Therap.*, **19**, 276–283.

Rawlins, M. D., Collste, P., Bertilsson, L. & Palmér, L. (1975) Distribution and elimination kinetics of carbamazepine in man. *Europ. J. Clin. Pharmacol.*, **8**, 91–96.

Reizenstein, P. & Lund, L. (1973) Effects of anticonvulsive drugs on folate absorption and the cerebrospinal fluid folate pump. *Scand. J. Haemat.*, **11**, 158–165.

Reynolds, E. H. (1973) Discussion, in *Tegretol in epilepsy*, ed. Wink, C. A. S. Manchester: C. Nicholls and Co. 118–122.

Reynolds, E. H. (1975) Neurotoxicity of carbamazepine, in Penry, J. K. & Daly, D. D. *Advances in neurology*. Vol. 11. New York. Raven Press. 345–353.

Richens, A. & Houghton, G. W. (1975) Effect of drug therapy on the metabolism of phenytoin, in *Clinical pharmacology of anti-epileptic drugs*, ed. Schneider, H., Janz, D., Gardner-Thorpe, C., Meinardi, H. and Sherwin, A. L. Berlin: Springer. 87–95.

Rylance, G. W., Butcher, G. M. & Moreland, T. (1977) Saliva carbamazepine levels in children. *Brit. Med. J.*, **ii**, 1481.

Schauf, C. L., Davis, F. A. & Marder, J. (1974) Effects of carbamazepine on the ionic conductances of Myxicola giant axons. *J. Pharmacol. exp. Therap.*, **189**, 538–543.

Schneider, H. (1975-a) General discussion, in *Clinical pharmacology of antiepileptic drugs*, ed. Schneider, H., Janz, D., Gardner-Thorpe, C., Meinardi, H. and Sherwin, A. L. Berlin: Springer. 207–209.

Schneider, H. (1975-b) Carbamazepine: an attempt to correlate serum levels with anti-epileptic and side effects, in *Clinical pharmacology of anti-epileptic drugs*, ed. Schneider, H., Janz, D., Gardner-Thorpe, C., Meinardi, H. and Sherwin, A. L. Berlin: Springer. 151–158.

Schneider, H. (1975-c) Carbamazepine: the influence of other anti-epileptic drugs on its serum level, in *Clinical pharmacology of anti-epileptic drugs*, ed. Schneider, H., Janz, D., Gardner-Thorpe, C., Meinardi, H. and Sherwin, A. L. Berlin: Springer. 189–195.

Shibasaki, H., Tabira, T., Inoue, N., Goto, I. & Kuroiwa, Y. (1973) Carbamazepine for painful crises in Fabry's disease. *J. Neurol. Sci.*, **18**, 47–51.

Simonsen, N., Olsen, P. Z., Kühl, V., Lund, M. & Wendelboe, J. (1975) A double blind study of carbamazepine and diphenylhydantoin in temporal lobe epilepsy. *Acta Neurol. Scandinav.* Suppl., **60**, 39–42.

Simpson, J. R. (1966) Collagen disease due to carbamazepine (Tegretol). *Brit. med. J.*, **ii**, 1434.

Starreveld-Zimmerman, A. A. E., van der Kolk, W. J., Meinardi, H. & Elshove, J. (1973) Are anticonvulsants teratogenic. *Lancet*, **ii**, 48–49.

Stephens, W. P., Espir, M. L. E., Tattersall, R. B., Quinn, N. P., Gladwell, S. R. F., Galbraith, A. W. & Reynolds, E. H. (1977) Water intoxication due to carbamazepine. *Brit. med. J.*, **i**, 754–755.

Theobald, W. & Kunz, H. A. (1963) Zur Pharmakologie des Antiepilepticums 5-Carbamyl-5H-dibenzo[b,f]azepin. *Arzneim.-Forsch.*, **13**, 122–125.

Thomas, T. H., Ball, S. G., Wales, J. K. & Lee, M. R. (1978) Effects of carbamazepine on plasma and urine arginine-vasopressin. *Clin. Sci. Molec. Med.*, **54**, 419–424.

Troupin, A. S. & Friel, P. (1975) Anticonvulsant levels in saliva, serum, and cerebrospinal fluid. *Epilepsia* (Amst.), **16**, 223–227.

Wada, J. A. (1977) Pharmacological prophylaxis in the kindling model of epilepsy. *Arch. Neurol.* (Chic.), **34**, 389–395.

Wada, J. A., Sato, M., Walke, A., Green, J. R. & Troupin, A. S. (1976) Prophylactic effects of phenytoin, phenobarbital, and carbamazepine examined in kindling cat preparations. *Arch. Neurol.* (Chic.), **33**, 426–434.

Wales, J. K. (1975) Treatment of diabetes insipidus with carbamazepine. *Lancet*, **4**, 948–956.

Weist, F. & Zicha, L. (1967) Dünnschichtchromatographische Untersuchungen uber 5-Carbamyl-5H-dibenzo(b,f)azepin and Harn und Liquor bir neuen Indikationsgebieten. *Arzneim. Forsch.*, **17**, 874–875.

Westernberg, H. G. M., van der Kleijn, E., Oei, T. T. & de Zeeuw, R. A. (1978) Kinetics of carbamazepine and carbamazepine-epoxide, determined by use of plasma and saliva. *Clin. Pharmacol. Therap.*, **23**, 320–328.

Windorfer, A. Jr. & Sauer, W. (1977), Drug interactions during anticonvulsant therapy in childhood: Diphenylhydantoin, primidone, phenobarbitone, clonazepam, nitrazepam, carbamazepine and dipropylacetate. *Neuropadiatrie*, **8**, 29–41.

Winek, C. L. (1976) Tabulation of therapeutic, toxic, and lethal concentrations of drugs and chemicals in blood. *Clin. Chem.* **22**, 832–836.

Wohlfahrth, E. (1972) Diabetes insipidus gedämpft: Erfolgreiche Langzeittherapie mit Carbamyldibenzolazepin. *Praxis—Kurier*, **10**, 10.

8

Barbiturate and chemically related anticonvulsants

Most barbiturates possess anticonvulsant activity although a few are convulsants (Shulman, 1970). However the general sedative properties of this family of drugs make most of them unsuitable for long-term anticonvulsant therapy in man. In at least three barbituric acid derivatives sedative properties are sufficiently slight relative to anticonvulsant effects to permit the drugs to be given for periods of years to treat epilepsy. These three derivatives are phenobarbitone, methylphenobarbitone and primidone (desoxyphenobarbitone). Phenobarbitone is extensively used throughout the world and methylphenobarbitone enjoys popularity in certain quarters. Primidone, a congener of phenobarbitone, is in part oxidized to phenobarbitone in man, and is a fairly widely used anticonvulsant. The clinically relevant pharmacology of phenobarbitone, methylphenobarbitone and primidone will be considered in the present chapter. Amylobarbitone will also be reviewed, though briefly. This substance, given parenterally, may be effective against status epilepticus. However, it it too sedative for continued use in epilepsy prophylaxis. A new barbiturate anticonvulsant, dimethoxymethylphenobarbitone, will be mentioned briefly.

PHENOBARBITONE (PHENOBARBITAL)

Common proprietary names: Luminal, Gardenal
Phenobarbitone was introduced into therapeutics as an anticonvulsant by Hauptmann (1912). It remains in widespread use more than 65 years later. The drug is effective in all varieties of epilepsy except *petit mal* absence seizures. For many years phenobarbitone was extensively prescribed as a sedative and minor tranquilizer, but for these purposes it is now superseded by more efficient and less toxic drugs.

CHEMISTRY

Phenobarbitone (5-ethyl-5-phenylbarbituric acid) is a white crystalline material with a somewhat bitter taste. It is poorly soluble in water but dissolves in organic solvents such as ethanol, diethylether and chloroform. Phenobarbitone has a molecular weight of 232·23 and a pKa value of 7·2 (Waddell and Butler, 1957). It is sometimes administered as its more water-soluble sodium salt.

PHARMACODYNAMICS

ACTIONS IN MAN

Anticonvulsant actions
Given orally or parenterally, phenobarbitone has some effect in the various types of myoclonic epilepsy, particularly in those varieties which develop in adolescence or early adult life. It is often effective against the convulsive seizures of generalized epilepsy and against all varieties of partial epilepsy. Phenobarbitone is of little use for absence seizures of generalized epilepsy.

Other actions
Phenobarbitone has a widespread depressant effect on neural function which may lead to a sedative effect. Some individuals, particularly children, become irritable and hyperactive when taking the drug.

ACTIONS IN ANIMALS

Anticonvulsant action

Models of generalized epilepsy
Phenobarbitone prevents photic seizures in the baboon, Papio papio (Stark, Killam and Killam, 1970; Meldrum, Horton and Toseland, 1975). The drug is effective in protecting against generalized myoclonic seizures induced by systemic injection of the following chemicals: pentylenetetrazole (Swinyard and Castellion, 1966), strychnine (Blum, Haefely, Jalfre, Polc and Schaerer, 1973; Loescher and Frey, 1977), thiosemicarbazide and 2,4-dimethyl-5-hydroxymethylpyrimidine (Banziger and Hane, 1967), local anaesthetics such as procaine, cocaine and lignocaine (Sanders, 1967) and also bicuculline (Blum, Haefely, Jalfre, Polc and Schaerer, 1973).

The drug either protects against, or modifies, maximum electroshock convulsions in various animal species (Goodman, Swinyard, Brown, Schiffman, Grewal and Bliss, 1954) and also prevents minimum electroshock seizures (Blum, Haefely, Jalfre, Polc and Schaerer, 1973).

Thus phenobarbitone is an effective anticonvulsant in animal models of generalized epilepsy of myoclonic or convulsive type.

Models of partial epilepsy
Phenobarbitone will suppress electrically-kindled seizures of amygdaloid origin in several animal species (Wada, 1977). The drug will also protect against

chemically-induced partial seizures (e.g. those arising from a stropanthin-produced focus in rabbit cerebral cortex, according to Petsche, 1972).

MECHANISMS OF ACTION

Neuron pools
There has been some difference between various workers' findings for the effects of phenobarbitone on spike activity at induced cortical epileptic foci. Morrell, Bradley and Ptashne (1959) noted that the drug caused a modest decrease in spiking at a freezing-induced cortical focus. Edmonds, Stark and Holliger (1974) found that the drug did not alter the frequency of spike discharges in a cortical focus produced by intracerebral penicillin injection in rats. Dow, Forfar and McQueen (1973) showed that phenobarbitone administration increased the frequency and duration of spiking at cobalt-induced cortical foci in these animals.

Phenobarbitone raises the threshold for the electrical induction of after-discharges in the hippocampus and amygdala of cats (Strobos and Spudis, 1960) and in the intralaminar thalamic nuclei and neocortex (Schallek and Kuehn, 1963). The drug does not alter after-discharging from a penicillin-induced cortical focus in rats (Edmonds, Stark and Hollinger, 1974).

Monosynaptic and polysynaptic transmission in the spinal cord is suppressed by phenobarbitone (Esplin, 1963). The drug has no clear-cut effect on post-tetanic potentiation (Fromm and Landgren, 1963; Kutt, 1974).

Single neurons
Even at concentrations 10 to 100 times greater than those at which the drug has an anticonvulsant effect, phenobarbitone produces only slight hyperpolarization of the neuronal resting membrane in the invertebrate Aplysia (Chalazonitis and Arvanitaki, 1973). Action potentials are altered only at supra-therapeutic phenobarbitone concentrations (e.g. 5×10^{-2} M, according to Rosenberg and Bartels, 1967).

From the data discussed above it would seem more likely that phenobarbitone has its anticonvulsant effect by altering synaptic transmission than by altering the electrical properties of axons.

Biochemical effects

Effects on energy production
At concentrations (10^{-3} M), about 10 times those at which it exerts its anticonvulsant effect, phenobarbitone inhibits terminal mitochondrial oxidation (Cowger and Labbe, 1967). Kyogaku and Yu (1968) raised the possibility that this inhibition might be due to phenobarbitone forming strong specific proton bonds with the adenine portion of flavine adenine dinucleotide. Given to cats, even in anaesthetic does, the drug does not block mitochondrial electron transport between NADH and cytochrome a_1, a_3. However it does reduce NAD^+ concentrations in the cerebral cortex, suggesting that cerebral oxygen consumption may be decreased (LaManna, Cordingley and Rosenthal, 1977). Despite its action in depressing oxidative metabolism in the brain, phenobarbitone enhances the transport of

glucose from blood to brain. This effect, however, occurs at phenobarbitone concentrations (0.25×10^{-3} M) which are at least twice those necessary for a therapeutic effect (Bachelard, 1976). Phenobarbitone inhibits cytochrome oxidase in rats, when given in therapeutic concentrations (Constantinescu, Hategan and Kriendler, 1973). In this species the drug also reduces brain succinate dehydrogenase activity (Leznicki and Dymecki, 1974). Phenobarbitone inhibits anaerobic glycolysis (Bachelard, 1976).

Thus at high therapeutic and supratherapeutic concentrations phenobarbitone begins to inhibit several biochemical mechanisms involved in glucose utilization and energy supply in neural tissue. Such actions might explain the cerebral depressant action of the drug, but whether they contribute to its anticonvulsant action is uncertain.

Effects on inorganic ions

Na^+. Phenobarbitone reduces intraneuronal Na^+ concentrations (Pincus, Grove, Marino and Glaser, 1970). It decreases Na^+ flux across cell membranes (Bunker and Vandam, 1965; Neuman and Frank, 1977). Formby (1970) found that phenobarbitone did not activate the sodium pump, the enzyme Na^+, K^+ linked adenosine triphosphatase. However Leznicki and Dymecki (1974) obtained a contrary result.

K^+. Bunker and Vandam (1965) found that phenobarbitone caused a decreased flux of K^+ across cell membranes while Neuman and Frank (1977) found that the drug did not alter K^+ conductance. In contrast Prichard (1972), found that the drug selectively and reversibly increased leech neuronal permeability to K^+.

Ca^{++}. Phenobarbitone, at a therapeutically relevant concentration (0.4×10^{-4} M) inhibited Ca^{++} influx into depolarized synaptosomes from rabbit cerebral cortex (Sohn and Ferendelli, 1976).

It is difficult to correlate these findings for the effect of phenobarbitone on small inorganic cations with the electrophysiological actions of the drug, and thereby to explain its anticonvulsant action.

Effects on synaptic transmitters

Acetylcholine. Phenobarbitone inhibits acetylcholine biosynthesis (Mori, 1974), and alters acetylcholine release (Tower and Elliott, 1953).

Serotonin. Phenobarbitone causes increased brain levels of serotonin in rats (Bonnycastle, Paasonen and Giarman, 1957). The drug does not inhibit brain monoamine oxidase, the enzyme responsible for serotonin degradation (Lezkicki and Dymecki, 1974).

Noradrenaline. Lidbrink and Farnebo (1973) showed that a wide range of phenobarbitone concentrations did not alter the *in vitro* uptake, storage or release of noradrenaline by rat cerebral cortex. Subsequently Weinberger, Nicklas and Berl (1976) found that (10^{-3}–10^{-4} M) phenobarbitone did inhibit noradrenaline uptake into rat brain synaptosomes.

Dopamine. We have not found information as to the effects of phenobarbitone on brain dopamine.

Gamma-aminobutyrate. Mouse brain GABA levels are raised by phenobarbitone (Saad, El Masry and Scott, 1972). At high therapeutic and supratherapeutic concentrations $(10^{-3}-10^{-4}$ M) the drug increases GABA uptake into rat brain synaptosomes (Weinberger, Nicklas and Berl, 1976). At supratherapeutic concentrations $(10^{-3}$ M) only, phenobarbitone inhibits mouse brain GABA transaminase and succinic semialdehyde dehydrogenase (Sawaya, Horton and Meldrum, 1975).

Some of the alterations in synaptic transmitters described above might contribute to the anticonvulsant action of phenobarbitone. However, sufficient knowledge is not yet available for a full explanation of the biochemical mode of action of the drug.

Effects on folates
Phenobarbitone is an anticonvulsant which causes folate depletion (Reynolds, 1976). The anti-epileptic effects and pathogenesis of such folate depletion have been discussed in greater detail in relation to phenytoin. One factor in phenobarbitone-induced folate deficiency may be the action of the drug in inhibiting the enzyme folate reductase (Lacy and Smith, 1973). This enzyme catalyses the biotransformation of folate to folinate (i.e. tetrahydrofolate).

Effects on macromolecules
Phenobarbitone $(10^{-3}$ M) decreases the incorporation of labelled leucine into rat brain protein (Swaiman and Stright, 1973). However lower phenobarbitone concentrations $(10^{-4}$ M), which are closer to those encountered therapeutically, do not have a definite effect on leucine incorporation. Smith, Liu, Leonard, Duceman and Vesell (1976) showed that phenobarbitone altered RNA synthesis in rat brain and decreased the activity of RNA polymerase II.

Despite the various data described above, it is still not possible to provide any adequate interpretation of the electrical and biochemical mechanisms involved in the anti-epileptic actions of phenobarbitone.

PHARMACOKINETICS

Although phenobarbitone has been extensively used for many years relatively little pharmacokinetic information is available regarding the drug.

ABSORPTION AND BIOAVAILABILITY

Oral administration
It is believed that after oral administration phenobarbitone absorption from the alimentary tract is reasonably complete, though direct data demonstrating this are lacking (Maynert, 1972). Following a single oral 750 mg phenobarbitone dose Lous (1954a) found that maximum plasma drug levels did not occur for 6 to 18 hours. This finding has sometimes been considered to suggest that phenobarbitone absorption from the human alimentary tract is relatively slow. However the rather late T_{max} for this drug may be due to its slow elimination, without its absorption necessarily being relatively slow. Boreus, Jalling and Kallberg (1975) stated that

the T_{max} after oral administration in neonates was 3 to 6 hours. In a single patient (Fig. 8.1) given a 240 mg oral dose of the drug Eadie, Lander, Hooper and Tyrer (1976) calculated that the absorption rate constant was 0.505 hour^{-1} (absorption half-time 1.37 hours) which suggests reasonably rapid absorption. Peak plasma level in this subject occurred 8 hours after dosage. Bioavailability could not be calculated as no intravenous or other reference preparation was given.

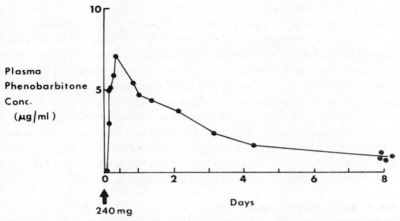

Fig. 8.1 Time course of plasma phenobarbitone concentrations in a patient given a single oral 240 mg phenobarbitone dose (Eadie, Lander, Hooper and Tyrer, 1976).

Rectal administration
Boyd and Singh (1967) stated that phenobarbitone absorbed well after rectal administration.

Intramuscular administration
In neonates Boreus, Jalling and Kallberg (1975) found that peak plasma phenobarbitone levels occurred 1–2 hours after intramuscular injection of the drug. Since the T_{max} after oral administration was 3–6 hours, the drug appeared to absorb faster after parenteral than after oral administration. Graham (1978) carried out a cross-over study of phenobarbitone absorption in adult subjects. Plasma phenobarbitone levels were measured during the first four or five hours after the drug was given orally or intramuscularly on different occasions, though in the same dose. There appeared little difference in either the mean peak plasma drug level or in the mean time to achieve this level. Peak levels occurred 2–3 hours from dosage in most subjects.

DISTRIBUTION

V_d
Hvidberg and Dam (1976) quoted the V_d of phenobarbitone as 0.7–1.0 litres kg^{-1}. In the neonate Painter, Pippinger, Carter and Pitlick (1977) found the V_d was 0.97 ± 0.20 litres kg^{-1} whilst Pitlick, Painter and Pippinger (1978) quoted a V_d

value of $0 \cdot 97 \pm 0 \cdot 15$ litres kg^{-1} for this age group. In the single personally studied patient referred to above the V_d was $0 \cdot 42$ litres kg^{-1}.

Plasma protein binding

About 50 per cent of phenobarbitone in plasma is bound to plasma protein (Waddell and Butler, 1957; Goldbaum and Smith, 1954; Lous, 1954 a and b; Svensmark, Schiller and Buchthal, 1960; Johanessen and Strandjord, 1975). Baumel, Gallagher and Mattson (1972) quoted a figure of 60 per cent for phenobarbitone binding to plasma protein in man, and McAuliffe, Sherwin, Leppik, Fayle and Pippenger (1977) a figure of 59 per cent. Waddell and Butler (1957) found that a 4 per cent solution of bovine albumin at pH 7·6 bound 46 per cent of the phenobarbitone which was introduced into the system. They also found that human serum albumin behaved like bovine albumin in this regard and that percentage binding of the drug did not vary over the phenobarbitone concentration range 20–100 μg/ml. There has been little recent interest in this matter and we are not aware of information on the effects of temperature, disease and the presence of other drugs on the plasma protein binding of phenobarbitone in man. However, binding of the drug is said to be reduced in the human neonate (Ehrnebo, Agurell, Jalling and Boreus, 1971).

Concentrations in various body fluids

Phenobarbitone concentrations in various body fluids, relative to simultaneously measured plasma phenobarbitone levels, reflect differences in protein contents and pH values of the fluids. Since phenobarbitone is an acid with a pKa of 7·2 it is significantly ionized at plasma pH (7.4). The fraction ionized in saliva (pH 6·2) would be appreciably less.

Cerebrospinal fluid

Johanessen and Strandjord (1975) found that CSF phenobarbitone levels averaged $52 \cdot 3 \pm 4 \cdot 4$ per cent of plasma levels, while Vajda, Williams, Davidson, Falconer and Breckenridge (1974) quoted a figure of 46 per cent, Houghton, Richens, Toseland, Davidson and Falconer (1975) a figure of 43 per cent, and Schmidt and Kupferberg (1975) a figure of 47 per cent.

Saliva

McAuliffe, Sherwin, Leppik, Fayle and Pippenger (1977) applied a correction for the pH difference between saliva and plasma when correlating phenobarbitone levels in the two fluids. With this correction, salivary and plasma water phenobarbitone levels were similar, the salivary level being $43 \cdot 1 \pm 5 \cdot 2$ per cent of the whole plasma level. Other authors who did not apply such a correction obtained figures for saliva: plasma phenobarbitone ratios of approximately $0 \cdot 3 : 1 \cdot 0$ (Cook, Amerson, Poole, Lesser and O'Tauma, 1975), $0 \cdot 32 – 0 \cdot 38 : 1 \cdot 0$ (Schmidt and Kupferberg, 1975) and $0 \cdot 31 – 0 \cdot 37 : 1 \cdot 0$ (Horning, Brown, Nowlin, Letratanangkoon, Kellaway and Zion, 1977).

Milk

Coradello (1973) stated that he could find no phenobarbitone in the milk of lactating women taking this drug. On theoretical grounds one would suspect the accuracy of this finding.

Concentrations in tissues
When phenobarbitone has had time to distribute through the animal body its concentrations in whole blood, plasma and in various tissues have been found generally similar (Goldbaum and Smith, 1954).

Brain
Phenobarbitone is not selectively accumulated in any brain region in cats (Domek, Barlow and Roth, 1960). However Pertschuk, Ford, Rainford and Brigati (1976) found that the drug tended to accumulate especially in neurons of the limbic system, caudate nucleus, cerebellum, cervical cord and trigeminal ganglia when mice were overdosed with the drug. Buchthal and Svensmark (1959) noted that brain and serum phenobarbitone concentrations were similar. More recently this question has been reinvestigated in man by Sherwin, Eisen and Sokolowski (1973), Vajda, Williams, Davidson, Falconer and Breckenridge (1974) and Houghton, Richens, Toseland, Davidson and Falconer (1975). These workers have found brain to plasma phenobarbitone ratios of $0.91 \pm 0.08:1$, $0.59 \pm 0.21:1$ and $1.13:1$, respectively.

Fetal tissues
Melchior, Svensmark and Trolle (1967) showed that phenobarbitone concentrations in umbilical cord serum from neonates were 95 per cent of the concentrations in maternal serum.

ELIMINATION

Elimination rate
It seems generally accepted that phenobarbitone elimination is a monoexponential process. However Wilson and Wilkinson (1973) suggested that the process might become rate-limited at phenobarbitone concentrations above 70 μg/ml. Authors have not usually published figures for the elimination rate constant of phenobarbitone. Instead they have quoted half-life values. In adults the half-life is 3·4 days (Mark, 1963) or 4 days (Buchthal and Lennox-Buchthal, 1972). Van der Kleijn, Guelen, van Wijk and Baars (1975) gave a value of 0·058 hour^{-1} for the elimination rate constant of the drug in humans, and 120 hours for the half-life. In one adult studied personally (Fig. 8.1) the elimination rate constant was 0·014 hour^{-1}, corresponding to a half-life of 48·7 hours. Garrettson and Dayton (1970) showed that the mean half-life of phenobarbitone was shorter in children (37 hours) than in adults (73 hours). Boreus, Jalling and Kallberg (1975) noted that in neonates phenobarbitone half-life was inversely related to plasma phenobarbitone level. This phenomenon does not seem to have been noted in adults. Pitlick, Painter and Pippenger (1978) found that the half-life of phenobarbitone decreased exponentially in the first four weeks of post-natal life (from a mean of 115 hours at the end of the first week to a mean of 67 hours at the end of the fourth week).

Clearance

Guelen, van der Kleijn and Woudstra (1975) quoted a value of 0.0053 ± 0.0038 litres kg^{-1} $hour^{-1}$ for the relative clearance of phenobarbitone. The relative clearance declined from values of about 0.012 litres kg^{-1} $hour^{-1}$ in young children to values of about 0.004 litres kg^{-1} $hour^{-1}$ by the age of 12 to 15 years, but thereafter did not change with age. In the one adult subject studied personally (Fig. 8.1) the clearance was 0.006 litres kg^{-1} $hour^{-1}$.

Per cent excreted unchanged

Figures for the percentage of a phenobarbitone dose excreted unchanged have varied from author to author, e.g. 10–30 per cent (Lous, 1966), about 67 per cent (Butler, Makafee and Waddell, 1954) and less than 50 per cent (Kallberg, Agurell, Ericcson, Bucht, Jalling and Boreus, 1975). Recently Whyte and Dekaban (1977) in a detailed study of 8 subjects found an average of 25 per cent of a phenobarbitone dose was excreted unchanged in urine. Therefore biotransformation appears to be the major avenue of elimination of phenobarbitone.

Biotransformation pattern

The biotransformation pathway for phenobarbitone appears to be as set out in Fig. 8.2.

In the study of Whyte and Dekaban (1977) a mean of only 42 per cent of a phenobarbitone dose was accounted for in urine as unchanged drug or indentified metabolites (mainly p-hydroxyphenobarbitone). Since phenobarbitone absorbs well there were probably unidentified phenobarbitone metabolites in urine, and these metabolites might have played a quantitatively important role in the drug's elimination. The finding of Tang, Inaba and Kalow (1977) suggested that perhaps 30 per cent of a phenobarbitone dose in man might be excreted in urine as the N-hydroxide of the drug, a previously unidentified metabolite. This would mean that most of the phenobarbitone dose can now be accounted for.

Excretion

Change in urine pH may alter the excretion of unmetabolized phenobarbitone. As urine becomes more alkaline more phenobarbitone within the renal tubular lumen will ionize, and therefore will be excreted. The mechanisms of renal excretion of phenobarbitone and its metabolites do not appear to have been studied in detail, though in two human subjects Waddell and Butler (1957) found renal phenobarbitone clearances of between 2 and 3 ml/minute, when urine flow rates were between 0.8 and 1.2 ml/minute.

CLINICAL PHARMACOKINETICS

Time course of plasma drug levels

Single dose

As indicated earlier, after oral or intramuscular administration of a single dose of the drug, plasma phenobarbitone levels rise to a peak somewhere between 2 and 18

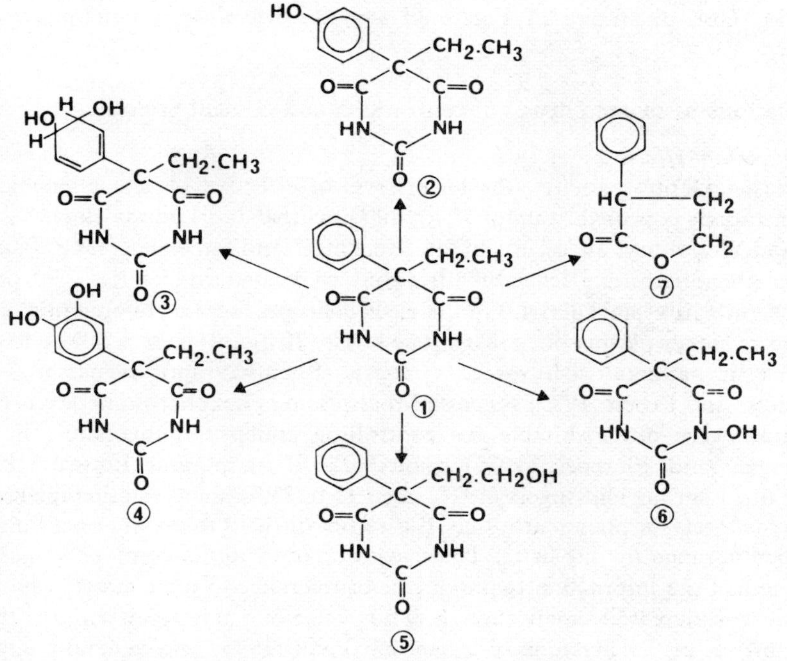

Phenobarbitone biotransformation

Fig. 8.2 Known biotransformation products of phenobarbitone.

1. phenobarbitone
2. p-hydroxyphenobarbitone, described by Butler (1956). Whyte and Dekaban (1977) found that 8 per cent of a phenobarbitone dose appeared in urine as this metabolite, and 17 per cent as the glucuronide conjugate of the metabolite. Neonates are able to form and conjugate the glucuronide conjugate of the metabolite. Neonates are able to form and conjugate p-hydroxyphenobarbitone (Boreus, Jalling and Kallberg, 1975). Craig, Hirano and Shideman (1960) stated that p-hydroxyphenobarbitone had weak anticonvulsant activity.
3. a dihydrodiol metabolite [5-(3,4-dihydroxy-1,5-cyclohexadiene-1-yl)-5-ethylbarbituric acid] (Harvey, Glazener, Stratton, Nowlin, Hill and Horning, 1972).
4. a catechol metabolite (Horning, Butler, Nowlin and Hill, 1975)
5. a hydroxyethyl metabolite (Glazko, 1975)
6. N-hydroxyphenobarbitone (Tang, Inaba and Kalow, 1977)
7. α-phenyl-γ-butyrolactone (Andresen, Davis and Templeton, 1976)

hours from dosage. Thereafter the levels decline slowly, typically with a half-life of 3–4 days in adults, and of about 2 or 3 days in children.

Repeated doses
With repeated doses of the drug, plasma phenobarbitone levels might be expected to achieve a steady state after about 3 weeks in adults (Svensmark and Buchthal, 1963) and after about 1½ weeks in children. Once a steady state is attained there should be relatively little fluctuation in plasma drug levels across a dosage interval, even if the drug were given only once a day. Since phenobarbitone has a 3–4 day half-life, plasma drug levels in the steady state might be expected to fluctuate through only 10–15 per cent of the mean level over a 24 hour dosage interval. Data

such as those illustrated in Fig. 6.13 suggest that these predictions apply in practice.

Correlations of plasma drug concentrations and clinical effects

Anticonvulsant effects

For most epileptic patients, the lower level of effective plasma phenobarbitone concentrations is probably about 10 μg/ml (Buchthal and Lennox-Buchthal, 1972; Aird and Woodbury, 1974). Buchthal, Svensmark and Simonsen (1968) found that plasma phenobarbitone levels of 10 μg/ml were associated with a 90 per cent decrease in paroxysmal activity in the electroencephalograms of epileptic patients. However, higher plasma phenobarbitone levels (20 μg/ml) were required to control seizures in patients with severe epilepsy (Buchthal and Svensmark, 1959). Pippenger and Rosen (1975) suggested that plasma phenobarbitone levels of 15 to 30 μg/ml were often suitable for controlling epilepsy in neonates. Feldman, Pippenger, and Florence (1975) quoted 15–40 μg/ml and Loiseau, Brachet-Liermain, Legroux and Jogeix (1977) cited 15 to 25 μg/ml as the therapeutic range of plasma levels for phenobarbitone. It is rather difficult to set an upper limit to the therapeutic range for the drug. Toxic manifestations often commence insidiously and one had the impression that a degree of tolerance to toxic effects can occur if drug dose is increased slowly enough. Thus while one may agree with the figure of 30 μg/ml set by Livingstone, Berman and Pauli (1975) as a generally applicable upper limit for the therapeutic range, one must admit that some patients tolerate higher plasma phenobarbitone levels without obvious undesirable effects, and with better control of epilepsy.

In a special situation (viz. children with febrile convulsions) it appears that 15 μg/ml is the threshold value of plasma phenobarbitone levels for protection against seizures (Faero, Kastrup, Lykkegaard Nielsen, Melchior and Thorn, 1972; Thorn, 1975). Heckmatt, Houston, Clow, Stephenson, Dodd, Lealman and Logan (1976) challenged this assertion, but inspection of their data suggests that these tended to support the idea of a 15 μg/ml threshold, though the evidence was not statistically significant.

Unwanted effects

As mentioned above, within limits the threshold for development of the sedative effects of phenobarbitone varies from person to person. To some extent it appears related to the rate at which phenobarbitone doses have been increased. Livingstone, Berman and Pauli (1975) considered that most persons taking phenobarbitone became drowsy when plasma drug levels were in the range 30–50 μg/ml. With levels above 70 μg/ml there was likely to be severe drowsiness, or coma. Winek (1976) regarded plasma phenobarbitone levels of 80–150 μg/ml as lethal.

Plasma level—dose correlations in treated populations

Relatively few data are available correlating plasma phenobarbitone concentrations in the steady state with oral dosage of the drug (e.g. Lous, 1954a; Plaa and Hine, 1960). For adult populations Buchtal and Lennox-Buchthal (1972) quoted oral doses of 1 mg/kg/day as yielding steady state plasma phenobarbitone levels of about 10 μg/ml, doses of 2 mg/kg/day producing levels around 20 μg/ml and doses of 3 mg/kg/day levels around 30 μg/ml. Plaa and Hine (1960) found the levels corresponding to the same doses were about 20 per cent lower than those cited above. The data of Eadie, Lander, Hooper and Tyrer (1976—Fig. 8.3) showed a less steep rate of rise in mean plasma drug level relative to dose than that quoted above. However these results were based on both adult patients and children. There was a considerable scatter of data points about the regression line. The mean drug dose required to produce a plama phenobarbitone level of 15 μg/ml was 1·75 mg/kg/day.

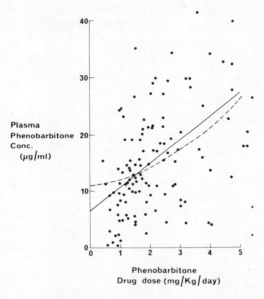

Fig. 8.3 Correlation between steady-state plasma phenobarbitone level and phenobarbitone dose in 121 patients. Linear and parabolic regressions of best fit are shown (Eadie, Lander, Hooper and Tyrer, 1977).

Effects of age

As might be expected from the half-life data, children require higher doses than adults, relative to body weight, to achieve the same plasma phenobarbitone levels. Svensmark and Buchthal (1964) found that children 1 to 14 years of age required doses (on a body weight basis) 2–3 times those of adults. However there was more variation between individual children than between individual adults. In neonates Pippenger and Rosen (1975) stated that phenobarbitone doses of 5–6 mg/kg/day kept plasma phenobarbitone levels in the range 15–30 μg/ml. Painter, Pippenger, Carter and Pitlick (1977) in neonates found that, after loading doses, a daily phenobarbitone dose of 5 mg/kg produced mean plasma drug levels of 28·0 ± 4·6 μg/ml on days 1 to 4, mean levels 33·5 ± 8·6 μg/ml on days 5–10 and mean levels of 30·3 ± 7·2 μg/ml on days 10–20, with mean levels falling to 17·4 ± 3·5 μg/ml after day 20. These findings would be consistent with increasing excretory capacity for the drug as the neonates grew older. However time-related auto-induction of biotransformation capacity is an alternative interpretation. In children in their first five post-natal days Ouvrier and Goldsmith (1977) found that a phenobarbitone dose of 7 mg/kg/day produced an average apparent steady state plasma drug level of 19 μg/ml. In general the phenobarbitone doses required by neonates appear comparable with the doses required by older children, and more than double the doses, on a weight basis, required by adults.

Eadie, Lander, Hooper and Tyrer (1976, 1977) studied the relation between plasma phenobarbitone level and drug dose in persons of various ages, other than neonates. Using linear regression techniques they were able to define four age groups in each of which the relation between plasma phenobarbitone level and drug dose per unit body weight differed to a statistically significant degree from the neighbouring age groups (Fig. 8.4). In general the drug dose required to produce a

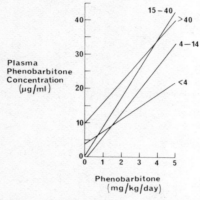

Fig. 8.4 Regressions for steady-state plasma phenobarbitone level on phenobarbitone dose in different age groups (Eadie, Lander, Hooper and Tyrer, 1977).

particular plasma phenobarbitone level fell with age. Thus to produce a mean plasma phenobarbitone level of 15 μg/ml a daily dose of 3·1 mg/kg was required in children under 4 years, a dose of 2·3 mg/kg in children 4–14 years, a dose of 1·75 mg/kg in persons 15–40 years and a dose of 0·90 mg/kg in persons over 40 years of age.

Effect of sex
Travers, Reynolds and Gallagher (1972) found a (non-statistically significant) tendency for females to have lower plasma phenobarbitone levels than males, relative to dose. Eadie, Lander, Hooper and Tyrer (1976, 1977) showed that, on a body weight basis, females required lower phenobarbitone doses than males to produce the same steady-state plasma drug levels (Fig. 8.5). This difference between the sexes could not be demonstrated in the age groups 4–14 years, 15–40 years and over 40 years. The difference was found only in children younger than 4 years, in whom females required substantially lower doses than males. This finding has not been explained. Even though the result was statistically significant, it needs confirmation.

Effect of pregnancy
Phenobarbitone dosage requirement to maintain plasma phenobarbitone levels

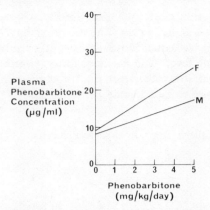

Fig. 8.5 Effect of sex on the regression for steady-state plasma phenobarbitone concentration on phenobarbitone dose (Eadie, Lander, Hooper and Tyrer, 1977).

rises as pregnancy progresses, and falls again in the puerperium (Lander, Edwards, Eadie and Tyrer, 1977: Fig. 6.20 and Fig. 8.6). Mygind, Dam and Christiansen (1976) and Dam, Mygind and Christiansen (1976) found no significant increase in phenobarbitone clearance in pregnancy.

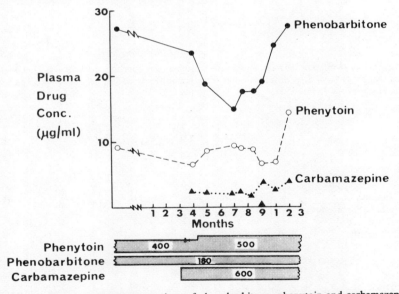

Fig. 8.6 Time-course of plasma concentrations of phenobarbitone, phenytoin and carbamazepine during a pregnancy in one subject. Despite a constant phenobarbitone dose throughout, plasma phenobarbitone levels fell progressively during pregnancy and rose again in the puerperium (Lander, Edwards, Eadie and Tyrer, 1977).

Plasma level—dose relationship in treated individuals

It has been stated that there is a simple linear relation between plasma phenobarbitone level and drug dose in the treated individual (Richens, 1974). At the time of writing the previous edition of this book (1973) we also believed this. With increasing experience we no longer do. The relation (Figs. 8.7 and 8.8) appears to be curvilinear. Successive equal dose increments produce increased rises in steady-state plasma drug level. The mechanisms responsible for this finding have not yet been elucidated, but the effect is of obvious clinical significance when phenobarbitone doses are to be adjusted.

Effects of disease

We have not seen data indicating how disease has affected the pharmacokinetics of phenobarbitone.

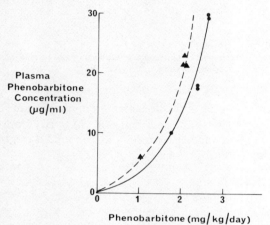

Fig 8.7 Curvilinear relation between steady-state plasma phenobarbitone levels and phenobarbitone doses in two patients who, at different times, received different daily phenobarbitone doses (Eadie, Lander, Hooper and Tyrer, 1977).

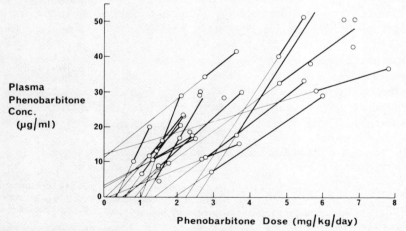

Fig. 8.8 Linear regressions for steady-state plasma phenobarbitone level on phenobarbitone dose in 17 subjects who received different daily phenobarbitone doses at different times. When the regressions were back-extrapolated a statistically significant excess number of the lines intercepted the 'x' axis. Since the true regressions must pass through the origin, this finding suggests that the relation between plasma phenobarbitone level and drug dose in the individual is curvilinear, and of a shape similar to those shown in Fig. 8.7. (Eadie, Lander, Hooper and Tyrer, 1977).

INTERACTIONS

PHARMACODYNAMIC

When phenobarbitone is given together with other anticonvulsants both the anti-epileptic and the sedative effects of the drug may be increased. To the writers' knowledge possible pharmacokinetic interactions have not been excluded in these circumstances.

PHARMACOKINETIC

Phenobarbitone affecting other substances

Plasma protein binding
Phenobarbitone does not appear to alter the plasma protein binding of phenytoin *in vitro* (Kristensen, Hansen and Skovsted, 1969; Lunde, Rand, Yaffe, Lund and Sjoqvist, 1970; Hooper, Sutherland, Bochner, Tyrer and Eadie, 1973), or that of carbamazepine (Hooper, Dubetz, Bochner, Cotter, Smith, Eadie and Tyrer, 1975).

Effects as an enzyme inducer
Phenobarbitone is a prototype for substances which induce enzymes of the hepatic microsomal mixed-oxidase system. This system is responsible for the metabolism of naturally occurring substances including bilirubin and endogenous steroids, and also many drugs (e.g. phenytoin, dicoumarol). Such enzyme induction has been the subject of several reviews (e.g. Gillette, 1963; Conney, 1967). Phenobarbitone administration in man for more than 7 days has been shown by liver biopsy to lead to increased formation of liver microsomal protein, with increased activity of hexobarbitone oxidase and cytochrome P_{450} (Lecamwasam, Franklin and Turner, 1975). There is a concurrent increase in urinary excretion of D-glucaric acid. Phenobarbitone intake also increases hepatic blood flow (Nies, Shand and Branch, 1974).

Chronic phenobarbitone administration in man leads to a fall in the plasma levels of certain endogenous substances and administered chemicals. It seems likely that these effects of the drug are the results of hepatic enzyme induction, though this has rarely been proven. Substances which have been recorded as having their plasma levels reduced, and/or their eliminations increased, by phenobarbitone include the following:

1 Endogenous substances
   bile salts, cholesterol and lipids (Linarelli, Hengstenberg and Drash, 1973)
   bilirubin (Thompson, Eddleston and Williams, 1969)
   cortisol (Burstein and Klaiber, 1965)
   folate (Davis and Woodliffe, 1971)

2 Exogenous substances
   aminopyrine (Vessell and Page, 1969)
   antipyrine (Conney, 1967)
   bishydroxycoumarin (Cucinell, Conney, Sansur and Burns, 1965)

carbamazepine (see page 154)
chloramphenicol-in neonates (Windorfer and Pringshein, 1977)
dicophane, i.e. D.D.T. (Davies, Edmundson, Carter and Barquet, 1969)
digitoxin (Conney, 1967)
dipyrone (Conney, 1967)
doxycycline, but not other tetracylines (Neuvonen and Penttila, 1974; Neuvonen, Penttila, Lehtovarra and Aho, 1975)
griseofulvin (Conney, 1967)
nortriptyline (Braithwaite, Flanagan and Richens, 1975)
phenylbutazone (Levi, Sherlock and Walker, 1968)
phenytoin (see page 89)
valproate (Takeda, Goto, Amano and Kukino, 1976)
warfarin (Cucinell, Conney, Sansur and Burns, 1965)

The effects of phenobarbitone on carbamazepine and phenytoin have been discussed elsewhere in this book (pages 154 and 89 respectively). Although the interaction of phenobarbitone with griseofulvin has been listed here as though its mechanism is enzyme induction, there is some evidence that this is not the case (Riegelman, Rowland, and Epstein, 1970). Possibly phenobarbitone impairs the absorption of griseofulvin.

Perry, Hansen and MacLean (1976) noted that phenobarbitone caused raised blood and CSF levels of glutamine and ornithine in some infants. The mechanisms involved are obscure.

Other substances affecting phenobarbitone

Plasma protein binding
We have not traced reports of other substances altering the plasma protein binding of phenobarbitone *in vitro*, apart from the report of Jordan, Shillingford and Steed (1977) that valproate slightly decreased phenobarbitone binding.

Other anticonvulsants
Phenytoin. Morselli, Rizzo and Garattini (1971), Lambie, Nanda, Johnson and Shakir (1976) and Windorfer and Sauer (1977) all found that phenytoin therapy tended to cause a rise in plasma phenobarbitone levels. Rizzo, Morselli and Garattini (1972) showed that phenytoin administration raised plasma and brain phenobarbitone concentrations in rats.

Carbamazepine. Cereghino, Brock, Van Meter, Penry, Smith and White (1975) found that carbamazepine had little effect on plasma phenobarbitone concentrations.

Clonazepam. This drug does not alter plasma phenobarbitone concentrations (Johanessen, Strandjord and Munthekaas, 1977).

Valproate. Valproate therapy tends to cause a considerable rise in plasma phenobarbitone level (Schobben, van der Kleijn and Gabreels, 1975; Vakil, Critchley, Philip, Fahim, Haydock, Cocks and Dyer, 1975; Adams, Luders and Pippenger, 1978). Another source of increased plasma levels of short-chain fatty acids (*viz.* the ketogenic diet) also causes raised plasma phenobarbitone levels (Livingstone, 1972).

Phenylacetylurea. Huisman, Van Heycop ten Ham and Van Zijl (1970) found that phenylacetylurea therapy caused raised plasma phenobarbitone levels.

Eadie, Lander, Hooper and Tyrer (1977) used multiple variable linear regression techniques to seek evidence of interactions in which the presence of other anticonvulsants altered plasma phenobarbitone levels in a population of 121 patients. They found no statistically significant evidence of an effect of phenytoin, carbamazepine or suthiame dose on the relation between plasma phenobarbitone level and phenobarbitone dose. They found the tendency of phenytoin was, if anything, to reduce mean plasma phenobarbitone level, in contrast to the findings of other workers as outlined above.

Other substances

Baylis, Crowley, Pruce, Sylvester and Marks (1971) found that folic acid therapy did not alter plasma phenobarbitone levels. This result is contrary to the finding of Mattson, Gallagher, Reynolds and Glass (1973) and of Fig. 6.30. Pyridoxine (Hansson and Sillanpaa, 1976), dicoumarol (Cucinell, Conney, Sansur and Burns, 1965) and phenylbutazone (Conney, 1967) lower plasma phenobarbitone levels. Frusemide slightly raises plasma phenobarbitone levels (Ahmad, Clarke, Hewett and Richens, 1976), but methylphenidate has no effect on them (Kupferberg, Jeffrey and Hunninghake, 1972).

TOXICITY

LOCAL EFFECTS

Phenobarbitone is nearly always given orally and rarely produces local irritation in the alimentary tract. Reactions at intramuscular injection sites also are uncommon.

DOSE DETERMINED SYSTEMIC EFFECTS

Nervous system

In the first few days of regular administration, phenobarbitone may make some patients drowsy. This drowsiness usually passes off without any reduction in phenobarbitone dosage. Such an effect suggests the possible development of a degree of tolerance. Because of the delay of two or three weeks in achieving plateau plasma and tissue levels of the drug it seems likely that this increased tolerance to the sedative effect of phenobarbitone may occur while plasma levels of the drug are still increasing. If plasma phenobarbitone levels finally become high enough (e.g. over 30 μg/ml according to Buchthal and Lennox-Buchthal, 1972) drowsiness may develop again. However, as mentioned earlier, patients not infrequently tolerate much higher plasma phenobarbitone levels without apparent ill-effect, so long as these levels are not achieved too rapidly. Phenobarbitone may produce irritability and hyperactivity in some children, possibly due to depression of higher inhibitory centres. Confusion may occur, particularly in the aged. Although phenobarbitone may appear to have no obvious adverse effect on cerebral functioning it is not uncommon to find that several months after a child begins phenobarbitone therapy there is a decline in scholastic performance. Schoolwork may improve if another anticonvulsant is substituted. Personality changes and insidious blunting of intellectual function may be problems in patients taking phenobarbitone. Reynolds and Travers (1974) have demonstrated a statistical correlation between increasing plasma phenobarbitone level (below the conventional toxic range) and psychomotor slowing and personality change in epileptic patients.

In overdosage, phenobarbitone rarely produces asterixis (Chadwick, Reynolds and Marsden, 1976).

Folate deficiency
The question of anticonvulsant-induced folate depletion has been discussed in Chapter 6 in connection with phenytoin. Here it should suffice to point out that in many instances of such folate deficiency the affected persons have been receiving multiple anticonvulsants, including phenobarbitone or substances metabolized to phenobarbitone. However, phenobarbitone administration alone may produce folate deficiency, with or without macrocytic anaemia (Chanarin, Mollin and Anderson, 1958; Davis and Woodliff, 1971).

Hypocalcaemia and osteomalacia
There have been reports of this complication in patients taking long-term anticonvulsants, usually in combination and including phenobarbitone or substances which are metabolized to it. The matter has been considered in more detail in Chapter 6 in relation to phenytoin.

Dupuytren's contracture
Critchley, Vakil, Hayward and Owen (1976) noted a 56 per cent incidence of Dupuytren's contracture in chronic epileptics in a residential centre. They regarded the abnormality as a probable sequel of chronic phenobarbitone use.

IDIOSYNCRATIC EFFECTS

These are uncommon and usually involve the skin. The rash is typically a fine punctate erythema but may consist of larger erythematous macules more closely resembling morbilli. Rarely exfoliative dermatitis may occur (McGeachy and Bloomer, 1953). Agranulocytosis and aplastic anaemia are very rare, as are jaundice and hepatitis (Welton, 1950).

EFFECTS ON THE FETUS AND NEONATE

The question of a possible dysmorphogenic effect of phenobarbitone in animals and man was reviewed by Staples (1972). He considered that 'it cannot be concluded that phenobarbital is teratogenic in any of the laboratory species to date.' However there have been reports of children with cleft palate or hare-lip being born to mothers who took anticonvulsants, including phenobarbitone, during pregnancy (Meadow, 1970). The matter has been discussed further in Chapter 6 where it is pointed out that the investigation of Shapiro, Hartz, Siskind, Mitchell, Slone, Rosenberg, Monson, Heinonen, Idänpään-Heikkila, Harö and

Saxen (1976) suggested that phenobarbitone itself was not dysmorphogenic in humans.

Mountain, Hirsch and Gallus (1970) obtained some evidence that anticonvulsant therapy during pregnancy, particularly therapy with barbiturate-type drugs, frequently caused blood coagulation defects in the new-born. These defects sometimes led to a clinical bleeding tendency. This may be overcome by the prophylactic use of vitamin K_1. The matter has been considered further in Chapter 6.

Erith (1975) reported the occurrence of a phenobarbitone-withdrawal syndrome in infants born to mothers who had taken the drug in pregnancy. The infants were hypotonic and irritable in their first three post-natal days, and tended to vomit.

PREPARATIONS AVAILABLE

These include:

Tablets (phenobarbitone)	—	15 mg, 30 mg, 60 mg, 100 mg
Tablets (phenobarbitone sodium)	—	15 mg, 30 mg, 60 mg, 100 mg
Ampoules (phenobarbitone sodium)	—	200 mg

METHYLPHENOBARBITONE (MEPHOBARBITAL)

Common proprietary names: 'Prominal', 'Phemitone'
Methylphenobarbitone is the N-methyl derivative of phenobarbitone. It was introduced into therapeutics by Blum (1932). The drug enjoys some popularity as an anticonvulsant, and has a similar range of antiepileptic action to phenobarbitone.

CHEMISTRY

Methylphenobarbitone (5-ethyl-1-methyl-5-phenylbarbituric acid) is a white crystalline powder, molecular weight 246.26. Its pKa value is approximately 7.6 (Waddell and Butler, 1957). The drug is more lipid soluble than phenobarbitone itself.

PHARMACODYNAMICS

In man and animals methylphenobarbitone is biotransformed to phenobarbitone.

Methylphenobarbitone, as distinct from the phenobarbitone produced from it, has been subject of little pharmacodynamic study. However, Craig and Shideman (1971) in a careful investigation showed that unmetabolized methylphenobarbitone was an anticonvulsant in its own right. It protected against maximum electroshock seizures in mice. In the absence of further knowledge about the actions of methylphenobarbitone itself, it may be that the chronic effects of the drug are largely mediated by the phenobarbitone produced from it. Yet methylphenobarbitone is more than a mere pro-drug for phenobarbitone, as will also be apparent from its pharmacokinetics.

PHARMACOKINETICS

ABSORPTION AND BIOAVAILABILITY

Methylphenobarbitone is given by mouth. There is indirect evidence, based on plasma levels of drug and metabolite relative to drug dosage, which suggests that methylphenobarbitone may be poorly absorbed from the alimentary tract (Maynert, 1972; Meinardi, Van der Kleijn, Meijer and Van Rees, 1975). In practice 2 mg methylphenobarbitone is often taken as approximately equivalent to 1 mg of phenobarbitone. It has been suggested that the eliminations of methyl-phenobarbitone and phenobarbitone follow similar pathways. If this is so, the most simple explanation for the dose difference is incomplete absorption of methyl-phenobarbitone.

In a study of the pharmacokinetics of the drug Eadie, Bochner, Hooper and Tyrer (1978) were unable to measure absorption parameters of methylphenobar-bitone accurately. They had available no intravenous preparation of the drug to permit determination of bioavailability. However, in 7 of their 8 subjects peak plasma methylphenobarbitone levels occurred within 8 hours of oral dosage. This suggests that absorption was moderately rapid since the drug was not rapidly eliminated. While this result cannot be taken as evidence of complete bioavailability, the slow absorption that is often associated with incomplete bioavailability of a drug did not appear to apply for methylphenobarbitone.

DISTRIBUTION

Eadie, Bochner, Hooper and Tyrer (1978) found the V_d of the drug averaged 130 litres in adults. In one subject in whom pharmacokinetic parameters for phenobar-bitone were determined, the V_d of phenobarbitone was 25·9 litres while the V_d of methylphenobarbitone was 246 litres. It would seem that methylphenobarbitone probably undergoes more extensive tissue binding than phenobarbitone. This finding may relate to the greater lipid solubility of methylphenobarbitone.

No information about the plasma protein binding of the drug is available. Coradello (1973) was unable to find the drug in milk from patients taking methylphenobarbitone.

ELIMINATION

Elimination rate

Eadie, Bochner, Hooper and Tyrer (1978) obtained evidence that methylphenobarbitone was more rapidly eliminated in subjects who were taking drugs which might have induced their liver mixed-oxidase systems than in patients who had taken no such drugs in the weeks prior to a methylphenobarbitone dose. In 'non-induced' patients the elimination rate constant for methylphenobarbitone was 0.0155 ± 0.0047 hour^{-1} and the half-life 49.0 ± 18.8 hours. In 'induced' patients the elimination rate constant was 0.0375 ± 0.0104 hour^{-1} and the half-life 19.6 ± 8.0 hours. The only other figures available for methylphenobarbitone elimination are half-life values of 34 and 47 hours in two subjects (Horning, Nowlin, Butler, Letratangangkoon, Sommer and Hill, 1975).

Clearance

Methylphenobarbitone clearance was 1.85 ± 0.70 litres hour^{-1} in 'non-induced' subjects, and 5.08 ± 2.70 litres hour^{-1} in 'induced' subjects (Eadie, Bochner, Hooper and Tyrer, 1978).

Per cent excreted unchanged

In three subjects Eadie, Bochner, Hooper and Tyrer (1978) found only 1.7 to 3.0 per cent of a dose of methylphenobarbitone was excreted unchanged in urine. Therefore elimination of the drug would seem to be chiefly by means of biotransformation.

Biotransformation pattern

It is known that methylphenobarbitone is oxidatively demethylated in the liver, forming phenobarbitone (Butler, 1952). The phenobarbitone is further biotransformed to p-hydroxyphenobarbitone and to a dihydrodiol metabolite (Harvey, Glazener, Stratton, Nowlin, Hill and Horning, 1972).

In one patient Eadie, Bochner, Hooper and Tyrer (1978) calculated that 52 per cent of a methylphenobarbitone dose was converted to phenobarbitone. Most of the remainder of the dose was not accounted for. In three patients, between 9 per cent and 24 per cent of a methylphenobarbitone dose was excreted as phenobarbitone. Therefore metabolites other than phenobarbitone account for a significant portion of a methylphenobarbitone dose.

Excretion

No information is available as to the factors involved in the renal excretion of methylphenobarbitone. One would expect the renal excretion of derived phenobarbitone to be pH dependent (see page 170).

CLINICAL PHARMACOKINETICS

Time course of plasma drug levels

Single dose

Eadie, Bochner, Hooper and Tyrer (1978) showed that, after oral administration, plasma levels of methylphenobarbitone attained a peak within 8 hours of dosage, and then declined monoexponentially. The rate of decline was more rapid in 'induced' subjects and peak plasma methylphenobarbitone levels tended to be lower in these subjects (Fig. 8.9). After a mean interval of 16 hours in 'non-induced' subjects, but more rapidly in 'induced' subjects (mean delay 5 hours) phenobarbitone appeared in plasma. Its levels increased to a peak after a mean time 87 hours from methylphenobarbitone intake. Thereafter plasma phenobarbitone

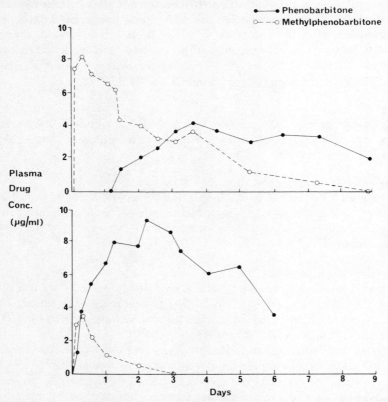

Fig. 8.9 Time-courses of plasma concentrations of methylphenobarbitone and derived phenobarbitone in two patients given their first doses of methylphenobarbitone orally. The subject illustrated in the upper panel had taken no previous anticonvulsants, while the subject illustrated in the lower panel had received other anticonvulsants and may have had his hepatic drug-metabolizing enzymes induced (Eadie, Bochner, Hooper and Tyrer, 1978).

levels declined with mean apparent half-life values of 146 hours in 'non-induced' subjects, and 63 hours in 'induced' subjects. However, these latter values are unlikely to be valid half-lives since phenobarbitone may have still been forming from residual methylphenobarbitone during the apparent phenobarbitone elimination phase.

Multiple doses

With regular administration of the drug once a day, or more often, one might expect plasma methylphenobarbitone levels to achieve a steady state some 8–10 days after therapy began. Derived phenobarbitone might induce the biotransformation of methylphenobarbitone, hence hastening its elimination and reducing the delay till steady state conditions apply. However, since the derived phenobarbitone is 2 or 3 times more slowly eliminated than methylphenobarbitone, it may take 3 or 4 weeks for plasma phenobarbitone levels to reach steady-state values. These phenobarbitone levels are usually a good deal higher than simultaneous plasma methylphenobarbitone levels. As illustrated in Fig. 8.10, steady-state plasma levels of both drug and its active metabolite are likely to show relatively little fluctuation over a dosage interval.

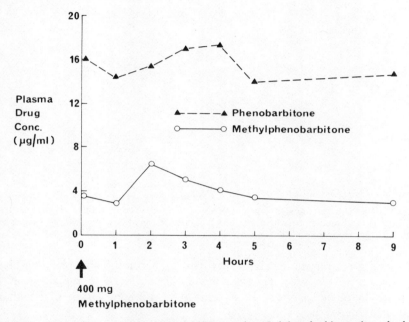

Fig. 8.10 Steady-state plasma levels of phenobarbitone and methylphenobarbitone showed relatively little fluctuation over a 9 hour period in a patient given an unusually large single dose of methylphenobarbitone (400 mg) at the start of the study.

Correlations of plasma drug levels and clinical effects
No data are available correlating plasma methylphenobarbitone levels with clinical effects. The more relevant correlations are those between the derived phenobarbitone and clinical effects. As far as one can judge, the ordinary correlations between the two still largely apply when phenobarbitone is derived from methylphenobarbitone.

Plasma level—dose correlations in treated populations
Eadie, Bochner, Hooper and Tyrer (1978) showed that steady-state plasma concentrations of both methylphenobarbitone and phenobarbitone correlate with methylphenobarbitone dose (Fig. 8.11). However, in the same subjects plasma phenobarbitone levels correlated better with methylphenobarbitone dose than did plasma methylphenobarbitone levels. The relation between simultaneously meas-

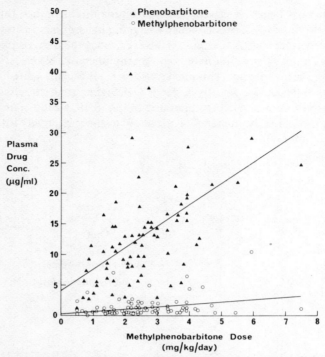

Fig. 8.11 Correlation between simultaneous steady-state plasma concentrations of phenobarbitone (solid triangles) and methylphenobarbitone (open circles) and methylphenobarbitone dose in patients (Eadie, Bochner, Hooper and Tyrer, 1978).

ured steady-state plasma levels of methylphenobarbitone and phenobarbitone is shown in Fig. 8.12. With plasma phenobarbitone levels in the range of 10–20 μg/ml, methylphenobarbitone levels tended to 1/7th to 1/10th of simultaneous phenobarbitone levels.

Effects of age
Eadie, Lander, Hooper and Tyrer (1977) showed that steady-state plasma phenobarbitone levels tended to be lower relative to methylphenobarbitone dose (per unit body weight) in children under 14 years than in persons between 15 to 40 years. Levels were lower relative to dose in persons 15 to 40 years of age than in older persons (Fig. 8.13).

Effects of sex
Eadie, Lander, Hooper and Tyrer (1977) found that males tended to require lower methylphenobarbitone doses than females to achieve the same steady-state plasma phenobarbitone levels (Fig. 8.14). This effect of sex was not detected in children, but occurred in persons over 15 years of age.

Effect of pregnancy
Plasma phenobarbitone levels tend to fall in pregnancy when the phenobaritone is derived from methylphenobarbitone (Lander, Edwards, Eadie, and Tyrer, 1977).

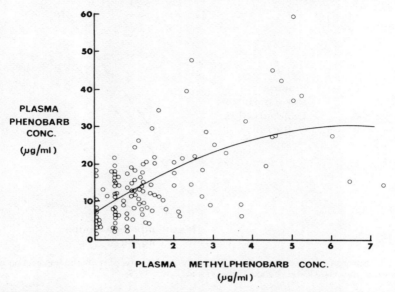

Fig. 8.12 The relation between simultaneous steady-state plasma concentrations of phenobarbitone and methylphenobarbitone in patients taking methylphenobarbitone (Eadie, Bochner, Hooper and Tyrer, 1978).

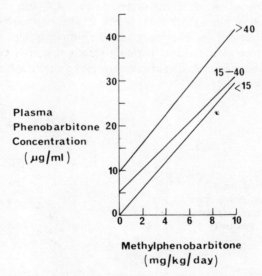

Fig. 8.13 Effect of age on the regression for steady-state plasma phenobarbitone level on methyl-phenobarbitone dose (Eadie, Lander, Hooper and Tyrer, 1977).

Plasma level–dose relationship in treated individuals

In the few individual subjects studied, steady-state plasma methylphenobarbitone levels appear to increase in direct proportion to drug dose. Plasma levels of derived phenobarbitone levels also appear to increase in direct proportion to drug dose

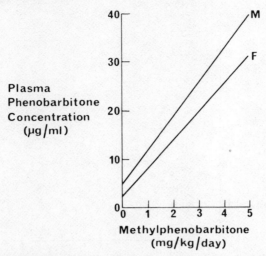

Fig. 8.14 Effect of sex on the regression for steady-state plasma phenobarbitone level on methyl-phenobarbitone dose (Eadie, Lander, Hooper and Tyrer, 1977).

(Figs 8.15 and 8.16). This is unlike the situation which applies when steady-state plasma phenobarbitone levels are measured in individuals given different phenobarbitone doses at different times (Figs. 8.7 and 8.8). The different behaviour of plasma phenobarbitone levels in the two circumstances is unexplained. The behaviour of plasma phenobarbitone levels relative to methyl-phenobarbitone dose in individual patients means that it is easier to manipulate plasma phenobarbitone levels if patients are given methylphenobarbitone rather than phenobarbitone.

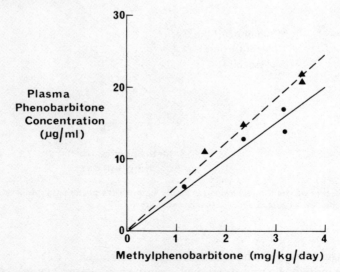

Fig. 8.15 Linear relationship between steady-state plasma levels of phenobarbitone and methylphenobarbitone dose in two patients who received different daily methylphenobarbitone doses at different times (Eadie, Lander, Hooper and Tyrer, 1977).

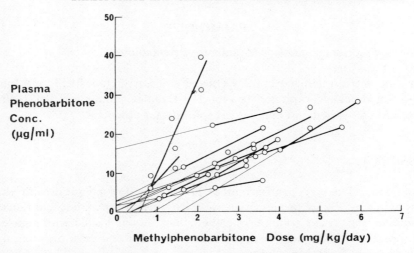

Plasma
Phenobarbitone
Conc.
(µg/ml)

Methylphenobarbitone   Dose (mg/kg/day)

Fig. 8.16 Individual regression lines for steady-state plasma phenobarbitone level on methylphenobarbitone dose in 14 patients. Equal numbers of back-extrapolated regressions intersect the 'x' and the 'y' axes, a finding consistent with the relations between phenobarbitone level and methylphenobarbitone dose being a linear one, with the regression line passing through the origin (Eadie, Lander, Hooper and Tyrer, 1977). This finding differs from that which applies when plasma phenobarbitone levels are derived from phenobarbitone (Fig. 8.8).

Effects of disease

No data are available regarding the effects of disease on methylphenobarbitone pharmacokinetics.

INTERACTIONS

The only information available regarding this matter is based on a multiple variable linear regression analysis on population data carried out by Eadie, Lander, Hooper and Tyrer (1977). This showed that phenytoin, carbamazepine and sulthiame had no statistically significant effect on the relation between plasma methylphenobarbitone or derived phenobarbitone levels and methylphenobarbitone dose.

TOXICITY

The unwanted effects of methylphenobarbitone are essentially those of the phenobarbitone derived from it.

PREPARATIONS AVAILABLE

These include:
Tablets (methylphenobarbitone)—30 mg; 60 mg; 200 mg

PRIMIDONE

Common proprietary names: 'Mysoline', 'Primacolone'

Primidone was synthesized in 1949 (Bogue and Carrington, 1953) and found a place as an anticonvulsant after the report of Handley and Stewart (1952). It may be useful in all varieties of epilepsy except *petit mal* absences.

CHEMISTRY

Primidone (2-desoxyphenobarbitone) has a structure identical with that of phenobarbitone, except for reduction of the carbonyl group at the 2 position of the pyrimidine ring. It is a white, crystalline, almost tasteless solid with a molecular weight of 218.25. The drug is poorly soluble in water and most organic solvents and is virtually neutral in solution.

PHARMACODYNAMICS

In man primidone is biotransformed to phenobarbitone. Many of the apparent actions of primidone, particularly when the drug is used long term, may depend on the phenobarbitone produced from it.

ACTIONS IN MAN

Primidone has the same spectrum of anticonvulsant action as phenobarbitone. It is useful in partial epilepsy and in convulsive seizures which occur as part of generalized epilepsy. The drug is less useful in myoclonic epilepsies, and is of little or no use in the absence seizures of primary generalized epilepsy.

ACTIONS IN ANIMALS

Goodman, Swinyard, Brown, Schiffman, Grewal and Bliss (1953) showed that in mice, before there was time for significant phenobarbitone formation, primidone prevented generalized seizures induced by systemic pentylenetetrazole administration. However, Baumel, Gallagher, Di Micco and Goico (1973) found that primidone did not protect against pentylenetetrazole seizures in rats. Primidone itself also appears to protect against maximum electroshock seizures in mice (Goodman, Swinyard, Brown, Schiffman, Grewal and Bliss, 1953). Frey and Hahn

(1960) found that primidone had little anticonvulsant activity against experimental seizures in guinea pigs. These animals could not biotransform the drug to phenobarbitone.

MECHANISMS OF ACTION

No information is available as to the electrophysiological and biochemical mechanisms of action of primidone itself.

PHARMACOKINETICS

ABSORPTION AND BIOAVAILABILITY

The drug is given by mouth. Little information is available about the bioavailability of primidone. However Kaufmaun, Habersang and Lansky (1977) recovered a mean of 92 per cent of a primidone dose in urine as unchanged drug or metabolites. This suggests that the bioavailability is reasonably complete. The only information relating to primidone absorption is that the T_{max} averages 2·7 hours with a range of 0·5 to 7·0 hours (Gallagher, Baumel and Mattson, 1972), has a mean value of 3 hours (Booker, Hosokowa, Burdette and Darcey, 1970) or $3·2 \pm 1·0$ hours (Gallagher and Baumel, 1972) or a range of 4–6 hours (Kaufmann, Habersang and Lansky, 1977). Gallagher and Baumel (1972) stated that absorption slowed after repeated doses of the drug. However they based this view on alterations in the T_{max} and ignored the fact that the half-life of the drug had also increased, which itself would have prolonged the T_{max}.

DISTRIBUTION

V_d
Van der Kleijn, Guelen, Van Wijk and Baars (1975) quoted a value of 0·60 litres kg^{-1} for the V_d of primidone. This is compatible with a drug distribution through body water.

Plasma protein binding
Neither primidone, nor its metabolite phenylethylmalonamide, is said to bind to any significant extent to plasma protein (Baumel, Gallagher and Mattson, 1972; Gallagher and Baumel, 1972). Troupin and Friel (1975) appeared to find that 25 per cent of primidone in serum was protein bound, but they expressed a lack of confidence in the accuracy of their measurement. Phenobarbitone, the other major metabolite of primidone, binds to plasma protein (page 168).

Concentrations in various body fluids
Since primidone is, for practical purposes, not significantly bound to plasma proteins and not ionized under physiological conditions, one would expect its concentrations in plasma and various body fluids to be very similar. Data are available mainly for CSF and saliva.

Cerebrospinal fluid

CSF levels of primidone averaged 68 per cent (Troupin and Friel, 1975), 80 per cent (Schmidt and Kupferberg, 1975) or 81 per cent (Houghton, Richens, Toseland, Davidson and Falconer, 1975) of plasma primidone levels. Schottelius and Fincham (1977) claimed that the CSF to plasma ratio of primidone was 0·6 if the measurements were carried out 2 to 4 hours after a drug dose, but 0·997 when measured 7 hours after a dose. Findings such as the above might suggest that the whole matter of the plasma protein binding of primidone should be reinvestigated.

Saliva

Mean values for salivary primidone levels relative to simultaneous plasma primidone levels were as follows: 75 per cent (McAuliffe, Sherwin, Leppik, Fayle and Pippenger, 1977), 85 per cent (Horning, Brown, Nowlin, Letratanangkoon, Kellaway and Zion, 1977), 96–97 per cent (Schmidt and Kupferberg, 1975) or 108 per cent (Troupin and Friel, 1975). This scatter in findings is disquieting and perhaps casts doubt on the drug assay methods used.

Milk

Coradello (1973) could not find primidone in the milk of patients taking the drug.

Concentrations in tissues

Van der Kleijn, Guelen, Van Wijk and Baars (1975) found that whole body autoradiography of experimental animals showed that primidone had a similar pattern of distribution to that of phenobarbitone. There were no particular differences in tissue and regional brain distribution. Since the the distribution of radioactivity derived from primidone was studied, it seems possible that to some extent the distribution of derived phenobarbitone may have been demonstrated simultaneously and may have influenced the findings.

Primidone is said to cross the placenta (Martinez and Snyder, 1973).

Brain

Houghton, Richens, Toseland, Davidson and Falconer (1975) measured brain primidone concentrations in human temporal lobectomy specimens. Brain primidone levels averaged 87 per cent of plasma levels in the same subject.

ELIMINATION

Elimination Rate

Van der Kleijn, Guelen, Van Wijk and Baars (1975) gave a value of 0·107 hour^{-1} for the elimination rate constant of primidone in humans. This value corresponds to a half-life of 6·5 hours. Other values quoted for the half-life of the drug are 10–12 hours (Booker, Hosokowa, Burdette and Darcey, 1970), 6·5 ± 1·0 hours (Gallagher and Baumel, 1972), 4·5 to 11 hours (Kaufmann, Habersang and Lansky, 1977), and in a single overdosed patient 15 hours (Brillman, Gallagher and Mattson, 1974). Half-life figures for phenylethylmalonamide (in single cases) were 20 hours (Brillman, Gallagher and Mattson, 1974), 17 and 26 hours (Gallagher,

Baumel and Mattson, 1972) and 29 and 36 hours (Baumel, Gallagher and Mattson, 1972). These values may be overestimates since phenylethylmalonamide may have still been forming from primidone during the measurements.

Clearance
Van der Kleijn, Guelen, Van Wijk and Baars (1975) gave a value of 0·0637 litres kg^{-1} hour^{-1} for the clearance of primidone.

Per cent excreted unchanged
Urine excretion data in children show that 15–66 per cent of a primidone dose is excreted unchanged (Kaufmann, Habersang and Lansky, 1977). Therefore at times biotransformation may not be the major elimination pathway for primidone.

Biotransformation pattern
The known biotransformation pathways for the drug are set out in Fig. 8.17. (It seems likely that the phenobarbitone follows the usual biotransformation pathways for that substance.)

Butler and Waddell (1956) calculated that 15 per cent of a primidone dose was converted to phenobarbitone in humans, and Olesen and Dam (1967) that there was a 24·5 per cent conversion. It seems possible that both these groups of workers may have ignored differences in elimination rates of primidone and phenobarbitone in arriving at these figures. The urine excretion data of Kaufmann, Habersang and Lansky (1977) suggested that in children only 1–8 per cent of a

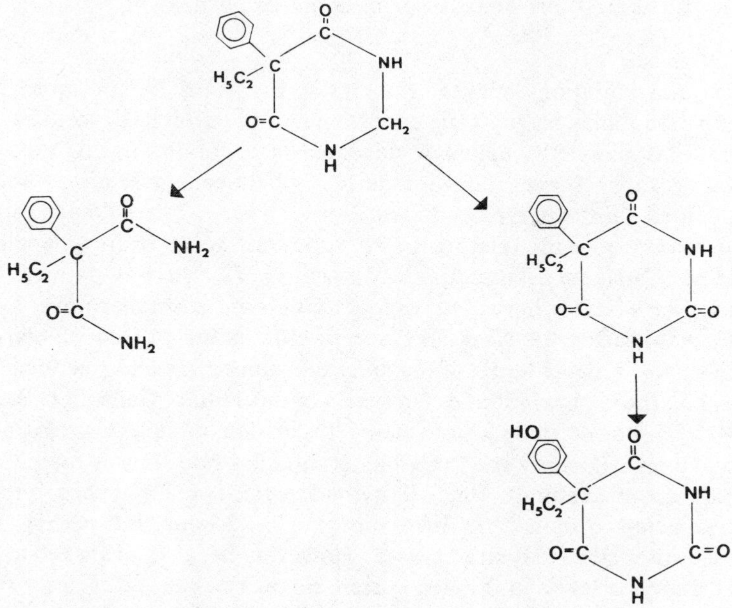

Fig. 8.17 Biotransformation pathways for primidone. The drug molecule may undergo ring scission to form phenylethylmalonamide, or it may be oxidized to form phenobarbitone, the benzene ring of which may then be oxidized to form p-hydroxyphenobarbitone.

primidone dose is converted to phenobarbitone, and that 16–65 per cent is converted to phenylethylmalonamide.

The urine excretion patterns of primidone and its metabolites are given above. At times most of a primidone dose is excreted unchanged in urine. The factors governing its renal excretion have not been studied in detail. However it is known that after overdosage primidone may crystallize out in human urine (Brillman, Gallagher and Mattson, 1974; Cate and Tenser, 1975).

CLINICAL PHARMACOKINETICS

Time course of plasma levels

Single dose
The time course of plasma primidone levels has been defined in the data discussed above. Peak plasma levels occur 2–6 hours after dosage. Plasma primidone levels then decline, apparently monoexponentially, with a half-life of about 5 to 10 hours. Phenylethylmalonamide, which in animals seems to be an anticonvulsant (Gallagher, Smith and Mattson, 1970), appears in the first 24 hours after primidone administration (Gallagher, Baumel and Mattson, 1972). Its level reaches a peak about 8 hours after primidone dosage. Phenylethylmalonamide levels decline more slowly than those of primidone, though few half-life data are available. Phenobarbitone is said not to appear till 2 or 4 days from a primidone dose (Huisman, 1969; Booker, Hosokawa, Burdette and Darcey, 1970; Gallagher and Baumel, 1972). Its levels first rise, and then decline with a half-life of about 4 days. However studies such as that illustrated in Fig. 8.18, suggest that phenobarbitone may sometimes appear within the first few hours of primidone administration.

Repeated doses
Theoretical considerations suggest that, after regular daily (or more frequent) dosage with primidone, steady-state conditions for the drug itself would apply after 1 or 2 days. For phenylethylmalonamide steady-state conditions might be expected to apply after about 1 week, and for derived phenobarbitone after about 3 or 4 weeks, provided elimination rates do not alter with time. There do not appear to be actual measurement data relating to this matter, apart from a single patient illustrated by Gallagher, Baumel and Mattson (1972). In this patient the above expectations were largely borne out, except that plasma phenobarbitone levels were reasonably stable after one week. Because of elimination rate considerations, one might expect steady-state levels of phenylethylmalonamide and phenobarbitone to be higher than those of primidone. However, in one patient Gallagher, Baumel and Mattson (1972) showed that plasma phenylethylmalonamide levels remained below primidone levels. (Possibly the available elimination rate figures for phenylethylmalonamide are inaccurate). Phenylethylmalonamide and phenobarbitone levels might be expected to show little fluctuation over a 12 hour, and perhaps over a 24 hour dosage interval in the steady state. However, because of its relatively short half-life, primidone levels in the steady-state might be expected to show significant variations over 8 to 12 hours, depending on when the measurements are taken in relation to the time of the last dose. This matter often seems to be ignored. Observations on the actual steady-state plasma levels of the three substances in

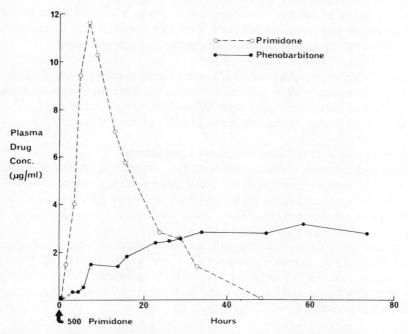

Fig. 8.18 Time-courses of plasma concentrations of primidone and derived phenobarbitone in a patient given his first dose of primidone (500 mg orally).

question over a dosage interval do not appear to be available. We can find no data on steady-state plasma phenylethylmalonamide levels. Booker, Hosokowa, Burdette and Darcey (1970) found that steady-state plasma primidone levels averaged 9·2 μg/ml when simultaneous phenobarbitone levels averaged 31 μg/ml. Gallagher and Baumel (1972) showed that plasma primidone and phenobarbitone levels were in an average ratio of 1:2·5 at a primidone dose of 10 mg/kg/day.

Relation of drug concentration to clinical effects

Anticonvulsant effect

Therapeutic ranges of plasma primidone concentration have been proposed (e.g. 8–12 μg/ml, as suggested by Van der Kleijn, Guelen, Van Wijk and Baars, 1975), while Winek (1976) quoted 10 μg/ml as a therapeutic concentration of primidone. Booker, Hosokowa, Burdette and Darcey (1970) suggested that primidone levels above 10 μg/ml are unlikely to produce further improvement in the control of epilepsy. Schottelius and Fincham (1977) considered that the upper limit of the therapeutic range was 12 μg/ml. Such recommendations seem to ignore the likely steady-state fluctuation in plasma primidone levels during a dosage interval, and also the fact that two other anticonvulsants, phenylethylmalonamide and phenobarbitone are simultaneously present. Phenylethylmalonamide levels are rarely measured, and phenobarbitone levels (which are likely to be in the therapeutic range for this substance) appear to be ignored. In such circumstances one wonders whether it is possible to make any valid recommendations about a therapeutic range of plasma primidone levels. From a clinical point of view it would seem that plasma phenobarbitone levels are more relevant. In practice they provide an adequate guide to primidone therapy in most instances.

Unwanted effects

Brillman, Gallagher and Mattson (1974) stated that depression of consciousness correlated better with plasma primidone level than with plasma phenobarbitone level in a case of primidone overdosage. Winek (1976) regarded plasma primidone levels of 50–80 μg/ml as toxic, and levels of 100 μg/ml as lethal.

Plasma level—dose correlations in treated population

Gallagher and Baumel (1972) published data correlating steady-state plasma primidone levels with primidone dose. There was a moderately wide scatter of data points. On the average, plasma primidone levels increased by 0·74 μg/ml for each 1 mg/kg/day of primidone given. There was a tendency for primidone levels to be disproportionately higher at higher primidone doses.

Plasma phenobarbitone level is proportionate to primidone dose (Gallagher and Baumel, 1972; Eadie, Lander, Hooper and Tyrer, 1977—Fig. 8.19). From Fig. 8.19 it may be seen that a primidone dose of 7·75 mg/kg/day produces an average plasma phenobarbitone level of 15 μg/ml, and a dose of 10 mg/kg/day an average plasma phenobarbitone level of 20 μg/ml.

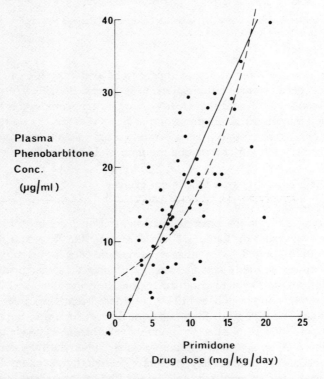

Fig. 8.19 Relation between steady-state plasma levels of derived phenobarbitone and dose of primidone in 58 patients. Linear and curvilinear regressions of best fit are shown (Eadie, Lander, Hooper and Tyrer, 1977).

Effect of age
No data appear to be available on the effect of age on the relation between plasma primidone level and drug dose. Eadie, Lander, Hooper and Tyrer (1977) could not detect an effect of age on the relation between plasma phenobarbitone levels and primidone dose in their patients.

Effects of sex
No data are available regarding the effect of sex on the relation between plasma primidone levels and drug dose. Sex did not alter the relation between plasma phenobarbitone level and primidone dose (Eadie, Lander, Hooper and Tyrer, 1977—Fig. 8.20).

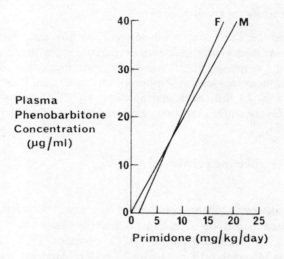

Fig. 8.20 Lack of a statistically significant effect of sex on the regressions for steady-state plasma level of derived phenobarbitone on dose of primidone (Eadie, Lander, Hooper and Tyrer, 1977).

Effects of pregnancy
Plasma levels of phenobarbitone, derived from biotransformation of primidone, may fall during pregnancy without primidone dose being changed (Lander, Edwards, Eadie and Tyrer, 1977).

Plasma level—dose relationships in treated individuals
No data are available as to the effects of dose increments on plasma primidone levels in patients treated with the drug. Our own data do not contain sufficient material on plasma phenobarbitone levels in patients given different doses of primidone at different times to permit the definition of a relation between plasma level and dose in individual patients.

Effects of disease
No data are available as to how disease affects primidone pharmacokinetics.

INTERACTIONS

PHARMACODYNAMIC INTERACTIONS

There may be additive pharmacodynamic anti-epileptic and sedative interactions between primidone and other anticonvulsants, and additive sedative interactions between primidone and various other drugs with cerebral depressant properties. However in such circumstances there is also the question that pharmacokinetic interactions may have been involved.

PHARMACOKINETIC INTERACTIONS

Primidone affecting other substances

It is difficult to be sure that such interactions do not represent effects of phenobarbitone or phenylethylmalonamide derived from primidone, rather than direct effects of primidone itself. However, primidone has been reported to decrease plasma phenytoin levels (Windorfer and Sauer, 1977) or leave these levels unaltered (Sherwin, Loynd, Bock and Sokolowski, 1974) and to decrease plasma carbamazepine levels while increasing carbamazepine -10, 11-epoxide formation (Schneider, 1975).

Other substances affecting primidone

Anticonvulsants

Phenytoin. Concurrent phenytoin therapy increases the biotransformation of primidone to phenobarbitone (Fincham, Schottelius and Sahs, 1974; Reynolds, Fenton, Fenwick, Johnson and Laundy, 1975; Schmidt, 1975; Callaghan, Feely, O'Callaghan and Duggan, 1976; Eadie, Lander, Hooper and Tyrer, 1977; Garrettson and Gomez, 1977; Windorfer and Sauer, 1977).

Carbamazepine. Eadie, Lander, Hooper and Tyrer (1977) and Windorfer and Sauer (1977) found that carbamazepine increased the formation of phenobarbitone from primidone. Cereghino, Van Meter, Brock, Penry, Smith and White (1973) thought carbamazepine might raise plasma primidone levels.

Ethosuximide. Schmidt (1975) found that ethosuximide did not alter plasma primidone levels.

Clonazepam. Nanda, Johnson, Keogh, Lambie and Melville (1977) found that clonazepam did not alter plasma primidone levels, while Windorfer and Sauer (1977) found that clonazepam raised plasma primidone levels.

Valproate. This drug may cause decreased plasma primidone levels (Windorfer and Sauer, 1977) or increased levels of both primidone and derived phenobarbitone (Adams, Luders and Pippenger, 1978).

Acetazolamide. Syversen, Morgan, Weintraub and Myers (1977) obtained evidence that acetazolamide sometimes reduced the absorption of primidone.

Other drugs
Isoniazid. Sutton and Kupferberg (1975) described one patient in whom

concurrent isoniazid intake increased plasma primidone levels and decreased plasma levels of phenylethylmalonamide and phenobarbitone. Interference with primidone biotransformation seemed the likely mechanism.

Methylphenidate. Kupferberg, Jeffrey and Hunninghake (1972) showed that methylphenidate did not alter plasma primidone levels.

Frusemide. This drug does not alter plasma primidone levels (Ahmad, Clarke, Hewett and Richens, 1976).

TOXICITY

The interpretation of primidone toxicity is complicated by the frequent impossibility of knowing whether toxic manifestations are due to the parent substance or to its metabolites phenobarbitone or phenylethylmalonamide. The known toxic manifestations of phenobarbitone may be expected to occur in persons receiving primidone. Little is known of the direct toxicity of phenylethylmalonamide in man (Booker, 1972).

LOCAL EFFECTS

Primidone is almost always administered by mouth but local alimentary tract side effects from the drug seem quite uncommon.

DOSE-DETERMINED SYSTEMIC EFFECTS

These include drowsiness, dizziness, ataxia, nystagmus and diplopia, asterixis (Chadwick, Reynolds and Marsden, 1976), megaloblastic erthyropoiesis and glossitis (Stein and Lewis, 1973) due to folic acid deficiency, vitamin K-dependent bleeding in the neonate, and possible incrimination in osteomalacia as mentioned in Chapter 6. The extent to which these effects depend on phenobarbitone and phenylethylmalonamide is uncertain.

As mentioned earlier, primidone crystalluria has been reported in over-dosed patients (Brillman, Gallagher and Mattson, 1974; Cate and Tenser, 1975).

IDIOSYNCRATIC EFFECTS

Skin rashes, usually maculo-papular but occasionally going on to epidermal necrolysis (Stuttgen, 1973) may occur after the onset of primidone therapy. There have been rare instances of leucopenia and thrombocytopenia, lymphadenopathy and a lupus erythematosus-like syndrome. Personality change occasionally develops after drug therapy is begun (Smith and Forster, 1954) and there has been a report of possible polyneuritis due to primidone (Verdura and Lupi, 1969). Sexual impotence is said to occur in a few patients (Livingstone, 1972). However Hierons and Saunders (1968) have reported instances of impotence apparently due to epilepsy, and improved by therapy with anticonvulsants, including primidone.

Occasional patients become exceedingly drowsy after their first dose of primidone. At one time this was ascribed to excessive metabolic oxidation of primidone to phenobarbitone (Plaa, Fujimoto and Hine, 1958). Data showing that phenobarbitone did not appear in plasma until 2 to 4 days after the administration of primidone (Gallagher and Baumel, 1972) made it likely that gross immediate drowsiness on commencing primidone therapy was due to the drug itself (Gallagher, Baumel, Mattson and Woodbury, 1973). However, findings such as those illustrated in Fig. 8.18 suggest that it may be premature to discard the increased biotransformation hypothesis.

EFFECTS ON THE FETUS AND NEONATE

What has been said regarding phenobarbitone dysmorphogenesis and neonatal coagulation defects might be expected to apply for primidone.

PREPARATIONS AVAILABLE

These include:
  Tablets — 250 mg
  Suspension — 25 mg per ml

DIMETHOXY-METHYLPHENOBARBITONE

There have been several recent publications concerning this substance, sometimes called 'Eterobarb'. It appears to be an anticonvulsant which, dose for dose, is less sedative than phenobarbitone (Gallagher, Baumel, Woodbury and Di Micco, 1975; Smith, Goldstein and Roomet, 1975). The drug is biotransformed to a monomethoxy-derivative, which is also an anticonvulsant in rats (Baumel, Gallagher, Di Micco and Dionne, 1976), and to phenobarbitone and methyl-phenobarbitone (Mattson, Williamson and Hanahan, 1976—Fig. 8.21). Whether dimethoxy-methylphenobarbitone has sufficient advantages to warrant marketing appears problematical.

AMYLOBARBITONE

Common proprietary name: Amytal

Amylobarbitone has been very widely used as a sedative and hypnotic. Its only use in connexion with epilepsy is as a parenteral anticonvulsant for status epilepticus. It will therefore be considered here only in outline.

CHEMISTRY

Amylobarbitone (amobarbital; 5-ethyl-5-isopentyl-barbituric acid) has a M.W. of 226·27. It is white, crystalline material which is poorly soluble in water at pH 7·0.

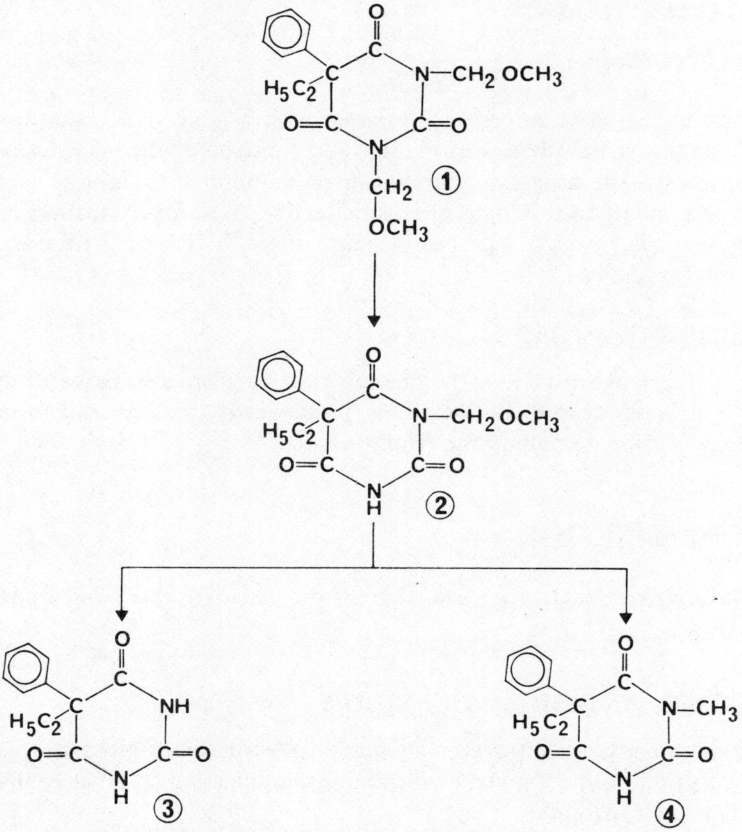

Fig. 8.21 Biotransformation pathway for 'Eterobarb'

1. N,N^1 – dimethoxy-methylphenobarbitone
2. N – monomethoxy-methylphenobarbitone
3. phenobarbitone
4. N – methylphenobarbitone

For parenteral use the drug is given as its sodium salt, which is more water soluble.

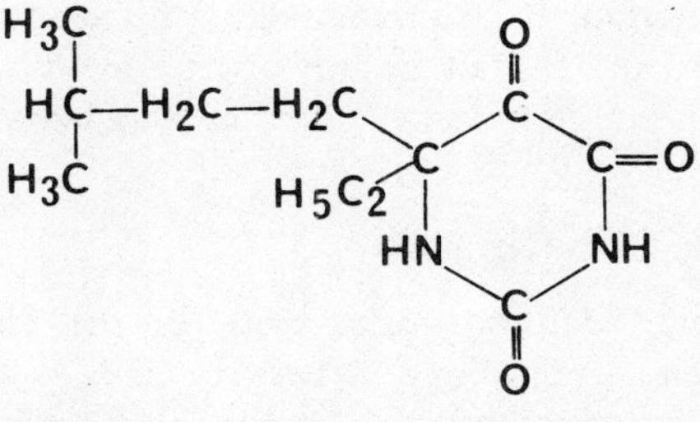

Fig. 8.22 Amylobarbitone

PHARMACODYNAMICS

ACTIONS IN MAN

Amylobarbitone is a sedative and hypnotic with a general depressant effect on neural function. It first depresses higher level function of the nervous system. As dose is increased the drug can depress central autonomic functions.

Given parenterally, the drug is often an effective agent for controlling convulsive status epilepticus, though in excessive dose there is risk of cardiovascular and respiratory depression.

MECHANISM OF ACTION

Biochemically, amylobarbitone is one of the classical agents used to inhibit terminal mitrochondrial oxidation. This action leads to decreased formation of high energy phosphate (adenosine triphosphate).

PHARMACOKINETICS

Some pharmacokinetic data are available for the drug (Inaba, Tang, Endrenyi and Kalow, 1976).

ABSORPTION AND BIOAVAILABILITY

Amylobarbitone is given intravenously for status epilepticus. No data are available for its absorption profile if given by intramuscular injection. If given orally, it has a 99 per cent bioavailability.

DISTRIBUTION

The V_d of the drug is $0 \cdot 5 - 1 \cdot 1$ litre kg^{-1}. Salivary amylobarbitone levels average 36 per cent of serum levels (Inaba and Kalow, 1975).

ELIMINATION

Elimination follows monoexponential kinetics, with a half-life of $23 \cdot 8 \pm 6 \cdot 7$ hours, and a clearance of $2 \cdot 2 \pm 0 \cdot 6$ litres $hour^{-1}$. Elimination is almost exclusively by means of biotransformation. Balasubramanian, Lucas, Mawer and Simons (1970) showed that less than 1 per cent of an amylobarbitone dose was excreted in urine unchanged, though 36 per cent was excreted as 3-hydroxyamylobarbitone.

CLINICAL PHARMACOKINETICS

No data are available relating to the drug in the circumstances in which amylobarbitone is used in neurology. When the drug is given intravenously the anti-epileptic effect may occur while the drug is still in a distributional phase. If so, definitive equilibria between plasma and brain may not yet be established.

INTERACTIONS

Amylobarbitone is likely to interact additively with sedatives or ethyl alcohol to produce an enhanced cerebral depressant effect.

If the drug is given on a long term basis it may induce the hepatic mixed oxidase system, but this is not a relevant consideration in connexion with its mode of use in status epilepticus.

TOXICITY

Local unwanted effects at the sites of parenteral amylobarbitone administration are not common.

In overdosage the drug produces considerable sedation. If dosage is increased further, coma, cardiac and respiratory depression and death may ensure. Drug-withdrawal convulsions may occur if a continued high dose intake of amylobarbitone is ceased abruptly.

PREPARATIONS AVAILABLE

Amylobarbitone sodium — 250 mg; 500 mg ampoules
(The contents of the ampoule must be dissolved in water or saline just before administration. The solution is stable for a few hours only.)

REFERENCES

Adams, D. J., Luders, H. & Pippenger, C. (1978) Sodium valproate in the treatment of intractable seizure disorders: A clinical and electoencephalographic study. *Neurology* (Minneap.), **28**, 152–157.

Ahmad, S., Clarke, L., Hewett, A. J. & Richens, A. (1976) Controlled trial of frusemide as an antiepileptic drug in focal epilepsy. *Brit. J. clin. Pharmacol*, **3**, 621–625.

Aird, R. B. & Woodbury, D. M. (1974) *The management of epilepsy.* Springfield. Charles C. Thomas.

Andresen, B. D., Davis, F. T. & Templeton, J. L. (1976) Synthesis and characterization of alpha phenyl gamma butyrolactone, a metabolite of glutethimide, phenobarbital and primidone, in human urine. *Res. Commun. Chem. Path. Pharmacol.*, **15**, 21–30.

Bachelard, H. S. (1976) Carbohydrate and energy metabolism in relation to mechanisms of epilepsy, in Bradford, H. F. and Marsden, C. D. *Biochemistry and Neurology.* London: Academic Press. 233–246.

Balasubramaniam, K., Lucas, S. B., Mawer, G. E. & Simons, P. T. (1970) The kinetics of amylobarbitone metabolism in healthy men and women. *Brit. J. Pharmacol.*, **39**, 564–572.

Banziger, R. & Hane, D. (1967), Evaluation of a new convulsant for anticonvulsant screening. *Arch. int. Pharmacodyn.*, **167**, 245–249.

Baumel, I. P., Gallagher, B. B., Di Micco, J. & Dionne, R. (1976) Metabolism, distribution and anticonvulsant properties of N,N -dimethoxymethylphenobarbital in the rat. *J. Pharmacol. exp. Therap.*, **196**, 180–187.

Baumel, I. P., Gallagher, B. B., Di Micco, J. & Goico, H. (1973) Metabolism and anticonvulsant properties of primidone in the rat. *J. Pharmacol. exp. Therap.*, **186**, 305–314.

Baumel, I. P., Gallagher, B. B. & Mattson, R. H. (1972) Phenylethylmalonamide (PEMA). An important metabolite of primidone. *Arch. Neurol.* (Chic.), **27**, 34–41.

Baylis, E. M., Crowley, J. M., Preece, J. M., Sylvester, P. E. & Marks, V. (1971) Influence of folic acid on blood-phenytoin levels. *Brit. Med. J.*, **1**, 62–64.

Blum, E. (1932) Die Bekampfung epileptischer Anfalle und iher Folgeer scheimungen mit Prominal. *Deutsch. med. Wschr.* **58**, 230–236.

Blum, J. E., Haefely, W., Jalfre, M., Polc, P. & Schärer, K. (1973) Pharmakologie und Toxicologie des Antiepileptikums Clonazepam. *Arzneim.-Forsch.*, **23**, 377–389.

Bogue, J. Y. & Carrington, H. C. (1953) The evaluation of Mysoline^R—A new anticonvulsant drug. *Brit. J. Pharmacol.*, **8**, 230–235.

Bonnycastle, D. D., Paasonen, M. K. & Giarman, N. J. (1956), Diphenylhydantoin and brain-levels of 5-hydroxytryptamine. *Nature*, **178**, 990–991.

Booker, H. E. (1972) Primidone. Toxicity, in *Antiepileptic drugs* ed. Woodbury, D. M., Penry, J. K. and Schmidt, R. P. Raven Press: New York, 377–383.

Booker, H. E., Hosokowa, K., Burdette, R. K. & Darcey, B. (1970) A clinical study of serum primidone levels. *Epilepsia* (Amst.), **11**, 395–402.

Boreus, L. O., Jalling, B. & Kallberg, N. (1975) Clinical pharmacology of phenobarbital in the neonatal period, in *Basic and therapeutic aspects of perinatal pharmacology* ed. Morselli, P. L., Garrattini, S. and Sereni, F. New York: Raven Press, 331–340.

Boyd, E. M. & Singh, J. (1967) Acute toxicity following rectal thiopental, phenobarbital and leptazole. *Anesth. Analg.*, (Cleve.), **46**, 395–399.

Brillman, J., Gallagher, B. B. & Mattson, R. H. (1974) Acute primidone intoxication. *Arch. Neurol.* (Chic.), **30**, 255–258.

Braithwaite, R. A., Flanagan, R. J. & Richens, A. (1975) Steady state plasma nortriptyline concentrations in epileptic patients. *Brit. J. clin. Pharmacol.*, **2**, 469–471.

Buchthal, F. & Lennox-Buchthal, M. A. (1972) Phenobarbital. Relation of serum concentration to control of seizures, in *Antiepileptic drugs* ed. Woodbury, D. M., Penry, J. K. and Schmidt, R. P. New York: Raven Press. 335–343.

Buchthal, F. & Svensmark, O. (1959), Aspects of the pharmacology of phenytoin (Dilantin) and phenobarbital relevant to their dosage in the treatment of epilepsy. *Epilepsia* (Amst.), **1**, 373–384.

Buchthal, F., Svensmark, O. & Simonsen, H. (1968) Relation of EEG and seizures to phenobarbital in serum. *Arch. Neurol.* (Chic.), **19**, 567–572.

Bunker, J. P. & Vandam, L. D. (1965) Effect of anaesthesia on metabolism and cellular functions. *Pharmacol. Rev.*, **17**, 183–263.

Burstein, S. & Klaiber, E. L. (1965) Phenobarbital induced increase in 6-betahydroxycortisol excretion: clue to its significance in human urine. *J. Clin. Endocrinol. Metab.*, **25**, 293.

Butler, T. C. (1952) Quantitative studies on the metabolic fate of mephobarbital (n-methyl phenobarbital). *J. Pharmacol. exp. Therap.*, **106**, 235–245.

Butler, T. C. (1956) The metabolic hydroxylation of phenobarbital. *J. Pharmacol. exp. Therap.*, **116**, 326–336.

Butler, T. C., Makaffee, C. & Waddell, W. J. (1954) Phenobarbital: Studies of elimination, accumulation, tolerance and dosage schedules. *J. Pharmacol. exp. Therap.*, **111**, 425–435.

Butler, T. C. & Waddell, W. J. (1956) Metabolic conversion of primidone (Mysoline) to phenobarbital. *Proc. Soc. Exptl. Biol. & Med.*, **93**, 544–546.

Callaghan, N., Feely, M., O'Callaghan, M. & Duggan, B. (1976), A survey of some anticonvulsant drug interactions. *Irish J. Med. Sci.*, **145**, 138.

Cate, J. C. IV & Tenser, R. (1975) Acute primidone overdosage with massive crystalluria. *Clin. Toxicol.*, **8**, 385–389.

Cereghino, J. J., Brock, J. T., Van Meter, J. C., Penry, J. K., Smith, L. D. & White, B. G. (1975) The efficacy of carbamazepine combinations in epilepsy. *Clin. Pharmacol. Therap.*, **18**, 733–741.

Cereghino, J. J., Van Meter, J. C., Brock, J. T., Penry, J. K., Smith, L. D. & White, B. G. (1973) Preliminary observations of serum carbamazepine concentration in epileptic patients. *Neurology* (Minneap.), **23**, 357–366.

Chadwick, D., Reynolds, E. H. & Marsden, C. D. (1976) Anticonvulsant-induced dyskinesias: a comparison with dyskinesias induced by neuroleptics. *J. Neurol. Neurosurg. Psychiat.*, **39**, 1210–1218.

Chalazonitis, N. & Arvanitaki, A. (1973) Convulsants and anticonvulsants on single neurons, in *International Encyclopaedia of Pharmacology and Therapeutics* ed. Mercier, J. Section 19 Vol. 2. Oxford. Pergamon Press. 401–354.

Chanarin, I., Mollin, D. L & Anderson, B. B. (1958) Folic acid deficiency and the megaloblastic anaemias. *Proc. roy. Soc. Med.*, **51**, 757.

Conney, A. H. (1967) Pharmacological implications of microsomal enzyme induction. *Pharmacol. Rev.*, **19**, 317–366.

Constantinescu, E., Hategan, D. & Kreindler, A. (1973) Effects of convulsant and anticonvulsant drugs on the activity of some enzymes in the rat brain. *Rev. Roum. Neurol.*, **10**, 353–358.

Cook, C. E., Amerson, E., Poole, W. K., Lesser, P. & O'Tauma, L. (1975) Phenytoin and phenobarbital concentrations in saliva and plasma measured by radioimmunoassay. *Clin. Pharmacol. Therap.*, **18**, 742–747.

Coradello, H. (1973) Ueber die Ausscheidung von Antiepileptika in die Muttermilch. *Wein. Klin.*

Wschr., **85**, 695–697.

Cowger, M. L. & Labbe, R. F. (1967) The inhibition of terminal oxidation by porphyrinogenic drugs. *Biochem. Pharmacol.*, **16**, 2189–2199.

Craig, C. R., Hirano, K. & Shideman, F. E. (1960) Anticonvulsant activity of a metabolite of phenobarbital. *Fed. Proc.*, **19**, 280.

Craig, C. R. & Shideman, F. E. (1971) Metabolism and anticonvulsant properties of mephobarbital and phenobarbital in rats. *J. Pharmacol. exp. Therap.*, **176**, 35–41.

Critchley, E. M. R., Vakil, S. D., Hayward, H. W. & Owen, V. M. H. (1976) Dupuytren's contracture in epilepsy: result of prolonged administration of anticonvulsants. *J. Neurol. Neurosurg. Psychiat.*, **39**, 498–503.

Cucinell, S. A., Conney, A. H., Sansur, M. & Burns, J. J. (1965) Drug interactions in man. 1. Lowering effect of phenobarbital on plasma levels of biohydroxycoumarin (Dicumarol) and diphenylhydantoin (Dilantin). *Clin. Pharmacol. Therap.*, **6**, 420–429.

Dam, M., Mygind, K. I. & Christiansen, J. (1976) Antiepileptic drugs: plasma clearance during pregnancy, in *Epileptology* ed. Janz, D. Stuttgart. Thieme. 179–183.

Davies, J. E., Edmundson, W. F., Carter, C. H. & Barquet, A. (1969) Effect of anticonvulsant drugs on dicophane (D.D.T.) residues in man. *Lancet* ii, 7–9.

Davis, R. E. & Woodliff, H. J. (1971) Folic acid deficiency in patients receiving anticonvulsant drugs. *M. J. Australia* **2**, 1070–1072.

Domek, N. S., Barlow, C. F. & Roth, L. J. (1960) An ontogenic study of phenobarbital-C^{14} in cat brain. *J. Pharmacol. exp. Therap.*, **130**, 285–293.

Dow, R. C., Forfar, J. C. & McQueen, J. K. (1973) The effects of some anticonvulsant drugs on cobalt induced epilepsy. *Epilepsia* (Amst.), **14**, 203–212.

Eadie, M. J., Bochner, F., Hooper, W. D. & Tyrer, J. H. (1978), Preliminary observations on the pharmacokinetics of methylphenobarbitone. *Clin. Exptl. Neurol.*, **15**, 131–144.

Eadie, M. J., Lander, C. M., Hooper, W. D. & Tyrer, J. H. (1976) The effects of phenobarbitone dose on plasma phenobarbitone levels in epileptic patients. *Proc. Aust. Assoc. Neurol.*, **13**, 89–96.

Eadie, M. J., Lander, C. M., Hooper, W. D. & Tyrer, J. H. (1977) Factors influencing plasma phenobarbitone levels in epileptic patients. *Brit. J. clin. Pharmacol.*, **4**, 541–547.

Edmonds, H. L., Stark, L. G. & Hollinger, M. A. (1974) The effect of diphenylhydantoin, phenobarbital and diazepam on the penicillin-induced epileptogenic focus in the rat. *Exp. Neurol.*, **45**, 377–386.

Ehrnebo, M., Agurell, S., Jalling, B., & Boreus, L. O. (1971) Age differences in drug binding by plasma proteins; studies on human foetuses, neonates and adults. *Europ. J. clin. Pharmacol.*, **3**, 189–193.

Erith, M. J. (1975) Withdrawal symptoms in newborn infants of epileptic mothers. *Brit. Med. J.*, iii, 40.

Esplin, D. W. (1963) Criteria for assessing effects of depressant drugs on spinal cord synaptic transmission, with examples of drug selectivity. *Arch. Int. Pharmacodyn.*, **143**, 479–497.

Faero, O., Kastrup, K. W., Lykkegaard Neilsen, E., Melchior, J. C. & Thorn, I. (1972) Successful prophylaxis of febrile convulsions with phenobarbital. *Epilepsia* (Amst.), **13**, 279–285.

Feldman, R. G., Pippinger, C. E. & Florence, M. L. (1975) The relation of anticonvulsant drug levels to complete seizure control. *Epilepsia* (Amst.), **16**, 203–204.

Fincham, R. W., Schottelius, D. D. and Sahs, A. L. (1974) The influence of diphenylhydantoin on primidone metabolism. *Arch. Neurol.* (Chic.), **30**, 259–262.

Formby, B. (1970) The *in vivo* and *in vitro* effect of diphenylhydantoin and phenobarbitone on K^+-activated phosphorohydrolase and (Na^+, K^+)-activated ATPase in particulate membrane fractions from rat brain. *J. Pharm. Pharmac.*, **22**, 81–85.

Frey, H-H. & Hahn, I. (1960) Untersuchungen über die Bedeutung des durch Biotransformation gebildeten Phenobarbital für die anticonvulsive Wirkung von Primidon. *Arch. Int. pharmacodyn.*, **128**, 281–290.

Fromm, G. H. & Landgren, S. (1963) Effect of diphenylhydantoin on single cells in the spinal trigeminal nucleus. *Neurology* (Minneap.), **13**, 34–37.

Gallagher, B. B. & Baumel, I. P. (1972-a) Primidone. Absorption, distribution and excretion, in *Antiepileptic drugs* ed. Woodbury, D. M., Penry, J. K. and Schmidt, R. P. New York: Raven Press, 357–359.

Gallagher, B. B., Baumel, I. P. & Mattson, R. H. (1972) Metabolic disposition of primidone and its metabolites in epileptic subjects after single and repeated administration. *Neurology* (Minneap.), **22**, 1186–1192.

Gallagher, B. B., Baumel, I. P., Mattson, R. H. & Woodbury, S. G. (1973) Primidone, diphenylhydantoin and phenobarbital. Aspects of acute and chronic toxicity. *Neurology* (Minneap.), **23**, 145–149.

Gallagher, B. B., Baumel, I. P., Woodbury, S. G. & Di Micco, J. A. (1975) Clinical evaluation of eterobarb, a new anticonvulsant drug. *Neurology* (Minneap.), **25**, 399–404.

Gallagher, B. B., Smith, D. B. & Mattson, R. H. (1970) The relationship of the anticonvulsant properties of primidone to phenobarbital. *Epilepsia* (Amst.) **11**, 293–301.

Garrettson, L. K. & Dayton, P. G. (1970) Disappearance of phenobarbital and diphenylhydantoin from serum of children. *Clin. Pharm. Therap.*, **11**, 674–679.

Garrettson, L. K. & Gomez, M. (1977) Phenytoin-primidone interaction. *Brit. J. clin. Pharmacol.*, **4**, 693–695.

Gillette, J. R. (1963) Metabolism of drugs and other foreign compounds by enzymatic mechanisms. *Prog. Drug. Res.*, **6**, 11–73.

Glazko, A. J. (1975) Antiepileptic drugs: biotransformation, metabolism and serum half-life. *Epilepsia* (Amst.), **16**, 367–391.

Goldbaum, L. R. & Smith, P. K. (1954) The interaction of barbiturates with serum albumin and its possible relation to their disposition and pharmacological actions. *J. Pharmacol. exp. Therap.*, **111**, 197–209.

Goodman, L. S., Swinyard, E. A., Brown, W. C., Schiffman, D. O., Grewal, M. S. & Bliss, E. L. (1953) Anticonvulsant properties of 5-phenyl-5-ethyl-hexahydropyrimidine-4,6-dione (Mysoline), a new antiepileptic. *J. Pharmacol. exp. Therap.*, **108**, 428–436.

Graham, J. (1978) A comparison of the absorption of phenobarbitone given via the oral and the intramuscular route. *Clin. Exptl. Neurol.*, **15**, 154–158.

Guelen, P. J. M., Van der Kleijn, E. & Woudstra, U. (1975) Statistical analysis of pharmacokinetic parameters in epileptic patients chronically treated with antiepileptic drugs, in *Clinical pharmacology of anti-epileptic drugs* ed. Schneider, H., Janz, D., Gardner-Thorpe, C., Meinardi, H. and Sherwin, A. L. Berlin: Springer. 2–10.

Handley, R. & Stewart, A. S. R. (1952) Mysoline[R]: A new drug in the treatment of epilepsy. *Lancet*, i, 742–744.

Hansson, O. & Sillanpaa, M. (1976) Pyridoxine and serum concentrations of phenytoin and phenobarbitone. *Lancet*, i, 256.

Harvey, D. J., Glazener, L., Stratton, C., Nowlin, J., Hill, R. M. & Horning, M. G. (1972) Detection of a 5-(3,4-dihydroxy-1,5-cyclohexadiene-1-yl)-metabolite of phenobarbital and mephobarbital in rat, guinea pig and human. *Res. Commun. Chem. Pathol. & Pharmacol.*, **3**, 557–566.

Hauptmann, A. (1912) Luminal bei Epilepsie. *Munch. med. Wschr.*, **59**, 1907–1909.

Heckmatt, J. Z., Houston, A. B., Clow, D. J., Stephenson, J. B. P., Dodd, K. L., Lealman, G. T. & Logan, R. W. (1976) Failure of phenobarbitone to prevent febrile convulsions. *Brit. Med. J.*, i, 559–561.

Hierons, R. & Saunders, M. (1966) Impotence in patients with temporal-lobe lesions. *Lancet*, ii, 761–764.

Hooper, W. D., Dubetz, D. K., Bochner, F., Cotter, L. M., Smith, G. A., Eadie, M. J. & Tyrer, J. H. (1975) Plasma protein binding of carbamazepine. *Clin. Pharmacol. Therap.*, **17**, 433–440.

Hooper, W. D., Sutherland, J. M., Bochner, F., Tyrer, J. H. & Eadie, M. J. (1973) The effect of certain drugs on the plasma protein binding of diphenylhydantoin. *Aust. N.Z. J. Med.*, **3**, 377–381.

Horning, M. G., Brown, L., Nowlin, J., Letratanangkoon, K., Kellaway, P. & Zion, T. E. (1977) Use of saliva in therapeutic drug monitoring. *Clin. Chem.*, **23**, 157–164.

Horning, M. G., Butler, C. M., Nowlin, J. & Hill, R. (1975) Drug metabolism in the human neonate. *Life Science* **16**, 651–671.

Horning, M. G., Nowlin, J., Butler, C. M., Letratanangkoon, K., Sommer, K. & Hill, R. M. (1975) Clinical applications of gas chromatograph/mass spectrometer/computer systems. *Clin. Chem.*, **21**, 1282–1287.

Houghton, G. W., Richens, A., Toseland, P. A., Davidson, S. & Falconer, M. A. (1975) Brain concentrations of phenytoin, phenobarbitone and primidone in epileptic patients. *Europ. J. Clin. Pharmacol.* **9**, 73–78.

Huisman, J. W. (1969) Disposition of primidone in man: An example of auto-induction of a human enzyme system. *Pharm. Weekbl.*, **104**, 799–802.

Huisman, J. W., Van Heycop Ten Ham, M. W. & Van Zijl, C. W. H. (1970) Influence of ethylphenacetamide on serum levels of other anti-epileptic drugs. *Epilepsia* (Amst.), **11**, 207–215.

Hvidberg, E. F. & Dam, M. (1976) Clinical pharmacokinetics of anticonvulsants. *Clin. Pharmacokinetics*, **1**, 161–188.

Inaba, T. & Kalow, W. (1975) Salivary excretion of amobarbital in man. *Clin. Pharmacol. Therap.*, **18**, 558–562.

Inaba, T., Tang, B. K., Endrenyi, L., & Kalow, W. (1976) Amobarbital—a probe of hepatic drug oxidation in man. *Clin. Pharm. Therap.*, **20**, 439–444.

Johannessen, S. I. & Strandjord, R. E. (1975) Absorption and protein binding in serum of several anti-epileptic drugs, in *Clinical pharmacology of antiepileptic drugs* ed. Schneider, H., Janz, D.,

Gardner-Thorpe, C., Meinardi, H. and Sherwin, A. L. Berlin. Springer. 262–273.
Johanessen, S. I., Strandjord, R. E. & Munthekaas, A. W. (1977) Lack of effect of clonazepam on serum levels of diphenylhydantoin, phenobarbital and carbamazepine. *Acta neurol. Scandinav.*, **55**, 506–512.
Jordan, B. J., Shillingford, J. S. & Steed, K. P. (1976) Preliminary observations in the protein-binding and enzyme-inducing properties of sodium valproate (Epilim), in *Clinical and pharmacological aspects of sodium valproate (Epilim), in the treatment of epilepsy.* Tunbridge Wells. M.C.S. Consultants., 112–116.
Kållberg, N., Agurell, S., Ericcson, O., Bucht, E., Jalling, B. & Boreus, L. O. (1975) Quantitation of phenobarbital and its main metabolites in human urine. *Europ. J. Clin. Pharmacol.*, **9**, 161–168.
Kaufmann, R. E., Habersang, R. & Lansky, L. (1977) Kinetics of primidone metabolism and excretion in children. *Clin. Pharmacol. Therap.*, **22**, 200–206.
Kristensen, M., Hansen, J. M. & Skovsted, L. (1969) The influence of phenobarbital on the half-life of diphenylhydantoin in man. *Acta med. Scand.*, **185**, 347–350.
Kupferberg, H. J., Jeffrey, W. & Hunninghake, D. B. (1972) Effect of methylphenidate on plasma anticonvulsant level. *Clin. Pharmacol. Therap.*, **13**, 201–204.
Kutt, H. (1974) Mechanism of action of antiepileptic drugs, in *Handbook of clinical neurology* ed. Vinken, P. J. and Bruyn G. W. Amsterdam. North Holland Publishing Co. Vol. 15, 621–663.
Kyoguku, Y. & Yu, B. S. (1968) The specific hydrogen bonding of riboflavin derivatives to an adenine compound. *Bull. Chem. Soc. Jap.*, **31**, 1742–1772.
Lacy, J. R. & Smith, D. B. (1973) The effect of folic acid and citrovorum factor on the anticonvulsant activity of phenobarbital. *Epilepsia* (Amst.), **14**, 96.
La Manna, J. C., Cordingley, G. & Rosenthal, M. (1977) Phenobarbital action *in vivo*: effects on extracellular potassium activity and oxidative metabolism in cat cerebral cortex. *J. Pharmacol. exp. Therap.*, **200**, 560–569.
Lambie, D. G., Nanda, R. M., Johnson, R. H. & Shakir, R. A. (1976) Therapeutic and pharmacokinetic effects of increasing phenytoin in chronic epileptics on multiple drug therapy. *Lancet*, **vii**, 386–389.
Lander, C. M., Edwards, V. E., Eadie, M. J. & Tyrer, J. H. (1977) Plasma anticonvulsant concentrations during pregnancy. *Neurology* (Minneap.), **27**, 128–131.
Lecamwasam, D. S., Franklin, C. & Turner, P. (1975) Effect of phenobarbitone on hepatic drug metabolizing enzymes and urinary D-glucaric acid excretion in man. *Brit. J. clin. Pharmacol.*, **2**, 257–262.
Levi, A. J., Sherlock, S. & Walker, D. (1968) Phenylbutazone and isoniazid metabolism in patients with liver disease in relation to previous drug therapy. *Lancet*, **ii**, 1275–1279.
Leznicki, A. & Dymecki, J. (1974) The effect of certain anticonvulsants *in vivo* on enzyme activities in the rat's brain. *Neurol. Neurochir. Pol.*, **24**, 413–419.
Lidbrink, P. and Farnebo, L. O. (1973) Uptake and release of noradrenaline in rat cerebral cortex *in vitro*: no effect of benzodiazepines and barbiturates. *Neuropharmacology*, **12**, 1087–1095.
Linarelli, L. G., Hengstenberg, F. H. & Drash, A. L. (1973) Effect of phenobarbital on hyperlipemia in patients with intrahepatic and extrahepatic cholestasis. *J. Pediat.*, **83**, 291–293.
Livingstone, S. (1972) *Comprehensive management of epilepsy in infancy, childhood and adolescence.* Springfield, Charles C. Thomas.
Livingstone, S., Berman, W. & Pauli, L. L. (1975) Anticonvulsant drug blood levels. Practical applications based on 12 years' experience. *J. Amer. Med. Assoc.*, **232**, 60–62.
Loescher, W. & Frey, H. H. (1977) Effect of convulsant and anticonvulsant agents on level and metabolism of γ-aminobutyric acid in mouse brain. *Naunyn Schmied. Arch. Pharm.*, **296**, 263–269.
Loiseau, P., Brachet Liermain, A., Legroux, M. & Jogeix, M. (1977) Intérêt du dosage des anticonvulsivants dans le traitement des épilepsies. *Nouv. Presse Med.*, **6**, 813–817.
Lous, P. (1954-a) Blood serum and cerbrospinal fluid levels and renal clearance of Phenemal in treated epileptics. *Acta pharmacol. et toxicol.*, **10**, 166–177.
Lous, P. (1954-b) Plasma levels and urinary excretion of three barbituric acids after oral administration to man. *Acta pharmacol. et toxicol.*, **10**, 147–165.
Lous, P. (1966) Elimination of barbiturates, in *Barbiturate poisoning and tetanus* ed. Johansen, S. H. Boston. Little Brown and Co. 341–350.
Lunde, P. K. M., Rane, A., Yaffe, S. J., Lund, L. & Sjöqvist, F. (1970) Plasma protein binding of diphenylhydantoin in man. Interaction with other drugs and effect of temperature and plasma dilution. *Clin. Pharmacol. Therap.*, **11**, 846–855.
McAuliffe, J. J., Sherwin, A. L., Leppik, I. E., Fayle, S. A. & Pippenger, C. E. (1977) Salivary levels of anticonvulsants: a practical approach to drug monitoring. *Neurology* (Minneap.), **27**, 409–413.
McGeachy, T. E. & Bloomer, W. E. (1953) The phenobarbital sensitivity syndrome. *Am. J. Med.*, **14**, 600–604.
Mark, L. C. (1963) Metabolism of barbiturates in man. *Clin. Pharmacol. Therap.*, **4**, 504–530.

208   ANTICONVULSANT THERAPY

Martinez, G. & Snyder, R. D. (1973) Transplacental passage of primidone. *Neurology* (Minneap.), **23**, 381–383.
Mattson, R. H., Gallagher, B. B., Reynolds, E. H. & Glass, D. (1973) Folate therapy in epilepsy. A controlled study. *Arch. Neurol.* (Chic.), **29**, 78–81.
Mattson, R. H., Williamson, P. D. & Hanahan, E. (1976) Eterobarb therapy in epilepsy. *Neurology* (Minneap.), **26**, 1014–1017.
Maynert, E. W. (1972) Phenobarbital, mephobarbital and metharbital. Absorption, distribution and excretion, in *Antiepileptic drugs* ed. Woodbury, D. M., Penry, J. K. and Schmidt, R. P. New York: Raven Press, 303–310.
Meinardi, H., Van der Kleijn, E., Meijer, J. W. A. & Van Rees, H. (1975) Absorption and distribution of antiepileptic drugs. *Epilepsia* (Amst.), **16**, 353–365.
Meadow, S. R. (1970) Congenital abnormalities and anticonvulsant drugs. *Proc. Roy. Soc. Med.*, **63**, 48–49.
Melchior, J. C., Svensmark, O. & Trolle, D. (1967) Placental transfer of phenobarbitone in epileptic women, and elimination in newborns. *Brit. Med. J.*, ii, 860–861.
Meldrum, B. S., Horton, R. W. & Toseland, P. A. (1975) A primate model for testing anticonvulsant drugs. *Arch. Neurol.* (Chic.), **32**, 288–294.
Mori, A. (1974) Neuropharmacologic studies on anticonvulsants. *Brain Develop.*, **6**, 435–440.
Morrell, F., Bradley, W. & Ptashne, M. (1959) Effect of drugs on discharge characteristics of chronic epileptogenic lesions. *Neurology* (Minneap.) **9**, 492–498.
Morselli, P. L., Rizzo, M. & Garattini, S. (1971) Interaction between phenobarbital and diphenylhydantoin in animals and in epileptic patients. *Proc. N.Y. Acad. Sci.*, **179**, 88–107.
Mountain, K. R., Hirsch, J. & Gallus, A. S. (1970) Neonatal coagulation defect due to anticonvulsant drug treatment in pregnancy. *Lancet*, i, 265–268.
Mygind, K. I., Dam, M., & Christiansen, J. (1976) Phenytoin and phenobarbitone plasma clearance during pregnancy. *Acta neurol. Scandinav.*, **54**, 160–166.
Nanda, R. N., Johnson, R. H., Keogh, H. J., Lambie, D. G. & Melville, I. D. (1977) Treatment of epilepsy with clonazepam and its effect on other anticonvulsants. *J. Neurol. Neurosurg. Psychiat.*, **40**, 538–543.
Neuman, R. S. & Frank, G. B. (1977) Effects of diphenylhydantoin and phenobarbital on voltage clamped myelinated nerve. *Canad. J. Physiol.*, **55**, 42–47.
Neuvonen, P. J. & Penttilä, O. (1974) Interaction between doxycycline and barbiturates. *Brit. Med. J.* i, 535–536.
Neuvonen, P. J., Penttilä, O., Lehtovarra, R. & Aho, K. (1975) Effect of antiepileptic drugs on the elimination of various tetracycline derivatives. *Europ. J. clin. Pharmacol.*, **9**, 147–154.
Nies, A. S., Shand, D. G. & Branch, R. A. (1974) Hemodynamic drug interactions: the effects of altering hepatic blood flow on drug disposition, in Morselli, P. L., Garattini, S. and Cohen, S. N. *Drug interactions*. New York: Raven Press, 231–240.
Olesen, O. V. & Dam, M. (1967) The metabolic conversion of primidone (Mysoline) to phenobarbitone in patients under long-term treatment. *Acta neurol. Scandinav.*, **43**, 348–356.
Ouvrier, R. A. & Goldsmith, R. (1977) Phenobarbitone dosage in the neonate. *Clin. Exp. Neurol.*, **14**, 194–202.
Painter, M. J., Pippenger, C., Carter, G. & Pitlick, W. (1977) Metabolism of phenobarbital and phenytoin by neonates with seizures. *Neurology* (Minneap.), **27**, 370.
Perry, T. L., Hansen, S. & Maclean, J. (1976) Cerebro-spinal fluid and plasma glutamine elevation by anticonvulsant drugs: a potential diagnostic and therapeutic trap. *Clin. Chem. Acta*, **69**, 441–445.
Pertschuk, L. P., Ford, D. H., Rainford, E. A. & Brigati, D. J. (1976) Localization of phenobarbital in mouse control nervous system by immunofluorescence. *Acta. neurol. Scandinav.*, **53**, 325–334.
Petsche, H. (1972) Demonstration of cortical point of application of the benzodiazepine derivative clonazepam; (Ro 5–4023) *E.E.G. E.M.G.*, **3**, 145–153.
Pincus, J. H., Grove, I., Marino, B. B. & Glaser, G. E. (1970) Studies on the mechanism of action of diphenylhydantoin. *Arch. Neurol.* (Chic.), **22**, 566–571.
Pippenger, C. E. & Rosen T. S. (1975) Phenobarbital plasma levels in neonates. *Clinics in Perinatology*, **2**, 111–115.
Pitlick, W., Painter, M. & Pippenger, C. (1978) Phenobarbital pharmacokinetics in neonates. *Clin. Pharmacol. Therap.*, **23**, 346–350.
Plaa, G. L., Fujimoto, J. M. & Hine, C. H. (1958) Intoxication from primidone due to its biotransformation to phenobarbital. *J. Amer. med. Ass.*, **168**, 1769–1770.
Plaa, G. L. & Hine, C. C. (1960) Hydantoin and barbiturate blood levels observed in epileptics. *Arch. int. Pharmacodyn.*, **128**, 375–382.
Prichard, J. W. (1972) Effect of phenobarbital on a leech neuron. *Neuropharmacology*, **11**, 589–590.
Reynolds, E. H. (1976) Folate and epilepsy, in Bradford, H. F. and Marsden, C. D. *Biochemistry and*

Neurology. London: Academic Press, 247–252.

Reynolds, E. H., Fenton, G., Fenwick, P., Johnson, A. L. & Laundy, M. (1975) Interaction of phenytoin and primidone. *Brit. Med. J.*, ii, 594–595.

Reynolds, E. H. & Travers, R. D. (1974) Serum anticonvulsant concentrations in epileptic patients with mental symptoms. A preliminary report. *Brit. J. Psychiat.*, 124, 440–445.

Richens, A. (1974) Drug estimation in the treatment of epilepsy. *Proc. roy. Soc. Med.*, 67, 1227–1229.

Riegelman, S., Rowland, M. & Epstein, W. L. (1970) Griseofulvin phenobarbital interaction in man. *J. Amer. Med. Ass.*, 213, 426–431.

Rizzo, M., Morselli, P. L. & Garattini, S. (1972) Further observations on the interactions between phenobarbital and diphenylhydantoin during chronic treatment in the rat. *Biochem. Pharmacol.*, 21, 449–454.

Rosenberg, P. & Bartels, E. (1967) Drug effects on the spontaneous electrical activity of the squid giant axon. *J. Pharmacol. exp. Therap.*, 155, 532–544.

Saad, S. F., El Masry, A. M. & Scott, P. M. (1972) Influence of certain anticonvulsants on the concentration of γ aminobutyric acid in the cerebral hemispheres of mice. *Europ. J. Pharmacol.*, 17, 386–392.

Sanders, H. D. (1967) A comparison of the convulsant activity of procaine and pentylenetetrazole. *Arch. int. Pharmacodyn.*, 170, 165–177.

Sawaya, M. C. B., Horton, R. W. & Meldrum, B. S. (1975) Effects of anticonvulsant drugs on the cerebral enzymes metabolizing GABA. *Epilepsia* (Amst.), 16, 649–655.

Schallek, W. & Kuehn, A. (1963) Effects of trimethadione, diphenylhydantoin and chlordiazepoxide on after-discharges in brain of cat. *Proc. Soc. exp. Biol. N.Y.*, 112, 813–817.

Schmidt, D. (1975) The effect of phenytoin and ethosuximide on primidone metabolism in patients with epilepsy. *J. Neurol.*, 209, 115–123.

Schmidt, D. & Kupferberg, H. J. (1975) Diphenylhydantoin, phenobarbital and primidone in saliva, plasma and cerebrospinal fluid. *Epilepsia* (Amst.), 16, 735–741.

Schneider, H. (1975) Carbamazepine: the influence of other anti-epileptic drugs on its serum level, in *Clinical pharmacology of anti-epileptic drugs* ed. Schneider, H., Janz, D., Gardner-Thorpe, C., Meinardi, H. and Sherwin, A. L. Berlin: Springer. 189–195.

Schobben, E., Van der Kleijn, E. & Gabreels, F. J. M. (1975) Pharmacokinetics of di-N-propylacetate in epileptic patients. *Europ. J. Clin. Pharmacol.*, 8, 97–105.

Schottelius, D. D. & Fincham, R. W. (1977) Clinical application of serum primidone levels in Pippenger, G. E., Penry, J. K. and Kutt, H. *Antiepileptic drugs—quantitative analysis and interpretation*. New York: Raven Press. 273–282.

Shapiro, S., Hartz, S. C., Siskind, V., Mitchell, A. C., Slone, D., Rosenberg, L., Monson, R. R., Heinonen, O. P., Idanpaan-Heikkila, J., Haro, S. & Saxén, L. (1976) Anticonvulsants and parental epilepsy in the development of birth defects. *Lancet*, i, 272–275.

Sherwin, A. L., Eisen, A. A., & Sokolowski, C. D. (1973) Anticonvulsant drugs in human epileptogenic brain. *Arch. Neurol.* (Chic.), 29, 73–77.

Sherwin, A. L., Loynd, J. S., Bock, G. W. & Sokolowski, C. D. (1974) Effect of age, sex, obesity and pregnancy on plasma diphenylhydantoin levels. *Epilepsia* (Amst.), 15, 507–521.

Shulman, A. (1970) The pharmacology of barbiturates. *M. J. Australia*, 1, 1199–1204.

Smith, B., & Forster, F. M. (1954) Mysoline(R) and milontin (two new medicines for epilepsy). *Neurology* (Minneap.), 4, 137–142.

Smith, D. B., Goldstein, S. G. & Roomet, A. (1975) A comparison of the hypnotic effect of the anticonvulsant dimethoxymethylphenobarbital and sodium phenobarbital in normal human volunteers. *Epilepsia* (Amst.), 16, 201.

Smith, S. J., Lui, K. K., Leonard, T. B., Duceman, B. W. & Vesell, E. S. (1976) Molecular biology of phenobarbital actions and interactions. *Ann. N.Y. Acad. Sci.*, 281, 372–383.

Sohn, R. S. & Ferrendelli, J. A. (1976) Anticonvulsant drug mechanisms. Phenytoin, phenobarbital and ethosuximide and calcium flux in isolated presynaptic endings. *Arch. Neurol.* (Chic.), 33, 626–629.

Staples, R. E. (1972) Teratology, in *Antiepileptic Drugs* ed. Woodbury, D. M., Penry, J. K. and Schmidt, R. P. New York: Reven Press. 55–62.

Stark, L. G., Killam, K. F. & Killam, E. K. (1970) The anticonvulsant effects of phenobarbital, diphenylhydantoin and two benzodiazepines in the baboon, Papio papio. *J. Pharmacol. exp. Therap.*, 173, 125–132.

Stein, G. M. & Lewis, H. (1973) Oral changes in a folic acid deficient patient precipitated by anticonvulsant drug therapy. *J. Periodont.*, 44, 645–650.

Strobos, R. R. J. & Spudis, E. V. (1969) Effect of anticonvulsant drugs on cortical and subcortical seizure discharges in cats. *Arch. Neurol.*, (Chic.), 2, 399–406.

Stuttgen, G. (1973) Total epidermal necrolysis provoked by barbiturates. *Brit. J. Derm.*, 88, 291–293.

Sutton, G. & Kupferberg, H. J. (1975) Isoniazid as an inhibitor of primidone metabolism. *Neurology* (Minneap.), **25**, 1179–1181.

Svensmark, O. & Buchthal, F. (1963) Accumulation of phenobarbital in man. *Epilepsia* (Amst.), **4**, 199–206.

Svensmark, O. & Buchthal, F. (1964) Diphenylhydantoin and phenobarbital. Serum levels in children. *Amer. J. Dis. Child.*, **108**, 82–87.

Svensmark, O., Schiller, P. J. & Buchthal, F. (1960) 5,5-diphenylhydantoin (Dilantin^R) blood levels after oral or intravenous dosage in man. *Acta. pharmacol. et toxicol.*, **16**, 331–346.

Swaiman, K. F. & Stright, P. L. (1973) The effect of anticonvulsants on *in vitro* protein synthesis in immature brain. *Brain Res.* (Amst.), **58**, 515–518.

Swinyard, E. A. & Castellion, A. W. (1966) Anticonvulsant properties of some benzodiazepines. *J. Pharmacol. exp. Therap.*, **151**, 369–375.

Syversen, G. B., Morgan, J. P., Weintraub, M. & Myers, J. (1977) Acetazolamide induced interference with primidone absorption: case reports and metabolic studies. *Arch. Neurol.* (Chic.), **34**, 80–84.

Takeda, A., Goto, H., Amano Y. & Kukino, K. (1976) A study on serum and cerebrospinal fluid levels of sodium valproate (DPA), a new antiepileptic drug. *Brain Develop.*, **8**, 1401–408.

Tang, B. K., Inaba, T. & Kalow, W. (1977) N-hydroxyphenobarbital—The major metabolite of phenobarbital in man. *Fed. Proc.*, **36**, 966.

Thompson, R. H. P., Eddleston, A. L. W. F. & Williams, R. (1969) Low plasma-bilirubin in epileptics on phenobarbitone. *Lancet*, **i**, 21–22.

Thorn, I. (1975) A controlled study of prophylactic long-term treatment of febrile convulsions with phenobarbital. *Acta neurol. Scandinav. Suppl.*, **60**, 67–73.

Tower, D. B. & Elliott, K. A. C. (1953) Experimental production and control of an abnormality in acetylcholine metabolism present in epileptogenic cortex. *J. Appl. Physiol.*, **5**, 375–391.

Troupin, A. S. & Friel, P. (1975) Anticonvulsant levels in saliva, serum and cerbrospinal fluid. *Epilepsia* (Amst.), **16**, 223–227.

Vajda, F., Williams, F. M., Davidson, S., Falconer, M. A. & Breckenridge, A. (1974) Human brain, cerebrospinal fluid and plasma concentrations of diphenylhydantoin and phenobarbital. *Clin. Pharmacol. Therap.*, **15**, 597–603.

Vakil, S. D., Critchley, E. M. R., Philips, J. C., Fahim, Y., Haydock, C., Cocks, A. & Dyer, T. (1976) The effect of sodium valproate (Epilin) on phenytoin and phenobarbitone blood levels, in *Clinical and pharmacological aspects of sodium valproate (Epilim) in the treatment of epilepsy*. Tunbridge Wells: M.C.S. Consultants, 75–77.

Van der Kleijn, E., Guelen, P. J. M., Van Wijk, C. & Baars, I. (1975) Clinical pharmacokinetics in monitoring chronic medication with anti-epileptic drugs, in *Clinical pharmacology of antiepileptic drugs* ed. Schneider, H., Janz, D., Gardner-Thorpe, C., Meinardi, H. and Sherwin, A. L. Berlin: Springer. 11–33.

Verdura, G. & Lupi, G. (1969) La prevenzione e la terapia degli effetti neurotossici acuti da 'primidone'. *Aggiorw. Pediatr.*, **20**, 81–86.

Vesell, E. S. & Page, J. G. (1969) Genetic control of the phenobarbital-induced shortening of plasma antipyrine half-lives in man. *J. Clin. Invest.*, **48**, 2202–2209.

Wada, J. A. (1977) Pharmacological prophylaxis in the kindling model of epilepsy. *Arch. Neurol.* (Chic.), **34**, 389–395.

Waddell, W. J. & Butler, T. C. (1957) The distribution and excretion of phenobarbital. *J. Clin. Invest.*, **36**, 1217–1226.

Weinberger, J., Nicklas, W. J. & Berl, S. (1976) Mechanism of action of anticonvulsants. Role of the differential effects on the active uptake of putative neurotransmitters. *Neurology* (Minneap.), **26**, 162–166.

Welton, D. G. (1950) Exfoliative dermatitis and hepatitis due to phenobarbital. *J. Amer. med. Ass.*, **143**, 232–234.

Whyte, M. P. & Dekaban, A. S. (1977) Metabolic fate of phenobarbital. A quantitative study of p-hydroxyphenobarbital elimination in man. *Drug Metabolism Distribution*, **5**, 63–70.

Wilson, J. T. & Wilkinson G. R. (1973) Chronic and severe phenobarbital intoxication in a child treated with primidone and diphenylhydantoin. *J. Pediat.*, **83**, 484–489.

Windorfer, A. Jr. & Pringsheim, W. (1977) Studies on the concentrations of chloramphenicol in the serum and cerebrospinal fluid of neonates, infants and small children. Reciprocal reactions between chloramphenicol, penicillin and phenobarbitone. *Europ. J. Pediat.*, **124**, 129–138.

Windorfer, A. Jr. & Sauer, W. (1977) Drug interactions during anticonvulsant therapy in childhood: Diphenylhydantoin, primidone, phenobarbitone, clonazepam, nitrazepam, carbamazepine and dipropylacetate. *Neuropadiatrie*, **8**, 29–41.

Winek, C. O. (1976) Tabulation of therapeutic, toxic and lethal concentrations of drugs and chemicals in blood. *Clin. Chem.* **22**, 832–836.

9

Succinimides

Several succinimide derivatives have been used in the treatment of *petit mal* absences and certain other types of epilepsy. These drugs were introduced into therapeutics successively by Zimmermann (1951; 1956) and Zimmerman and Burgemeister (1958). One derivative, ethosuximide, has established itself as the contemporary treatment of choice for absence epilepsy. Two others, phensuximide and methsuximide, have come into more limited clinical use. They have been less extensively studied than their more effective congener ethosuximide.

ETHOSUXIMIDE

Common proprietary name: Zarontin

CHEMISTRY

Ethosuximide (2-ethyl-2-methylsuccinimide) is a white crystalline material (molecular weight $141 \cdot 2$) which is readily soluble in water and in the more polar organic solvents such as ethanol. It is a weak acid with a pKa value of $9 \cdot 3$.

PHARMACODYNAMICS

ACTIONS IN MAN

Ethosuximide is an effective anticonvulsant for the absence seizures of primary generalized epilepsy (i.e. *petit mal* attacks). The drug may have some protective action against myoclonic seizures of generalized epilepsy, particularly those varieties which appear to be of hereditary origin, though not associated with structural brain abnormalities. Ethosuximide is not useful in other varieties of epilepsy.

ACTIONS IN ANIMALS

Models of generalized epilepsy

Ethosuximide does not protect against photomyclonic seizures in the baboon Papio papio (Meldrum, Horton and Toseland, 1975). However the drug does offer protection against generalized myoclonic seizures induced by the systemically administered chemical convulsants pentylenetetrazole (Chen, Weston and Bratton, 1963) and penicillin (Guberman, Gloor and Sherwin, 1975). The drug provides only very incomplete protection against maximum electro-shock seizures in mice (U.S. Department of Health, Education and Welfare Report, 1976).

Models of partial epilepsy

Little information is available as to the actions of ethosuximide in these experimental preparations.

MECHANISMS OF ACTION

Neuron pools

Dow, Forfar and McQueen (1973) showed that ethosuximide did not suppress spike activity at a cobalt-induced epileptogenic focus in rat cerebral cortex.

Single neurons

Reports of the action of ethosuximide on single neurons are not available.

Biochemical

Effects on energy production
Ethosuximide facilitates glucose transport from blood to brain (Nahorski, 1972). When given chronically to rats the drug decreases succinate dehydrogenase activity (Leznicki and Dymecki, 1974). These two observations do not permit any coherent picture of the actions of the drug on energy availability, or explain its anticonvulsant action.

Effect on inorganic ions
Little information is available as to the effects of ethosuximide on the small inorganic cations which appear relevant to neuronal function. Leznicki and Dymecki (1974) showed that brain Na^+, K^+-adenosine triphosphate activity was decreased by long-term administration of ethosuximide to rats.

Effects on neurotransmitters
No data are available concerning the effects of ethosuximide on brain acetylcholine, serotonin or catecholamine concentrations. The drug does not inhibit monoamine oxidase in rat brain (Leznicki and Dymecki, 1974). Deitrich and Erwin (1975) showed that ethosuximide at therapeutically relevant concentrations ($K_i = 5.4 \times 10^{-4}$ M) inhibits brain aldehyde dehydrogenase so that it might have an indirect effect on brain noradrenaline levels.

Gamma-aminobutyrate: Ethosuximide (5×10^{-4} M), at concentrations within its therapeutic range of $2 \cdot 1 - 8 \cdot 5 \times 10^{-4}$ M,increases the release of GABA from slices of rat cerebral cortex (Tappax and Pacheco, 1973). Sawaya, Horton and Meldrum (1975) showed that the drug, at concentrations within its therapeutic range, slightly inhibited GABA transaminase in mouse brain but did not affect succinate semialdehyde dehydrogenase activity.

Insufficient information is available to allow one to explain the anticonvulsant action of ethosuximide in terms of altered synaptic transmitter activity.

Effects on folates
It is not known whether ethosuximide therapy alters folate levels in biological fluids. The drug is not often used as the sole anticonvulsant in humans.

Effects on macromolecules
No information is available regarding the effects of ethosuximide on the various types of biological macromolecule.

PHARMACOKINETICS

ABSORPTION AND BIOAVAILABILITY

Ethosuximide is given by mouth. The drug appears to be absorbed fairly rapidly from the alimentary tract though calculations of its absorption rate constant are not available. Hansen and Feldberg (1964), Dill, Peterson, Chang and Glazko (1965) and Wechselberg and Hübel (1967) found peak plasma levels 1 to 4 hours after a single oral dose of the drug. Glazko (1975) quoted $0 \cdot 5 - 2 \cdot 0$ hours for the T_{max} of the drug while Eadie, Tyrer, Smith and McKauge (1977) found that the T_{max} occurred within 3 hours of dosage. Buchanan, Fernandez and Kinkel (1969) showed that ethosuximide was absorbed faster from a syrup preparation than from capsules. If the results of animal studies (Chang, Dill and Glazko, 1972) are applicable to man, oral doses of ethosuximide should be almost completely absorbed from the alimentary tract. No human absolute bioavailability data for the drug are available.

DISTRIBUTION

V_d

Values for the V_d of ethosuximide are as follows: in adults approximately 50 litres (Buchanan, Kinkel and Smith, 1973), $0 \cdot 69$ litres kg^{-1} (Van der Kleijn, Guelen, Van Wijk and Baars, 1975) and $0 \cdot 67 \pm 0 \cdot 04$ litres kg^{-1} (Eadie, Tyrer, Smith and McKauge, 1977). These values are compatible with the drug's being distributed throughout body water, with perhaps a little tissue binding.

Plasma protein binding
In humans ethosuximide appears not to be bound (or is only minimally bound) to plasma proteins (Chang, Dill and Glazko, 1972; Sherwin and Robb, 1972; Glazko, 1975).

Drug concentrations in various body fluids

Because of its minimal plasma protein binding, acid nature and pKa well above physiological pH, ethosuximide might be expected to occur at similar concentrations in plasma and in various body fluids.

Cerebrospinal fluid

CSF and serum levels of ethosuximide are similar (Wechselberg and Hübel, 1967; Sherwin and Robb, 1972).

Saliva

Saliva and plasma ethosuximide levels are very similar (Fig. 9.1; Horning, Brown Nowlin, Letratanangkoon, Kellaway and Zion, 1977; McAuliffe, Sherwin, Leppik, Fayle and Pippenger, 1977).

Milk

Coradello (1973) failed to find ethosuximide in milk of patients taking the drug. One wonders whether this finding is valid.

Drug concentrations in tissues

Ethosuximide was reasonably uniformly distributed throughout the tissues of the rat (Dill, Peterson, Chang and Glazko, 1965). However, in adipose tissue, levels were lower than elsewhere and plasma and brain concentrations of the drug were similar. Patel, Levy and Rapport (1977) showed very little difference between ethosuximide concentrations in a number of different areas of rat brain; in general, brain levels of ethosuximide were about 90–94 per cent of plasma drug levels. No data for man are available.

ELIMINATION

Elimination rate

The only published figures for the elimination rate constant (in adults) that we have traced are $0 \cdot 023$ hour^{-1} and $0 \cdot 019$ hour^{-1} (Buchanan, Fernandez and Kinkel, 1969), and $0 \cdot 015 \pm 0 \cdot 006$ hour^{-1} (Eadie, Tyrer, Smith and McKauge, 1977). Published half-life values for adults include the following: 54 hours (Holmes and Lane, 1965), $55 \cdot 9$ hours (Buchanan, Kinkel and Smith, 1973); 56 hours (Glazko, 1975), 52–54 hours (Goulet, Kinkel and Smith, 1976) and $52 \cdot 7 \pm 24 \cdot 5$ hours (Eadie, Tyrer, Smith and McKauge, 1977). The half-life is shorter in children, being $33 \cdot 4$ hours for capsules, $29 \cdot 7$ hours for solution (Buchanan, Fernandez and Kinkel, 1969) and 29 hours (Buchanan, Kinkel, Turner and Heffelfinger, 1976).

Browne, Dreifuss, Dyken, Goode, Penry, Porter, White and White (1975) found an elimination half-life of $35 \cdot 5$ hours in a mixed group of patients and mentioned that the half-life was shorter in patients on lower drug doses. They showed that the half-life did not shorten during 8 weeks of ethosuximide therapy, suggesting that autoinduction of elimination capacity was unimportant over this period.

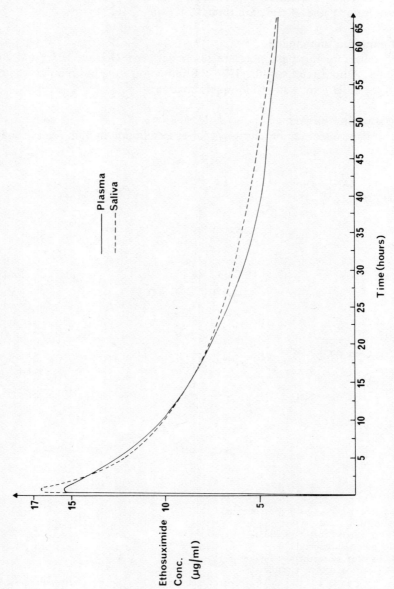

Fig. 9.1 The time-courses of plasma and salivary ethosuximide concentrations appear very similar in a patient following a single 500 mg oral dose of ethosuximide (Eadie, Tyrer, Smith and McKauge, 1977).

Clearance

Values for ethosuximide clearance include 0.016 and 0.013 litres kg^{-1} $hour^{-1}$ in two children (Buchanan, Fernandez and Kinkel, 1969) and 0.010 ± 0.004 litres kg^{-1} $hour^{-1}$ in adults (Eadie, Tyrer, Smith and McKauge, 1977).

Per cent excreted unchanged

Published values for this parameter are 17–38 per cent (Glazko, 1975) and 20 per cent (Goulet, Kinkel and Smith, 1976). Elimination of ethosuximide therefore appears to be chiefly by way of biotransformation.

Biotransformation pattern

The known biotransformation pathways for ethosuximide in man are as shown in Fig. 9.2.

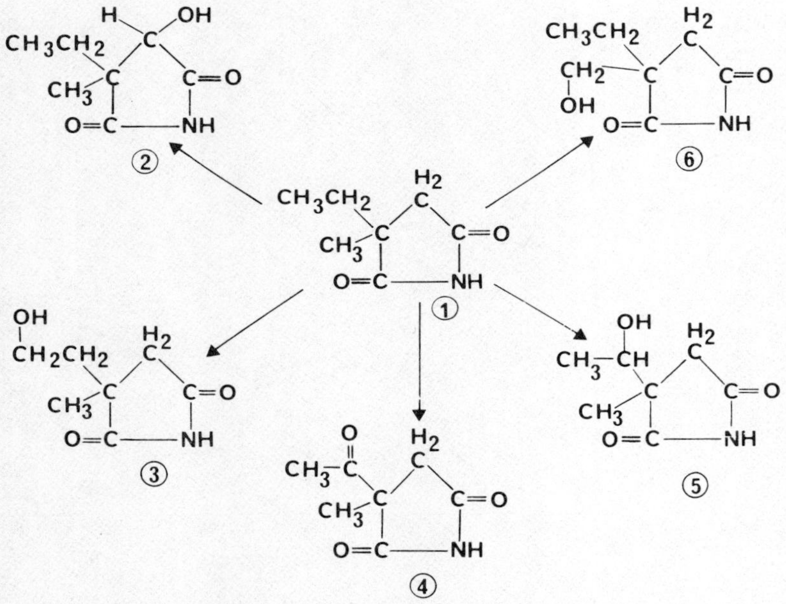

Fig. 9.2 Known metabolites of ethosuximide in man.

1. Ethosuximide (2-ethyl-2-methylsuccinimide)
2. 2-ethyl-2-methyl-3-hydroxysuccinimide
3. 2-(1-hydroxyethyl)-2-methylsuccinimide
4. 2-acetyl-2-methylsuccinimide
5. 2-(2-hydroxyethyl)-2-methylsuccinimide
6. 2-ethyl-2-(hydroxymethyl) succinimide

Metabolites, 2,3,4,5 and 6 were identified by Horning, Stratton, Nowlin, Harvey and Hill (1973), metabolites 3 and 4 by Chang, Burkett and Glazko (1972) and metabolite 2 by Preste, Westerman, Das, Wilder and Duncan (1974).

The various hydroxy compounds are conjugated with glucuronic acid prior to excretion in urine.

Excretion

The metabolites indicated in Fig. 9.2 have been found in human urine, together with unmetabolized ethosuximide. Goulet, Kinkel and Smith (1976) found that when 20 per cent of an ethosuximide dose was excreted unchanged in urine, 22 per cent of the dose was present in urine as isomer A and 33 per cent as isomer B of 2-(1-hydroxyethyl)-2-methylsuccinimide. Probably the other metabolites account for up to 25 per cent of the dose. The renal mechanisms involved in the excretions of these various substances have not been studied.

CLINICAL PHARMACOKINETICS

Time-course of plasma levels

Single dose

After oral administration of a single ethosuximide dose, plasma drug levels peak within 1 to 3 hours, and then decline with a mean half-life of about 30 hours in children, and about 55 hours in adults (Fig. 9.3).

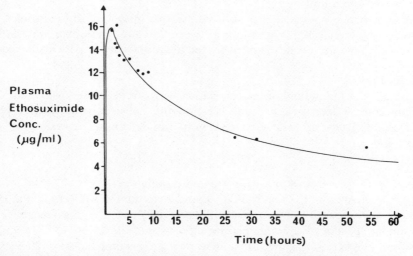

Fig. 9.3 Time-course of plasma ethosuximide levels in a patient following her first oral 500 mg dose of the drug (Eadie, Tyrer, Smith and McKauge, 1977).

Repeated doses

With repeated doses, steady-state conditions might be expected after the lapse of about 7 days in children, and after about 1½–2 weeks in adults.

Chang, Dill and Glazko (1972) quoted Holmes and Lane (1965) as stating that with repeated oral doses plasma ethosuximide concentrations took more than 7 days to reach a plateau, while Buchanan and Smith (1971) found that the plateau did not occur for 10 to 12 days. Because of the relatively long half-life of ethosuximide it should be possible to keep plasma levels of the drug relatively steady over 24 hours with once daily dosage. Buchanan and Smith (1971) showed that this is the case, the variation between maximum and minimum plasma levels over 24 hours being about 25 per cent of the minimum level. With more frequent drug administration less plasma level fluctuation occurs (Sherwin and Robb, 1972).

Correlation of plasma drug concentration and clinical effects

Anticonvulsant effects

Therapeutic response in *petit mal* absence epilepsy is easily determined in most cases. Therefore one might expect that the therapeutic range of plasma ethosuximide concentrations would have been determined accurately. Penry, Porter and Dreifuss (1972) considered that ethosuximide at plasma levels of 40–60 μg/ml gave complete control of absence epilepsy. Sherwin and Robb (1972) set the therapeutic range at 40–120 μg/ml, and Browne, Dreifuss, Dyken, Goode, Penry, Porter, White and White (1975) at 40–100 μg/ml. The latter authors found that plasma ethosuximide levels of 41–99 μg/ml were associated with a greater than 75 per cent reduction in seizure frequency in 79 per cent of a group of 39 previously untreated sufferers with absence epilepsy. Winek (1976) considered that the therapeutic range was 25–75 μg/ml.

Our experience has been that absence epilepsy may be fully controlled with plasma ethosuximide levels anywhere between 26 μg/ml and 180 μg/ml, and that these levels have been well tolerated by the great majority of patients concerned.

Unwanted effects

There has been little study of the correlation between plasma ethosuximide levels and unwanted effects of the drug. We find that most patients tolerate plasma ethosuximide levels up to at least 150 μg/ml without undue drowsiness or other undesirable effect.

Plasma level—dose correlations in treated populations

Haerer, Buchanan and Wiygul (1970) found that, for 21 subjects in the steady state, an average daily ethosuximide dose of $20 \cdot 7 \pm 5 \cdot 8$ mg/kg (range $12 \cdot 1$ to $35 \cdot 4$ mg/kg) produced a mean plasma ethosuximide level of $40 \pm 14 \cdot 9$ μg/ml. Solow and Green (1971) showed that an average ethosuximide dose of $20 \cdot 6$ mg/kg/ day produced a mean plasma ethosuximide concentration of $63 \cdot 2$ μg/ml. Penry, Porter and Dreifuss (1972) found an average ethosuximide dose of $21 \cdot 7$ mg/kg/day yielded an average steady state plasma ethosuximide level of $63 \cdot 5$ μg/ml. These workers noted wide variation in the relation between plasma level and dose in individual patients. Brown, Dreifuss, Dyken, Goode, Penry, Porter, White and White (1975) found that steady-state plasma ethosuximide levels in μg/ml averaged $2 \cdot 95$ times the daily drug dose expressed in mg/kg. Personal data (Fig. 9.4) are in general conformity with the above findings, and indicate that expressing doses on a body weight basis improves the fit of a regression line to the data. However, the position of the regression line for plasma level on dose to some extent depends on the size of the ethosuximide dose being considered. The reason for this will become apparent when the relation between plasma ethosuximide level and drug dose in the individual is dealt with below.

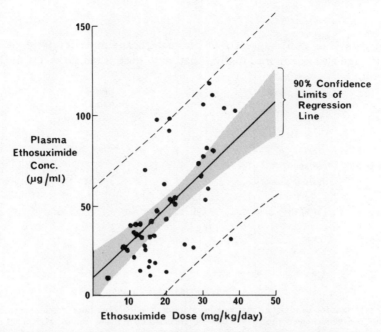

Fig. 9.4 Relation between steady-state plasma ethosuximide levels and ethosuximide dose. The 90 per cent confidence limits of the regression line are shaded, and the 90 per cent confidence limits for predicting a plasma ethosuximide level from the drug dose are shown as broken lines (Smith, McKauge, Dubetz, Tyrer and Eadie, 1979).

Effect of age

Sherwin and Robb (1972) and Browne, Dreifuss, Dyken, Goode, Penry, Porter, White and White (1975) found that plasma ethosuximide levels in the population increased more rapidly relative to dose in adults than in children. Personal data do not conform with this finding (Fig. 9·5).

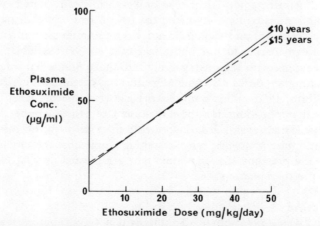

Fig. 9.5 Regression lines for steady-state plasma ethosuximide levels on drug dose in children under 10 years of age, and in persons over 15 years of age. There is no statistically significant difference between the two regression lines (Smith, McKauge, Dubetz and Eadie, 1979).

Effect of sex

Personal data (Fig. 9.6) suggest that plasma ethosuximide levels in the female population tend to rise more rapidly, relative to dose, than do levels in the male population.

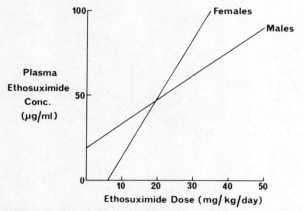

Fig. 9.6 Regression for steady-state plasma ethosuximide level on drug dose in males and females. Levels tend to rise more steeply relative to dose in females than in males (Smith, McKauge, Dubetz, Tyrer and Eadie, 1979).

Effect of pregnancy

Eadie, Lander and Tyrer (1977) found that, in the one woman they studied, it was necessary to increase ethosuximide dosage during pregnancy to maintain plasma ethosuximide levels. No further data are available.

Plasma level—dose correlations in treated individuals

Eadie (1976) illustrated a non-linear relation between steady-state plasma ethosuximide levels and ethosuximide dose in a treated patient. Further data have been collected which suggest that this non-linearity is a common phenomenon (Figs. 9.7 and 9.8). The explanation for the non-linearity is not yet available. However the finding is in keeping with the observation that ethosuximide half-life is shorter at lower than at higher doses (Browne, Dreifuss, Dyken, Goode, Penry, Porter, White and White, 1975). This non-linearity between plasma level and dose has obvious clinical implications for the adjustment of ethosuximide doses in individual patients. Thus several dose increments may fail to bring plasma ethosuximide levels into the therapeutic range. Another single dose increment of the same magnitude as the previous ones may then take the plasma drug level much of the way through the therapeutic range.

Effects of disease

Peterson and Zweig (1974) obtained some evidence that increased ethosuximide doses were necessary to obtain therapeutic results in patients who had undergone jejuno-ileal bypass procedures.

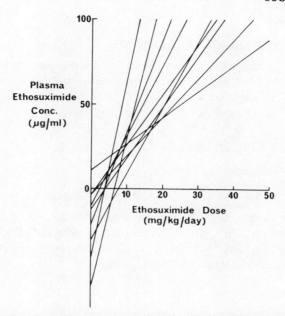

Fig. 9.7 Regression lines for 9 patients whose steady-state plasma ethosuximide levels were plotted against drug dose when they took different ethosuximide doses. Eight of the nine regressions had a negative intercept on the 'y' axis. This preponderance of negative intercepts is unlikely to be due to chance. Since the true regression must pass through the origin it seems likely that the relation between steady-state plasma ethosuximide level and the drug dose in the individual is curved (Smith, McKauge, Dubetz, Tyrer and Eadie, 1979.

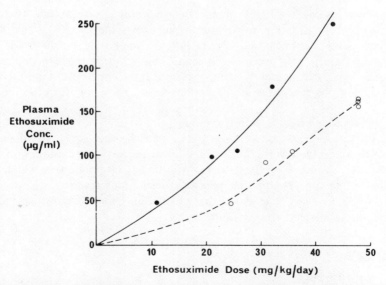

Fig. 9.8 Curvilinear relation between steady-state plasma ethosuximide levels and drug dose in two patients who received ethosuximide in, respectively, four and five different doses at different times (Smith, McKauge, Dubetz, Tyrer and Eadie, 1979).

INTERACTIONS

PHARMACODYNAMIC INTERACTIONS

Ethosuximide has sometimes been given in combination with troxidone or clonazepam to obtain better control of absence seizures. In these circumstances the possibility of pharmacokinetic interactions has not been ruled out, so that interpretation of the mechanism of action is uncertain.

PHARMACOKINETIC INTERACTIONS

Ethosuximide affecting other substances

Plasma protein binding

Ethosuximide does not alter the plasma protein binding of phenytoin (Lunde, Rane, Yaffe, Lund and Sjoqvist, 1970; Hooper, Sutherland, Bochner, Tyrer and Eadie, 1973; Patsalos and Lascelles, 1977), or carbamazepine (Hooper, Dubetz, Bochner, Cotter, Smith, Eadie and Tyrer, 1975).

Other anticonvulsants

Phenytoin. Frantzen, Hansen, Hansen and Kristensen (1967) reported that ethosuximide caused raised plasma phenytoin levels in man. Richens and Houghton (1975) could not confirm this interaction.

Primidone. Schmidt (1975) showed that ethosuximide did not alter the formation of phenobarbitone from primidone.

Other substances

Pyridoxine. Reinken (1973) found that long term succinimide therapy was associated with a fall in serum pyridoxal phosphate levels.

Gilbert, Scott, Galloway and Petrie (1974) found that ethosuximide did not increase D-glucaric acid excretion in man. This suggests that ethosuximide may not induce hepatic drug metabolizing enzymes. If so, one of the major mechanisms for producing pharmacokinetic interactions would not apply for ethosuximide.

Other substances affecting ethosuximide

We have found no reports of interactions in which other substances have altered plasma ethosuximide levels. Multivariate linear regression techniques on our own data revealed evidence of a statistically significant interaction in which methyl-phenobarbitone appeared to raise plasma ethosuximide levels relative to ethosuximide dose. There was no evidence that phenytoin, phenobarbitone, primidone or carbamazepine affected ethosuximide levels.

TOXICITY

LOCAL EFFECTS

Ethosuximide may cause local irritative effects on the stomach, with gastric discomfort, nausea, vomiting and anorexia.

DOSE-DEPENDENT SYSTEMIC EFFECTS

Dose-related side effects of ethosuximide include tiredness, headache and feelings of dysequilibrium. The relation between toxicity and plasma ethosuximide level is dealt with above.

IDIOSYNCRATIC EFFECTS

Idiosyncratic side effects of ethosuximide chiefly involve the skin and blood-forming tissues. Non-specific skin rashes occur rarely. There has been a report of erythema multiforme exudativum (Stevens-Johnson syndrome). Beernink and Miller (1973) found that the drug caused an increased incidence of antinuclear antibodies in children. There have been several reports that ethosuximide may produce systemic lupus erythematosus or related syndromes (Buchanan, 1972; Teoh and Chan, 1975; Singsen, Fishman and Hanson, 1976). Rare instances of leucopenia and pancytopenia associated with use of the drug have been reported (Kiørboe, Paludan, Trolle and Overvad, 1964; Cohn, 1968).

EFFECTS ON THE FETUS AND NEONATE

Dysmorphogenesis from the drug is unlikely to be a problem in contemporary Western society because the indication for the use of ethosuximide (*petit mal* absence epilepsy) has nearly always disappeared before the usual age of reproduction.

PREPARATIONS AVAILABLE

These include:
   Capsules—250 mg
   Suspension (for oral use)—250 mg per 5 ml

PHENSUXIMIDE

Common proprietary name: Milontin

Phensuximide (N-methyl-2-phenylsuccimide; MW 189·21) is a crystalline compound which is poorly soluble in water, though soluble in the more polar organic solvents, e.g. methanol, ethanol.

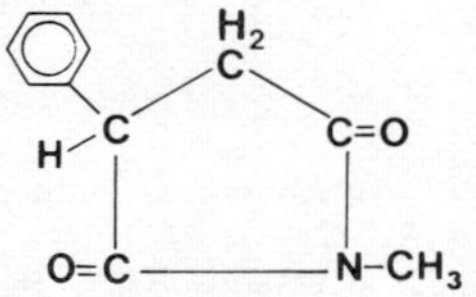

Fig. 9.9 Phensuximide

Phensuximide is less effective than ethosuximide against human absence epilepsy, and is relatively little used clinically. In man the drug forms an N-desmethyl metabolite. The half-life of the drug is 7·8 hours (range 4·5–12·0 hours) and that of its metabolite is similar (Porter, Penry, Lacy, Newmark and Kupferberg, 1977). Peak plasma levels occur $\frac{1}{2}$ to $1\frac{1}{2}$ hours after dosage (Kinkel, 1971). With regular dosage of 3000 mg per day steady-state plasma levels of phensuximide average 5·7 μg/ml, and levels of the metabolite 1·7 μg/ml.

Preparation available
  Phensuximide—500 mg capsule.

METHSUXIMIDE

Common proprietary name: Celontin

Methsuximide (N,2-dimethyl-2-phenylsuccinimide; MW 203·23) is a crystalline compound which is soluble in ethanol.

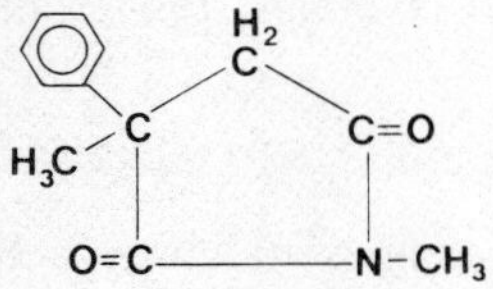

Fig. 9.10 Methsuximide

The drug is said to be useful in both absence seizures and in partial seizures of temporal lobe origin, but it appears to be little used for either. It undergoes N-desmethylation in both animals and man (Muni, Altschuler and Niecheril, 1973). Phenobarbitone facilitates this desmethylation (Barrow, Darcey and Booker, 1974). Methsuximide has a half-life of only 1·0–2·2 hours, but its N-desmethyl derivative has a much longer half-life of 36 hours (Porter, Penry, Lacy, Newmark and Kupferberg, 1977). Strong, Abe, Gibbs and Atkinson (1974) found that steady-state plasma levels of the N-desmethyl metabolite were 73 to 2800 times those of the parent substance. They suggested a provisional therapeutic range of 10–40 μg/ml for the metabolite.

Preparation available
  Methsuximide—300 mg capsules.

REFERENCES

Barrow, S. J., Darcey, B. A. & Booker, H. E. (1974) Metabolism and kinetics of methsuximide in man. *Neurology* (Mineap.), **24**, 386.

Beernink, D. H. & Miller, J. J. III (1973) Anticonvulsant induced antinuclear antibodies and lupus like disease in children. *J. Pediat.*, **82**, 113–117.

Browne, T. R., Dreifuss, F. E., Dyken, P. R., Goode, D. J., Penry, J. K., Porter, R. J., White, B. G. & White, P. T. (1975) Ethosuximide in the treatment of absence (*petit mal*) seizures. *Neurology* (Minneap.), **25**, 515–524.

Buchanan, R. A. (1972), Ethosuximide Toxicity, in *Antiepileptic Drugs* ed. Woodbury, D. M., Penry, J. K. and Schmidt, R. P. New York, Raven Press. 449–454.

Buchanan, R. A., Fernandez, L. & Kinkel, A. W. (1969) Absorption and elimination of ethosuximide in children. *J. Clin. Pharmacol.*, **9**, 393–398.
Buchanan, R. A., Kinkel, A. W. & Smith, T. C. (1973) The absorption and excretion of ethosuximide. *Int. J. Clin. Pharmacol.*, **7**, 213–218.
Buchanan, R. A., Kinkel, A. W., Turner, J. L. & Heffelfinger, J. C. (1976) Ethosuximide dosage regimens. *Clin. Pharmacol. Therap.*, **19**, 142–147.
Buchanan, R. A. & Smith, T. C. (1971) cited by Chang, T., Dill, W. A. and Glazko, A. J. (1972) *loc. cit.*
Chang, T., Burkett, A. R. & Glazko, A. J. (1972) Ethosuximide biotransformation, in *Antiepileptic Drugs* ed. Woodbury, D. M., Penry, J. K. and Schmidt, R. P. New York. Raven Press. 425–429.
Chang, R., Dill, W. A. & Glazko, A. J. (1972) Ethosuximide. Absorption, Distribution and Excretion, in *Antiepileptic Drugs* ed. Woodbury, D. M., Penry, J. K. and Schmidt, R. P. New York. Raven Press. 417–423.
Chen, G., Weston, J. K. & Bratton, A. C. Jr. (1963) Anticonvulsant activity and toxicity of phensuximide, methsuximide and ethosuximide., *Epilepsia* (Amst.), **4**, 66–76.
Cohn, R. (1968) A neuropathological study of a case of *petit mal* epilepsy. *Electroenceph. Clin. Neurophysiol.*, **24**, 282.
Coradello, H. (1973) Ueber die Ausscheidung von Antiepileptika in die Muttermilch. *Wein. Klin. Swchr.*, **85**, 695–697.
Deitrich, R. A. & Erwin, G. V. (1975) Involvement of biogenic amine metabolism in ethanol addiction. *Fed. Proc.*, **34**, 1962–1968.
Department of Health, Education & Welfare Publication No. (NIH) 76–1093 (1976), Anticonvulsant screening project.
Dill, W. A., Peterson, L., Chang, T. & Glazko, A. J. (1965), Physiologic disposition of a-methyl-a-ethyl succinimide (Ethosuximide; Zarontin) in animals and man. *Chem. Abstr.*, 149th Annual Meeting. 30 N.
Dow, R. C., Forfar, J. C. & McQueen, J. K. (1973) The effects of some anticonvulsant drugs on cobalt induced epilepsy. *Epilepsia* (Amst.), **14**, 203–212.
Eadie, M. J. (1976) Plasma level monitoring of anticonvulsants. *Clin. Pharmacokinetics* **1**, 52–66.
Eadie, M. J., Lander, C. M. & Tyrer, J. H. (1977) Plasma drug level monitoring in pregnancy. *Clinical Pharmacokinetics*, **2**, 427–436.
Eadie, M. J., Tyrer, J. H., Smith, G. A. & Mc Kauge, L. (1977) Pharmacokinetics of drugs used for petit mal absence epilepsy. *Clin. Exptl. Neurol.*, **14**, 172–183.
Frantzen, E., Hansen, J. M., Hansen, O. E. & Kristensen, M. (1976) Phenytoin (Dilantin[R]) intoxication. *Acta Neurol. Scandinav.*, **43**, 440–446.
Gilbert, J. C., Scott, A. K., Galloway, D. B. & Petrie, J. C. (1974) Ethosuximide: liver enzyme induction and D-glucaric acid excretion. *Brit. J. clin. Pharmacol.*, **1**, 249–252.
Glazko, A. J. (1975) Antiepileptic drugs: biotransformation, metabolism and serum half-life. *Epilepsia* (Amst.), **16**, 367–391.
Goulet, J. R., Kinkel, A. W. & Smith, T. C. (1976) Metabolism of ethosuximide. *Clin. Pharmacol. Therap.*, **20**, 213–218.
Guberman, A., Gloor, P. & Sherwin, A. L. (1975) Response of generalised penicillin epilepsy in the cat to ethosuximide and diphenylhydantoin. *Neurology* (Minneap.), **25**, 758–764.
Haerer, A. F., Buchanan, R. A. & Wiygul, F. M. (1970) Ethosuximide blood levels in epileptics. *J. Clin. Pharmacol.*, **10**, 370–374.
Hansen, S. E. & Feldburg, L. (1964) Absorption and elimination of Zarontin. *Dan. Med. Bull.*, **11**, 54–55.
Holmes, E. L. & Lane, A. Z. (1965) cited by Chang, T., Dill, W. A. and Glazko, A. J. (1972). *Loc. cit.*
Hooper, W. D., Dubetz, D. K., Bochner, F., Cotter, L. M., Smith, G. A., Eadie, M. J. & Tyrer, J. H. (1975) Plasma protein binding of carbamazepine. *Clin. Pharmacol. Therap.*, **17**, 433–440.
Hooper, W. D., Sutherland, J. M., Bochner, F., Tyrer, J. H. & Eadie, M. J. (1973), The effect of certain drugs on the plasma protein binding of diphenylhydantoin. *Aust. N. Z. J. Med.*, **3**, 1377–381.
Horning, M. G., Brown, L., Nowlin, J., Letratanangkoon, K., Kellaway, P. & Zion, T. E. (1977) Use of saliva in therapeutic drug monitoring. *Clin. Chem.*, **23**, 157–164.
Horning, M. G., Stratton, C., Nowlin, J., Harvey, D. J. & Hill, R. M. (1973), Metabolism of 2-ethyl-2-methylsuccinimide (Ethosuximide) in the rat and human. *Drug. Metabolism Distribution*, **1**, 569–576.
Kiørboe, E., Paludan, J., Trolle, E. & Overvad, E. (1964), Zarontin (ethosuximide) in the treatment of petit mal and related disorders. *Epilepsia* (Amst.), **5**, 83–89.
Kinkel, A. (1971) cited by Glazko, A. J. and Dill, W. A. (1972) Other succinimides. Methuximide and phensuximide, in *Antiepileptic drugs* ed. Woodbury, D. M., Penry, J. K. and Schmidt, R. P. New York. Raven Press. 455–464.

Leznicki, A. & Dymecki, J. (1974), The effect of certain anticonvulsants *in vivo* on enzyme activities in the rat's brain. *Neurol. Neurochir. Pol.*, **24**, 413–419.

Lunde, P. K. M., Rane, A., Yaffe, S. J., Lund, L. & Sjöquist, F. (1970), Plasma protein binding of diphenylhydantoin in man. Interaction with other drugs and the effect of temperature and plasma dilution. *Clin. Pharmacol. Therap.*, **11**, 846–855.

McAuliffe, J. J., Sherwin, A. L., Leppik, I. E., Fayle, S. A. & Pippenger, C. E. (1977) Salivary levels of anticonvulsants: a practical approach to drug monitoring. *Neurology* (Minneap.), **27**, 409–413.

Meldrum, B. S., Horton, R. W. & Toseland, P. A. (1975) A primate model for testing anticonvulsant drugs. *Arch. Neurol.* (Chic.), **32**, 288–294.

Muni, I. A., Altschuler, C. H. & Neicheril, J. C. (1973) Identification of blood metabolite of methsuximide by GLC-mass spectrometry. *J. Pharm. Sci.*, **62**, 1820–1823.

Nahorski, S. R. (1972) Biochemical effects of the anti-convulsants trimethadione, ethosuximide and chlordiazepoxide in rat brain. *J. Neurochem.*, **19**, 1937–1946.

Patel, I. H., Levy, R. H. & Rapport, R. L. (1977) Distribution characteristics of ethosuximide in discrete areas of rat brain. *Epilepsia* (Amst.), **18**, 533–541.

Patsalos, P. N. & Lascelles, P. T. (1977), Effect of sodium valproate on plasma protein binding of diphenylhydantoin. *J. Neurol. Neurosurg. Psychiat.*, **40**, 570–574.

Penry, J. K., Porter, R. J. & Dreifuss, F. E. (1972) Ethosuximide. Relation of plasma levels to clinical control, in *Antiepileptic drugs* ed. Woodbury, D. M., Penry, J. K. and Schmidt, R. P. New York. Raven Press. 431–441.

Peterson, D. I. & Zweig, R. W., (1974) Absorption of anticonvulsants after jujunoileal bypass. *Bull. Los Angeles Neurol. Soc.*, **39**, 51–55.

Porter, R. J., Penry, J. K., Lacy, J. R., Newmark, M. E. & Kupferberg, H. J. (1977) The clinical efficacy and pharmacokinetics of phensuximide and methsuximide. *Neurology* (Minneap.) **27**, 375.

Preste, P. G., Westerman, C. E., Das, N. P., Wilder, B. J. & Duncan, J. H. (1974), Identification of 2-ethyl-2-methyl-3-hydroxysuccinimide as a major metabolite of ethosuximide in humans. *J. Pharm. Sci.*, **63**, 467–469.

Reinken, L. (1973) Die Wirkung von Hydantoin und Succinimid auf den Vitamin B6 Stoffwechsel. *Clin. Chim. Acta.*, **48**, 435–436.

Richens, A. & Houghton, G. W. (1975) Effect of drug therapy on the metabolism of phenytoin, in *Clinical Pharmacology of Anti-epileptic drugs* ed. Schneider, H., Janz, D., Gardner-Thorpe, C., Meinardi, H. and Sherwin, A. L. Berlin, Springer. 87–95.

Sawaya, M. C. B., Horton, R. W. & Meldrum, B. S. (1975) Effects of anticonvulsant drugs on the cerebral enzymes metabolizing GABA. *Epilepsia* (Amst.), **16**, 649–655.

Schmidt, D. (1975) The effect of phenytoin and ethosuximide on primidone metabolism in patients with epilepsy. *J. Neurol.*, **209**, 115–123.

Sherwin, A. L. & Robb, J. P. (1972) Ethosuximide: Relation of plasma level to clinical control, in *Antiepileptic drugs* ed. Woodbury, D. M., Penry, J. K. and Schmidt, R. P. New York: Raven Press. 443–448.

Singsen, B. H., Fishman, L. & Hanson, V. (1976) Antinuclear antibodies and lupus like syndromes in children receiving anticonvulsants. *Pediatrics*, **57**, 529–534.

Smith, G. A., McKauge, L., Du Betz, D. K., Tyrer, J. H. & Eadie, M. J. (1979) Factors influencing plasma concentrations of ethosuximide. *Clin. Pharmacokinetics*, **4**, 38–52.

Solow, E. B. & Green, J. B. (1972) The simultaneous determination of multiple anticonvulsant drug levels by gas-liquid chromatography. Method and clinical application. *Neurology* (Minneap.), **22**, 540–550.

Strong, J. M., Abe, T., Gibbs, E. L. & Atkinson, A. J. Jr. (1974) Plasma levels of methsuximide and N-desmethylmethsuximide during methsuximide therapy. *Neurology* (Minneap.), **24**, 250–255.

Tappaz, M. & Pachelo, H. (1973) Effets de convulsivants et d'anticonvulsivants sur la capture de GABA. *J. Pharmacol.* (Paris), **4**, 259–306.

Teoh, P. C. & Chan, H. L. (1975) Lupus scleroderma syndrome induced by ethosuximide. *Arch. Dis. Childh.*, **50**, 658–661.

Van der Kleijn, E., Guelen, P. J. M., Van Wijk, C. & Baars, I. (1975) Clinical pharmacokinetics in monitoring chronic medication with anti-epileptic drugs, in *Clinical pharmacology of antiepileptic drugs* ed. Schneider, H., Janz, D., Gardner-Thorpe, C., Meinardi, H. and Sherwin, A. L. Berlin. Springer. 11–13.

Wechselberg, K. & Hübel, G. (1967) Zur Resorption und Verteilung von Methyl-Älthyl-Succinimid (MAS) im Serum und Liquor bei Kindern. *Z. Kinderheilkd.*, **100**, 10–19.

Winek, C. L. (1976), Tabulation of therapeutic, toxic, and lethal concentrations of drugs and chemical in blood. *Clin. Chem.*, **22**, 832–836.

Zimmerman, F. T. (1951) Use of methylphenylsuccinimide in treatment of *petit mal* epilepsy. *Arch. Neurol. Psychiat.*, **66**, 156–162.

Zimmerman, F. T. (1956) Evaluation of N-α-α-methylphenyl succinimide in the treatment of *petit mal* epilepsy. *N. Y. State J. Med.*, **56**, 1460–1465.

Zimmerman, F. T. & Burgemeister, B. B. (1958) A new drug for *petit mal* epilepsy. *Neurology* (Minneap.), **8**, 1769–1775.

10

Oxazolidinediones

TROXIDONE (TRIMETHADIONE): PARAMETHADIONE

Common proprietary names: Tridione; Paradione

Following the introduction of troxidone (Lennox, 1945), the oxazolidinedione family of anticonvulsants was used to treat absence seizures for over 25 years. These drugs are now declining in importance as more effective and less toxic substances are introduced. However two of these drugs remain in some clinical use, troxidone being employed occasionally and paramethedione being used rarely. Knowledge of the pharmacodynamics and clinical pharmacology of this group of drugs is confined largely to troxidone.

CHEMISTRY

The oxazolidinedione structure consists of a five-membered heterocyclic ring with substitutent alkyl side chains in the positions shown.

Troxidone (3,5,5-trimethyloxazolidine-2,4-dione) was synthesized by Spielman (1944). It is a white crystalline bitter-tasting substance (molecular weight 143.2) with a relatively low melting point (46°C). It is moderately soluble in water and in many common organic solvents (ethanol, chloroform and diethylether). Its ethylated homologue, paramethadione (3,5-dimethyl-5-ethyloxazolidine-2,4-dione), is a liquid at room temperature (molecular weight 157·2). It is less soluble in water than troxidone but dissolves readily in many organic solvents (ethanol, chloroform, diethylether). In the body, troxidone is demethylated at the 3 position to form

	R_1	R_2	R_3
Trimethadione	CH_3	CH_3	CH_3
Dimethadione	CH_3	CH_3	H
Paramethadione	CH_3	C_2H_5	CH_3

another anticonvulsant molecule (dimethadione) which, on a molar basis, in the mouse is 80 per cent as effective an anticonvulsant as troxidone itself (Frey, 1969). Unlike the essentially neutral troxidone, dimethadione is weakly acidic in aqueous solution. Its pKa is 6·13 at 37°C (Withrow and Woodbury, 1972). Paramethadione undergoes a dealkylation analogous to that of troxidone.

PHARMACODYNAMICS

ACTIONS IN MAN

Troxidone and paramethadione appear to be useful in the prophylaxis of absence seizures, and possibly in certain types of myoclonic generalized epilepsy.

ACTIONS IN ANIMALS

Models of generalized epilepsy

In various species troxidone will protect against generalized myoclonic seizures provoked by systemic administration of both pentylenetetrazole (Goodman, Grewal, Brown and Swinyard, 1953) and local anaesthetics such as procaine, lignocaine and cocaine (Sanders, 1967). The drug also offers a degree of protection against seizures provoked by thiosemicarbazide and 2,4-dimethyl-5-hydroxymethyl pyrimidine (Banziger and Hane, 1967). Troxidone modifies the pattern of seizures induced by bicuculline (Blum, Haefely, Jalfre, Polc and Scharer, 1973).

Troxidone offers some protection against maximum electroshock convulsions in various experimental animals (Goodman, Grewal, Brown and Swinyard, 1953), but is less effective than against chemically-induced generalized epilepsy.

Models of partial epilepsy

Troxidone has been little studied in such models. The drug was said to have little effect on electrically-induced spikes in the occipital cortex of the cat (Vastola and Rosen, 1960), but more recent work showed that it facilitated seizures in this experimental preparation (Ito, Hori, Yoshida and Shimizu, 1977).

MECHANISM OF ACTION

Neuron pools

Morrell, Bradley and Ptashne (1959) found that troxidone tended to prevent the spread into the thalamus of epileptogenic activity from a cortical focus produced by local freezing. However the drug did not prevent the local propagation within the cortex of activity arising in the focus. Troxidone raised the threshold for electrical activation of after-discharges in the amygdaloid nucleus, hippocampus and ectosylvian gyrus of cats (Strobos and Spudis, 1960) and in the intralaminar nuclei of the thalamus (Schallek and Kuehn, 1963). The latter authors showed that troxidone had less effect on after-discharges in the neocortex.

Troxidone does not alter the phenomenon of post-tetanic potentiation (Esplin and Curto, 1957; Woodbury, 1969).

Single neurons

There is virtually no information as to the actions of troxidone on single neurons.

Biochemical

Energy production

Troxidone facilitates glucose entry into the brain (Nahorski, 1972). The drug inhibits the increases in oxygen uptake and in anaerobic glycolysis that occur when brain slices are stimulated electrically (Mori, 1974). However these effects may be a result of the anticonvulsant action of the drug, rather than a cause of this action.

Effects on inorganic ions

In lobster nerve, troxidone reduces intracellular Na^+ concentration (Pincus, Grove, Marino and Glaser, 1970). The drug, and also its metabolite dimethadione, activate Na^+, K^+, Mg^{++}–linked adenosine triphosphatase (Brink and Freeman, 1972).

Dimethadione causes an increase in extraneuronal H^+ concentration, with intraneuronal accumulation of CO_2 (Butler, Kuroiwa, Waddell and Poole, 1966). Whether this pH change contributes to the anticonvulsant effect is uncertain.

Effect on synaptic transmitters

There are very few data available regarding the effect of troxidone on known or putative neurotransmitters. This lack of information probably reflects the declining importance of oxazolidinedione anticonvulsants at a time when there is increasing interest in neurotransmitter chemistry. Diaz (1974) showed that troxidone caused increased serotonin synthesis in rat brain.

Effect on folates

Whether administration of troxidone alters folate levels in biological fluids is unknown.

Effects on macromolecules

No data regarding this matter are available.

PHARMACOKINETICS

ABSORPTION AND BIOAVAILABILITY

In five men Booker (1972) found peak serum levels of troxidone 30 minutes after a single oral dose of the drug. In a study in dogs Frey and Schulz (1970) showed that peak serum levels of troxidone occured 1 to 3 hours after an oral dose of the drug. Thus in both species troxidone appears to be rapidly absorbed from the alimentary tract. No information as to the bioavailability of the drug is available.

Hoffman and Chun (1975) found that the T_{max} for paramethadione was 0·5 to 1·0 hour.

DISTRIBUTION

Little quantitative pharmacokinetic information in man is available. Taylor and Bertcher (1952) found in mice that troxidone concentrations were similar in blood, brain, muscle, kidney and liver, but the assay used was not specific. The data of Frey and Schultz (1970) suggested that troxidone was distributed fairly uniformly throughout body water in dogs. Dimethadione had a rather smaller volume of distribution than troxidone. Neither troxidone (Ferngren and Paalzow, 1969) nor dimethadione (Roos, 1965) appeared to undergo any selective regional concentration in the brain, and neither was bound significantly to plasma protein (Booker, 1972).

Data are not available for the distribution of paramethadione.

ELIMINATION

Elimination rate

The half-life of troxidone is 16 hours (Booker, 1972). Its metabolite dimethadione is very much more slowly eliminated, only about 6 per cent of a dose appearing in urine each day (Butler and Waddell, 1958; Jensen, 1962; Frey and Schulz, 1970).

Hoffman and Chun (1975) showed that paramethadione elimination followed a biexponential time course, with a β phase half-life of 16 hours. There was evidence that the N-desmethyl metabolite of paramethadione was very slowly eliminated, though exact data were not provided.

Clearance

Clearance data for the various oxazolidinedione drugs and their metabolites are not available.

Per cent excreted unchanged

Very little of a troxidone or paramethadione dose is excreted unchanged in man (Richards and Everett, 1946), while dimethadione is excreted largely unchanged.

Biotransformation pattern

In man troxidone is totally, or almost totally, N-demethylated to dimethadione (Butler, 1953). No other metabolic product appears to have been isolated. Paramethadione is similarly dealkylated (Butler, 1955). Most of the dealkylation occurs in the liver.

Excretion

The excretions of the acids, dimethadione and the analogous N-desmethyl derivative of paramethadione, are likely to be dependent on urine pH.

CLINICAL PHARMACOKINETICS

Time-course of plasma levels

Single dose

Booker (1972) found that after a single oral dose of 600 mg of troxidone a mean peak serum troxidone level of 14 μg/ml occurred after 30 minutes in five human subjects. Thereafter the serum level fell with a half-life in plasma of 16 hours. No information as to the rate of appearance of dimethadione is available.

Hoffman and Chun (1975) in 3 subjects showed that paramethadione plasma levels rose to a peak 30–60 minutes after intake, and then declined with a 16 hour half-life. Plasma levels of the N-desmethyl metabolite were still rising when the study was terminated, 2 days after drug administration.

Repeated doses

In so far as troxidone and paramethadione are concerned, steady-state conditions might be expected to apply after 3 to 4 days of regular oral therapy. However, though exact information is not available, it would probably take a good deal longer, perhaps about 2 weeks, for steady-state conditions to apply for their metabolites.

Booker and Darcey (1971) and Booker (1972) found that serum levels of dimethadione were about 20 times higher than troxidone levels in patients taking the latter drug on a long-term basis. Levels of troxidone tended to fall by 30 per cent overnight whereas dimethadione levels were virtually constant over 24 hours. These findings, and the half-life data, suggest that troxidone should have an adequate biological effect if given in sufficient dosage once a day. It seems likely that similar considerations would apply for paramethadione.

Correlations of plasma drug concentrations and clinical effects

Much of the apparent anticonvulsant effect of troxidone is probably produced by the dimethadione formed from it. Plasma dimethadione levels of 700 μg/ml or higher appear to provide the best chance of controlling the seizures of absence epilepsy (Jensen, 1962; Chamberlin, Waddell and Butler, 1965; Booker, 1972).

Plasma level—dose correlations

Booker (1972) found that for patients taking constant troxidone dosages at least up to 60 mg/kg/day there was a linear relation between serum levels of both troxidone and dimethadione and the troxidone dosage. For troxidone the serum level in μg/ml averaged 0·6 times the oral dose in mg/kg/day, whereas for dimethadione the serum level averaged 12 times the oral troxidone dose expressed on the same basis. Data are not available correlating the behaviour of plasma concentrations of troxidone and its metabolite with oral dosage increments of troxidone in the individual patient.

No data are available for paramethadione.

Effects of disease

No information is available as to the effects of disease on the pharmacokinetics of troxidone.

INTERACTIONS

PHARMACODYNAMIC INTERACTIONS

Before the newer anticonvulsants clonazepam and valproic acid became available troxidone was sometimes combined with ethosuximide to obtain an additional anticonvulsant effect against absence epilepsy. The possibility of a pharmacokinetic interaction in these circumstances was not excluded, and may have contributed toward any anticonvulsant effect which occurred.

PHARMACOKINETIC INTERACTIONS

It is know that troxidone slows the hepatic dealkylation of N-methyl-barbitone *in vitro* (Butler, Waddell and Poole, 1965) but whether troxidone inhibits other dealkylations is unknown. Paramethadione, but not troxidone, is said to induce liver drug-metabolizing enzymes (Conney, 1967).

Data concerning the direct effects of the oxazolidinediones on other drugs, or of other drugs on oxazolidinedione concentrations, are not available. It seems possible that changes in the pH of various tissue fluids could affect the distribution of dimethadione by altering its ionization (Butler, Kuriowa, Waddell and Poole, 1966), since only the non-ionized molecule of dimethadione is likely to pass through lipoidal cell membranes separating the various collections of body fluid.

TOXICITY

LOCAL EFFECTS

Local alimentary irritative effects from troxidone and paramethadione are not common. When they occur they are usually not severe.

DOSE–DEPENDENT SYSTEMIC EFFECTS

The dose-related side effects of troxidone include sedation, which is rarely a problem clinically, and glare phenomena, which are experienced by many people taking troxidone and which may be quite distressing (Sloan and Gilger, 1947). Paramethadione is believed to be less likely to produce this troublesome side effect (Davis and Lennox, 1949).

IDIOSYNCRATIC EFFECTS

Idiosyncratic effects include skin eruptions ranging in severity from erythematous rashes to exfoliative dermatitis. Nephrotic syndromes have been reported (Barnett, Simons and Wells, 1948; Heymann, 1967). There have been at least two reported cases of myasthenia (Peterson, 1966; Booker, Chun and Sanguino, 1970). Neutropenia occurs in about 20 per cent of persons taking troxidone (Davis and Lennox, 1947) and pancytopenia and fatal aplastic anaemia may occur occasionally (Wells, 1957). Beernick and Miller (1973) found an increased incidence of anti-nuclear antibodies in children taking troxidone.

EFFECTS ON THE FETUS AND NEONATE

Dysmorphogenesis from these drugs would seem unlikely to be a significant problem. Their use is decreasing, and the type of epilepsy for which they are useful is one which occurs mainly below the age of 15 years (below which age reproduction is relatively infrequent in contemporary Western society). However, in a study of a small group of women taking oxazolidinedione therapy during pregnancy, German, Kowal and Ehlers (1970) found a much greater incidence of maldeveloped babies than in epileptic mothers generally.

PREPARATIONS AVAILABLE

These include:

Troxidone   Paramethadione
Tablet—150 mg   Capsules—300 mg
Capsules—300 mg

REFERENCES

Banziger, R. & Hane, D. (1967) Evaluation of a new convulsant for anticonvulsant screening. *Arch. int. Pharmacodyn.*, **167**, 245–249.

Barnett, H. L., Simons, D. J. & Wells, R. E. Jr. (1948) Nephrotic syndrome occurring during Tridone[R] therapy. *Amer. J. Med.*, **4**, 760–764.

Beernink, D. H. & Miller, J. J. III (1973) Anticonvulsant induced anti-nuclear antibodies and lupus like disease in children. *J. Pediat.*, **82**, 113–117.

Blum, J. E., Haefely, W., Jalfre, M., Polc, P. & Scharer, K. (1973), Pharmakologie und Toxicologie des Antiepileptikums Clonazepam. Arzneim.-Forsch., **23**, 377–389.

Booker, H. E. (1972) Trimethadione and other oxazolidinediones. Relation of plasma levels to clinical control, in *Antiepileptic drugs* ed. Woodbury, D. M., Penry, J. K. and Schmidt, R. P. New York. Raven Press. 403–407.

Booker, H. E., Chun, R. W. M. & Sanguino, M. (1970) Myaesthenia gravis syndrome associated with trimethadione. *J. Amer. Med. Ass.*, **212**, 2262–2263.

Booker, H. E. & Darcey, B. (1971) Simultaneous determination of trimethadione and its metabolite, dimethadione, by gas-liquid chromatography. *Clin. Chem.*, **17**, 607–609.

Brink, J. J. & Freeman, E. A. (1972) Effects of 5-phenyl-oxazolidinedione on sodium-potassium-magnesium-activated adenosine triphosphatase activity in mouse brain. *J. Neurochem.*, **19**, 1783–1788.

Butler, T. C. (1953) Quantitative studies of the demethylation of trimethadione (Tridione[R]). *J. Pharmacol. exp. Therap.*, **108**, 11–18.

Butler, T. C. (1955) Metabolic demethylation of 3,5-dimethyl-5-ethyl 2,4-oxazolidinedione (paramethadione, Paradione[R]). *J. Pharmacol. exp. Therap.*, **113**, 178–185.

Butler, T. C., Kuroiwa, Y., Waddell, W. J. & Poole, D. T. (1966) Effects of 5,5-dimethyl-2,4-oxazolidinedione (DMO) on acid-base and electrolyte equilibria. *J. Pharmacol. exp. Therap.*, **152**, 62–66.

Butler, T. C. & Waddell, W. J. (1958) N-methylated derivatives of barbituric acids, hydantoin and oxazolidine used in the treatment of epilepsy. *Neurology* (Minneap.), **8**, Suppl. **1**, 106–112.

Butler, T. C., Waddell, W. J. & Poole, D. T. (1965) Demethylation of trimethadione and metharbital by rat liver microsomal enzymes: substrate concentration: yield relationships and competition between substrates. *Biochem. Pharmacol.*, **14**, 937–942.

Chamberlin, H. R., Waddell, W. J. & Butler, T. J. (1965) A study of the product of demethylation of Tridione in the control of *petit mal* epilepsy. *Neurology* (Minneap.), **15**, 449–454.

Conney, A. H. (1967) Pharmacological implications of microsomal enzyme induction. *Pharmacol. Rev.*, **19**, 317–366.

Davis, J. P. & Lennox, W. G. (1949) A comparison of paradione and tridione in the treatment of epilepsy. *J. Pediat.*, **34**, 273–278.

Diaz, P. M. (1974) Interaction of pentylenetetrazole and trimethadione on the metabolism of serotonin in brain and its relation to the anticonvulsant action of trimethadione. *Neuropharmacology*, **13**, 615–621.

Esplin, D. W. & Curto, E. W. (1957) Effect of trimethadione on synaptic transmission in the spinal cord: antagonism of trimethadione and pentylene-tetrazole. *J. Pharmacol. exp. Therap.*, 121, 457–467.

Ferngren, H. & Paalzow, L. (1969) High frequency electro-shock seizures and their antagonism during postnatal development in the mouse. II. Effects of phenobarbital, sodium methobarbital, trimethadione, dimethadione, ethosuximide and acetazolamide. *Acta Pharmacol. (Kbh).*, 28, 477–483.

Frey, H. -H. (1969) Determination of the anticonvulsant potency of unmetabolized trimethadione. *Acta pharmacol. et toxicaol.*, 27, 295–300.

Frey, H. -H. & Schulz, R. (1970) Time course of the demethylation of trimethadione. *Acta Pharmacol. Toxicol. (Kbh.)*, 28, 477–483.

German, J., Kowal, A. & Ehlers, K. H. (1970) Trimethadione and human teratogenesis. *Teratology*, 3, 349–362.

Goodman, L. S., Grewal, M. S., Brown, W. C. & Swinyard, E. A. (1953) Comparison of maximal seizures evoked by pentylenetetrazole (Metrazol) and electroshock in mice, and their modification by anticonvulsants. *J. Pharmacol. exp. Therap.*, 108, 168–176.

Heymann, W. (1967) Nephrotic syndrome after use of trimethadione and Paradione in *petit mal*. *J. Amer. Med. Ass.*, 202, 893–894.

Hoffman, D. J. & Chun, A. H. C. (1975) Paramethadione and metabolite serum levels in humans after a single oral paramethadione dose. *J. Pharm. Sci.*, 64, 1702–1703.

Ito, T., Hori, M., Yoshida, K. & Shimizu, M. (1977) Effect of anticonvulsants on cortical focal seizures in cats. *Epilepsia* (Amst.), 18, 63–71.

Jensen, B. N. (1962) Trimethadione in the serum of patients with *petit mal*. *Dan. Med. Bull.*, 9, 74–79.

Lennox, W. G. (1945) The *petit mal* epilepsies: their treatment with tridione. *J. Amer. med. Ass.*, 129, 1069–1074.

Mori, A. (1974) Neuropharmacologic studies on anticonvulsants. *Brain Develop.*, 6, 435–440.

Morrell, F., Bradley, W. & Ptashne, M. (1959), "Effect of drugs on discharge characteristics of chronic epileptogenic lesions. *Neurology* (Minneap.), 9, 492–498.

Nahorski, S. R. (1972) Biochemical effects of the anticonvulsants trimethadione, ethosuximide and chlordiazepoxide in rat brain. *J. Neurochem.*, 19, 1937–1946.

Peterson, H. DeC. (1966) Association of trimethadione therapy and myaesthenia gravis. *New Eng. J. Med.*, 274, 506–507.

Pincus, J. H., Grove, I., Marino, B. B. & Glaser, G. E. (1970) Studies on the mechanism of action of diphenylhydantoin. *Arch. Neurol.* (Chic.), 22, 566–571.

Richards, R. K. & Everett, G. M. (1946) Tridione[R]: a new anticonvulsant drug. *J. Lab. Clin. Med.*, 31, 1330–1336.

Roos, A. (1965) Intracellular pH and intracellular buffering power of the cat brain. *Am. J. Physiol.*, 209, 1233–1246.

Sanders, H. D. (1967) A comparison of the convulsant activity of procaine and pentylenetetrazole. *Arch. Int. Pharmacodyn.*, 170, 165–177.

Schallek, W. & Kuehn, A. (1963) Effects of trimethadione, diphenylhydantoin and chlordiazepoxide on after-discharges in brain of cat. *Proc. Soc. exp. Biol. N.Y.*, 112, 813–817.

Sloan, L. L. & Gilger, A. P. (1947) Visual effects of Tridione[R]. *Am. J. Ophthalmol.*, 30, 1387–1405.

Spielman, M. A. (1944) Some analgesic agents derived from oxazolidine-2,4-dione. *J. Amer. Chem. Soc.*, 66, 1244–1245.

Strobos, R. R. J. & Spudis, E. V. (1960) Effect of anticonvulsant drugs on cortical and subcortical seizure discharges in cats. *Arch. Neurol* (Chic.), 2, 399–406.

Taylor, J. D. & Bertcher, E. L. (1952) Determination and distribution of trimethadione (Tridione) in animal tissues. *J. Pharmacol. exp. Therap.*, 106, 277–285.

Vastola, E. F. & Rosen, A. (1960) Suppression by anticonvulsants of focal electrical seizures in the neocortex. *Electroenceph. clin. Neurophysiol.*, 12, 327–332.

Wells, C. E. (1957) Trimethadione: its dosage and toxicity. *Arch. Neurol. Psychiat.* (Chic.), 77, 140–155.

Withrow, C. D. & Woodbury, D. M. (1972) Trimethadione and other oxazolidine-diones. Absorption, distribution and excretion, in *Antiepileptic drugs* ed. Woodbury, D. M., Penry, J. K. and Schmidt, R. P. Raven Press: New York. 389–393.

Woodbury, D. M. (1969) Mechanism of action of anticonvulsants, in *Basic mechanisms of the epilepsies* ed. Jasper, H. H., Ward, A. A. and Pope, A. Boston. Little, Brown and Co., 647–681.

11

Benzodiazepine anticonvulsants

DIAZEPAM: NITRAZEPAM: CLONAZEPAM

Diazepam—common proprietary name: Valium
Nitrazepam—common proprietary name: Mogadon
Clonazepam—common proprietary names: Rivotril, Clonopin

The various benzodiazepine derivatives have been introduced into therapeutics only in comparatively recent times. However certain members of the group have attained an enormous popularity as minor tranquillizers. Many of the benzodiazepines have valuable anticonvulsant properties. Parenteral diazepam is commonly employed as the treatment of choice for status epilepticus. Oral nitrazepam till recently was the most effective remedy available for myoclonic seizures. The newer benzodiazepine derivative, clonazepam, is an effective oral anticonvulsant, unusual in that it appears active against all forms of epilepsy. In its parenteral form, clonazepam was found by Gastaut, Catier, Dravet and Roger (1970) and by Gastaut, Courjon, Poiré and Weber (1971) to be the most effective drug yet available against status epilepticus.

In the present Chapter only diazepam, nitrazepam and clonazepam are discussed in detail. Each of these substances is used as primary therapy for epilepsy. Other benzodiazepines, if used in epilepsy, are employed basically as adjuvants to other therapies (e.g. oxazepam) or else are still finding their places as anticonvulsants (e.g. lorazepam).

The three benzodiazepines here considered are important drugs. Many of their pharmacological properties are similar. Therefore, to emphasise common features and to reduce repetition, each aspect of the pharmacology of the drugs is dealt with comparatively, rather than the full pharmacology of one drug before that of the next.

CHEMISTRY

The chemistry of the benzodiazepines was described at length by Archer and Sternbach (1968).

Diazepam   (7-chlor-1-methyl-5-phenyl-1,3-dihydro-2H-1,4-benzodiazepine-2-one) was synthesized by Sternbach and Reeder (1961). It is a colourless crystalline basic compound (molecular weight 284·76). It is relatively insoluble in water but is soluble in organic solvents of medium polarity (e.g. diethyl ether). Diazepam has a pKa of 3·3. Camerman and Camerman (1970) remarked on a similarity in steric configuration between the molecule of phenytoin and that of diazepam. Blum, Haefely, Jalfre, Polc and Schaerer (1973) pointed out that most of the anticonvulsants, including benzodiazepines, contain a R_1—$\underset{\underset{R_2}{|}}{C}$—$\underset{\underset{O}{\|}}{C}$—$\underset{\underset{R_3}{|}}{N}$ grouping.

Nitrazepam (7-nitro-5-phenyl-3H-1,4-benzodiazepine-2-one) is a yellow crystalline materal (molecular weight 281·26). It is relatively insoluble in water but soluble in ethanol. The drug is basic and has pKa values of 3·4 and 10·8. It was synthesized by Sternbach, Fryer, Keller, Metlesics, Sach and Steiger (1963).

Clonazepam   (7-nitro-5-(2-chlorophenyl)-1,3-dihydro-2H-1,4-benzodiazepine-2-one) is also a yellowish-white crystalline compound. It is soluble in ethanol and hydrochloric acid. Its molecular weight is 315·72. It is a base with pKa values of 1·5 and 10·5.

	R_1	R_2	R_3
Diazepam	$-CH_3$	$-H$	$-Cl$
Nitrazepam	$-H$	$-H$	$-NO_2$
Clonazepam	$-H$	$-Cl$	$-NO_2$

PHARMACODYNAMICS

ACTIONS IN MAN

Anticonvulsant actions

Certain patterns of usage have evolved for the three benzodiazepines here discussed. Diazepam is now used chiefly as a parenteral anticonvulsant, though there is evidence that it has some effect in absence and myoclonic seizures when given as regular oral medication. Nitrazepam does not appear to be used parenterally but is a reasonably effective agent when given orally for myoclonic epilepsy. Clonazepam, which has been promoted primarily as an anticonvulsant, is useful parenterally in status epilepticus and useful orally in all varieties of generalized epilepsy. It is also useful in partial epilepsy, in particular in those varieties which originate in the temporal lobe (Fazio, Manfredi and Piccinelli, 1975).

Other actions
Diazepam is well known for its anti-anxiety and tranquillizing actions. It is also a hypnotic. Diazepam has been employed to relieve skeletal muscle spasm, and also spasticity (Cartlidge, Hudgson and Weightman, 1974). There is now evidence that clonazepam may also be effective for the latter purpose (Cendrowski and Sobczyk, 1977). Nitrazepam is a widely used and safe hypnotic. Clonazepam also possesses sedative properties. Clonazepam has proved useful in relieving the pain of tic douloureux (Chandra, 1976; Court and Kase, 1976), and in controlling certain dyskinesias including chorea (Pieris, Boralessa and Lionel, 1976) and intention myoclonus (Goldberg and Dorman, 1976).

ACTIONS IN ANIMALS

The anticonvulsant effects of various benzodiazepines in experimental epilepsy were studied by Swinyard and Castellion (1966).

Models of generalized epilepsy
Clonazepam, and to a lesser extent diazepam, prevent photomyoclonic seizures in the baboon Papio papio (Stark, Killam and Killam, 1970). Clonazepam protects against generalized myoclonic convulsions due to systemically administered pentylenetetrazole, strychnine, thiosemicarbazide, 2,4-dimethyl-5-hydroxypyrimidine, cocaine, procaine, lignocaine, bicuculline and bemegride (Blum, Haefely, Jalfe, Polc and Scharer, 1973). These authors reported that diazepam was effective against seizures induced by the first four of these convulsant agents, as well as against seizures induced by bicuculline (Ostrovskaya, Molodavkin, Porfireva and Zubovskaya, 1975). Diazepam is also effective against picrotoxin activated seizures (Loescher and Frey, 1977). Both diazepam and clonazepam protect against maximum and minimum electroshock seizures in mice (Blum, Haefely, Jalfre, Polc and Scharer, 1973).

Models of partial epilepsy
Diazepam is an effective anticonvulsant against electrically kindled seizures arising from the amygdaloid nucleus (Tanaka, 1972; Racine, Livingstone and Joaquin, 1975).
    Clonazepam prevents seizures originating from an experimentally-produced penicillin focus in rat cerebral cortex (Blum, Haefely, Jalfre, Polc and Scharer, 1973).

MECHANISMS OF ACTION

Neuron pools
Clonazepam (Guinta, Ottino, Rossi and Tercereo, 1970; Petsche, 1972) and diazepam (Celesia, Booker and Sato, 1973) failed to alter focal spiking at chemically-induced cortical zones of epileptogenesis in experimental animals. However clonazepam inhibited spread of activity from the foci (Giunta, Ottino, Rossi and Tercereo, 1970). Tsuchiya, Fukushima and Kitagawa (1976) claimed that diazepam, nitrazepam and clonazepam all shortened (though they did not

stop) the primary discharge at a penicillin-induced cortical focus. They also found these benzodiazepines inhibited seizure spread from the focus. The electrical after-discharge threshold in the cat cortex and thalamus is raised by clonazepam (Schallek, cited by Blum, Haefely, Jalfre, Polc and Scharer, 1973). Diazepam raises the after-discharge threshold in the thalamus, amygdala and hippocampus, but not in the neocortex (Boyer, 1966). Clonazepam does not influence the phenomenon of post-tetanic potentiation (Swinyard and Castellion, 1966). Diazepam selectively enhances GABA mediated pre- and post-synaptic inhibition in the cat cuneate nucleus (Polc and Haefely, 1976) and post-synaptic inhibition in pyramidal tract cortical neurons of cats (Raabe and Gumnit, 1977).

Single neurons

Little information has been traced regarding the effects of the benzodiazepines under discussion on single neurons. Diazepam and clonazepam decrease the firing rate of rat cerebellar Purkinje cells (Pieri and Haefely, 1976). Diazepam decreased the spontaneous firing of single hippocampal and amygdaloid neurons in cats (Chou and Wang, 1977), and single sensory and motor cortical neurons in rats (Ostrovskaya and Molodavkin, 1977). Curtis, Lodge, Johnston and Brand (1976) concluded that benzodiazepines neither mimic nor antagonize the actions of glycine or GABA on spinal or cerebellar neurons in cats.

Biochemical

Effects on energy production
No data are available to suggest that the benzodiazepines act by altering neural energy production.

Effects on inorganic ions
There do not appear to be reports of any effects of the benzodiazepines on inorganic ion concentrations in neural tissue. Diazepam inhibited the Mg^{++} linked adenosine triphosphatase of synaptic vesicles (Gilbert and Wyllie, 1976).

Effects on synaptic transmitters
   Acetylcholine. Consolo, Ladinsky, Peri and Garattini (1974) showed that diazepam raised acetylcholine levels in the cerebrum and diencephalon, but not in the cerebellum or mid-brain of mice. Zsilla, Cheney and Costa (1976) found that diazepam decreased acetylcholine turnover in the rat midbrain and cortex, but not in the striatum or hippocampus. Bianchi, Beani and Bertelli (1975) found that diazepam increased acetylcholine concentrations in the forebrain of the guinea pig.
   Serotonin. Clonazepam caused raised brain serotonin levels (Fennessy and Lee, 1972; Jenner, Chadwick, Reynolds and Marsden, 1975). Diazepam decreased serotonin synthesis in the telecephalon and diencephalon of mice (Dominic, Sinha and Barchas, 1975).
   Noradrenaline. Diazepam, nitrazepam and clonazepam all increase brain noradrenaline levels (Fennessy and Lee, 1972). Taylor and Laverty (1969) found that diazepam caused decreased noradrenaline turn-over in thalamus, mid-brain, cortex and cerebellum.

Dopamine. Clonazepam and nitrazepam, but not diazepam, have been found to raise brain dopamine levels (Fennessy and Lee, 1972). However diazepam decreased dopamine turn-over in the olfactory tubercle, nucleus accumbens and the neocortex (Fuxe, Agnati and Bolme, 1975).

Gamma-aminobutyrate (GABA). Diazepam inhibited mitochondrial GABA-transaminase activity and caused raised brain GABA levels (Ostrovoskaya, Molodaukin, Porfiryeau and Zubovskaya, 1975). The drug did not alter cerebellar GABA levels (Mao, Guidotti and Costa, 1975). Olsen, Lamar and Bayless (1977) found that diazepam inhibited GABA uptake by synaptosomes from mouse brain. Thus the drug might tend to potentiate the effects of GABA. Sawaya, Horton and Meldrum (1975) demonstrated that clonazepam had no effect on GABA transaminase, nor on succinic semialdehyde dehydrogenase, the two enzymes which catalyze the metabolic degradation of GABA.

Glycine. It has been suggested that benzodiazepines may act by mimicking the actions of the putative neurotransmitter glycine at its receptors in the central nervous system (Young, Zukin and Snyder, 1974). However Curtis, Game and Lodge (1976) and Curtis, Lodge, Johnston and Brand (1976) have obtained data incompatible with this hypothesis.

'Second Messengers'. The possibility that benzodiazepines may act by altering levels of serotonin or catecholamines is increased by the finding that certain of this family of drugs alter the activities of enzymes concerned with the function of the 'second messengers', cyclic adenosine monophosphate and cyclic guanosine monophosphate. Thus Dalton, Crowley, Sheppard and Schallek (1975) found that diazepam and to a lesser extent its metabolite nordiazepam inhibited cyclic AMP phosphodiesterase in cat brain. Mao, Guidotti and Costa (1975) found that diazepam caused a dose-dependent decrease in cerebellar cyclic guanosine monophosphate without alteration in cyclic adenosine monophosphate. Govoni, Fresia, Spano and Trabucchi (1976) confirmed these findings and showed that nordiazepam had a greater effect than diazepam on cyclic GMP.

Effects on folates. There is no evidence that benzodiazepines cause folate deficiency.

Effects on macromolecules. We have not seen reports that benzodiazepines affect macromolecule formation.

PHARMACOKINETICS

ABSORPTION AND BIOAVAILABILITY

Oral administration

Diazepam. Diazepam absorbs fairly rapidly after oral administration with a mean absorption half-time of 32 minutes (Eatman, Colburn, Boxenbaum, Posmanter, Weinfeld, Ronfeld, Weissman, Moore, Bigaldi and Kaplan, 1977). De Silva, Koechlin and Bader (1966) found peak plasma diazepam levels of 0·18–0·21 μg/ml one hour after a 10 mg oral dose in humans. Kaplan, Jack, Alexander and Weinfeld (1973) found a similar T_{max} value of 1·0–1·5 hours. Schwartz, Koechlin, Postma, Plamer and Krol (1963) showed that only 10 per cent of an oral diazepam dose was excreted in faeces. Thus the absorption of the drug appears reasonably complete.

Nitrazepam. Rieder (1973) calculated that orally administered nitrazepam had an absorption rate constant of $2\cdot16$ hour^{-1}, indicating rapid absorption. He found that the T_{max} was less than 2 hours, while the mean bioavailability of the drug was 78 per cent. Breimer, Bracht and De Boer (1977) found a T_{max} value of 81 ± 62 minutes.

Clonazepam. Kaplan, Alexander, Jack, Puglisi, De Silva, Lee and Weinfeld (1974) found the T_{max} of this drug was 1–2 hours. Sjo, Hvidberg, Naestoft and Lund (1975) determined a T_{max} value of 3 hours. Eadie, Tyrer, Smith and McKauge (1977) found the T_{max} was usually within 3 hours, and in two subjects found a mean bioavailability of 99 per cent.

Rectal administration

Diazepam. Agurell, Berlin, Ferngren and Hellstrom (1975) showed that diazepam absorbed better from the rectum if given in solution than if given in a suppository. In the former case the drug absorbed as rapidly as if given by intramuscular injection. Conchie and Lowis (1973) reported two instances in which diazepam, administered in suppositories, took 20 minutes to control severe convulsions.

Intramuscular administration

Diazepam. Hillestad, Hansen, Melsom and Driveness (1974) showed that in 9 subjects an intramuscular dose of 20 mg diazepam yielded a mean peak plasma diazepam level of 293 ng/ml after 60 minutes. When the same drug dose was given to the same subjects orally, the mean peak plasma level was higher (490 ng/ml) and occurred earlier (T_{max} = 30 minutes). Sturdee (1976) confimed these findings in healthy persons, but showed that after intramuscular injection the drug absorbed better than after oral administration when given to patients with pre-eclampsia.

Nitrazepam is not available for parenteral use and no data are yet available for clonazepam absorption after intramuscular injection.

DISTRIBUTION

V_d

Diazepam. Published values for the V_d of diazepam are as follows:

$1\cdot10$ litres kg^{-1}	in premature infants	Morselli, Principi,
$1\cdot99$ litres kg^{-1}	in children	Tognoni, Reali, Belvedere, Standen and Sereni (1973)
$1\cdot80 \pm 0\cdot29$ litres kg^{-1}	in premature infants	Morselli Mandelli,
$2\cdot60 \pm 0\cdot53$ litres kg^{-1}	in 4–8 year old children	Tognoni, Principi, Pardi and Sereni (1974)
$1\cdot16$ litres kg^{-1}		Andreasen, Hendel, Greisen and Hvidberg (1976)
$0\cdot32 \pm 0\cdot09$ litres kg^{-1}	Klotz, Antonin and Bieck (1976-a)	
$1\cdot04 \pm 0\cdot11$ litres kg^{-1}	Klotz, Antonin, Brügel and Bieck (1977)	

Nitrazepam. Iisalo, Kangas and Ruikka (1977) found that the V_d of nitrazepam in adults aged 21 to 38 years was $2\cdot4 \pm 0\cdot8$ litres kg^{-1}, and in adults 66 to 89 years $4\cdot8 \pm 1\cdot7$ litres kg^{-1}.

Clonazepam. Values for the V_d of clonazepam are 1·5–4·4 litres kg^{-1} (Berlin and Dahlstrom, 1975), 3·1 and 1·9 litres kg^{-1} (Knop, Van der Kleijn and Edmunds, 1975-a and -b) and 1·93 ± 0·32 litres kg^{-1} (Eadie, Tyrer, Smith and McKauge, 1977).

Plasma protein binding

Figures for the plasma protein binding of the benzodiazepines here considered are as set out in Table 11.1 Figures for the binding of these benzodiazepines to bovine serum albumin and to human serum albumin differ (Muller and Wollert, 1976).

Table 11.1. Plasma protein binding of various benzodiazepines

Author	% Bound			
	Diazepam	Nordiazepam	Nitrazepam	Clonazepam
Van der Kleijn (1969)	95%	–	–	–
Reider and Wendt (1971)	–	–	83–86%	–
Muller and Wollert (1973)	90%	–	55%	47%
Kanto, Kangas and Siirtola (1975)	98%	97%	–	–
Tsutsumi, Inaba, Mahon and Kalow (1975)	93·7 ± 0·8%	–	–	–
Van der Kleijn, Guelen, van Wijk and Baars (1975)	–	–	–	80%
Klotz, Antonin and Bieck (1976-a)	96·8%	96·6%	–	–
Thiessen, Sellers, Denbeigh and Dolman (1976)	98·5 ± 0·4%	–	–	–
Kangas, Kanto and Erkkola (1977)	–	–	88%	–

The percentage binding of diazepam to plasma protein does not vary with drug concentrations in the therapeutic range (Van der Kleijn, 1971). Free fatty acids, in particular lauric acid, displace diazepam from plasma protein binding sites (Tsutsumi, Inaba, Mahon and Kalow, 1975).

Entero-hepatic circulation

Diazepam. Mahon, Inaba, Umeda, Tsutsumi and Stone (1976) found no evidence that diazepam underwent an enterohepatic circulation in man.

Concentrations in various body fluids

Cerebrospinal fluid

Diazepam. Kangas, Kanto and Siirtola (1974) found that the CSF levels of diazepam and nordiazepam were 2 per cent and 3 per cent respectively of the plasma levels of these substances. This finding is in keeping with the high plasma protein binding of these drugs.

Saliva

Diazepam. Giles, Zilm, Frecker, Macleod and Sellers (1977) found that salivary diazepam levels were some 2 per cent of plasma levels of the drug.

Milk

Diazepam. Erkkola and Kanto (1972) in 3 women showed that maternal plasma levels of diazepam and nordiazepam were 491 ± 56 and 340 ± 59 ng/ml respectively, 4 days post partum. At the same time levels of the two substances in milk were 51 ± 2 and 28 ± 4 ng/ml respectively. Two days later the respective plasma levels were 601 ± 22 and 483 ± 22 ng/ml, and the milk levels 78 ± 18 and 52 ± 8 ng/ml. However Brandt (1976) stated that levels of nordiazepam are higher than levels of diazepam in human milk.

Concentrations in tissues

Diazepam. The whole body autoradiographic studies of van der Kleijn, van Rossum, Muskens and Rijntjes (1971) have shown that after injection of the drug into mice there is a rapid, fairly selective uptake of diazepam by adipose tissue and, in the nervous system, by the spinal cord, diencephalic grey matter and cerebral cortex. Diazepam itself is fairly rapidly eliminated but its metabolites persist in the gut, liver, and white matter of brain and spinal cord. The findings of Coutinho, Cheripko and Carbone (1970), also in mice, were similar. However in monkeys Idaenpaeaen Hiekkilae, Taska, Allen and Schoolar (1971) found that, in the nervous system, diazepam and its metabolites were at relatively high concentrations in the cerebral white matter, lateral geniculate body, optic tract, anterior commisure, corpus callosum, dentate nucleus, pons and medulla; the compounds were at relatively low levels in the hippocampus, cerebral grey matter, hypothalamus and caudate nucleus. Brain levels of diazepam were much higher than blood levels of the drug (Van der Kleijn, 1969). Celesia, Booker and Sato (1974) found that brain and serum diazepam levels were in a 2:1 ratio in cats.

Korttila, Mattila and Linnoila (1975), on the basis of pharmacokinetic studies in humans, obtained evidence that the tissue binding of nordiazepam was saturable. After 11 weeks of diazepam intake, but not earlier, Zingales (1973) found small amounts of diazepam and its metabolites were present in human erythrocytes. However simultaneous plasma levels of these substances were very much higher.

De Silva, D'Arconte and Kaplan (1964) found that maternal and fetal plasma levels of diazepam were similar. Mandelli, Morselli, Nordio, Pardi, Sereni and Tognoni (1975) confirmed this finding and showed that it also applied for nordiazepam levels. However, as time passed after a diazepam dose, umbilical cord plasma levels of the benzodiazepines rose relative to maternal plasma levels. These authors stated that nordiazepam levels were usually 2–3 times diazepam levels in fetal tissues. Erkkola, Kanto and Sellman (1974) found that, after continued maternal use of diazepam, early human fetal and maternal diazepam and nordiazepam levels were both in an approximate 0·4:1·0 ratio.

Nitrazepam. Rieder (1965) showed that in rats, after intraperitoneal injection, nitrazepam was concentrated in the stomach, gut and bladder. Small amounts occurred in other organs. In humans the drug and its metabolites passed through the placenta. Concentrations were similar in maternal and full term fetal blood, but were relatively lower in the 14–17 week fetus (Kangas, Kanto and Erkkola, 1977). The concentration of nitrazepam and metabolites in milk were about 50 per cent of those in plasma (Reider and Wendt, 1971).

Clonazepam. Knop, Van der Kleijn and Edmunds (1975-b) published whole

Table 11.2. Elimination parameters of diazepam and its metabolites

Author	Half-life (hours)			
	Diazepam	Nor-diazepam	Temazepam	Oxazepam
Van der Kleijn (1969)	9–24	25–50	–	–
Kaplan, Jack, Alexander & Weinfeld (1973)	27–36	50–99	–	–
Morselli, Mandelli, Tognoni, Principi, Pardi & Sereni (1974)	75 ± 37* 31 ± 2† 18 ± 3	–	–	–
Morselli, Principi, Tongoni, Reali, Belvedere Standen & Sereni (1973)	54†	–	–	–
Greenblatt & Shader (1974)	18*	–	–	3–21
Hillestad, Hansen & Melsom (1974)	54	92	–	–
Van der Kleijn, Guelen, Van Wijk and Baars (1975)	32	–	–	–
Andreasen, Hendel, Greisen and Hvidberg (1976)	32·1	–	–	–
Gamble, Dundee & Gray (1976)	48–96	96–192	–	–
Klotz, Antonin & Bieck (1976-b)	33·9 ± 10·6[1] 52·9 ± 17·4[2]	–	–	–
Klotz, Antonin, Brügel and Bieck (1977)	46·6 ± 14·2	50·9 6·2	–	–
Eatman, Colburn, Boxenbaum, Posmanter, Weinfeld, Ronfeld, Weissman, Moore, Gibaldi & Kaplan (1977)	57	–	–	–
Fuccella, Bolcioni, Tamassia, Ferrario & Tognoni (1977)	–	–	7·25–8·25	–

* in premature infants   [1] after the first dose
† in newborn infants   [2] after 6 days of therapy
‡ in children 3–7 years of age

body autoradiographs illustrating the distribution of clonazepam in mice and squirrel monkeys. High amounts of radioactivity occurred in the stomach, liver, gall bladder, spleen, intestine, kidney, urinary bladder and heart, relative to levels in the blood and the brain.

ELIMINATION

Elimination rate

Diazepam. Some published values for the elimination rate parameters of diazepam and its metabolites nordiazepam and oxazepam are set out in Table 11.2. The elimination rate is slower in premature infants than in older children. Klotz, Antonin and Bieck (1976-b) showed a statistically significant slowing in diazepam elimination after the drug was given in chronic dosage. They ascribed this effect to a slowing of diazepam metabolism as nordiazepam accumulated.

Nitrazepam. Rieder (1973) found a mean β phase half-life of 25·1 hours for nitrazepam. Van der Kleijn, Guelen, Van Wijk and Baars (1975) quoted a k value of 0·034 hour^{-1} ($T_{\frac{1}{2}} = 21$ hours). Iisalo, Kangas and Ruikka (1977) obtained β values of $0·0254 \pm 0·0074$ hour^{-1} and $0·0198 \pm 0·0080$ hour^{-1} (corresponding to half-lives of $28·9 \pm 7·4$ and $40·4 \pm 16·2$ hours) for healthy young adults, and people 66–89 years of age, respectively. Breimer, Bracht and De Boer (1977) found nitrazepam had a terminal half-life of 30 ± 5 hours.

Clonazepam. Published values for the elimination rate parameters of clonazepam are set out in Table 11.3.

Table 11.3 Half-life values for clonazepam

Author	Half-life (hours)
Naestoft, Lund, Larsen and Hvidberg (1973)	24–28
De Silva, Puglisi and Munno (1974)	47*
Kaplan, Alexander, Jack, Puglisi, de Silva, Lee and Weinfeld (1974)	26·4
Berlin and Dahlstrom (1975)	19–60
Dreifuss, Penry, Rose, Kupferberg, Dyken and Sato (1975)	22–33
Hvidberg and Sjo (1975)	22 and 38†
Knop, Van der Kleijn and Edmunds (1975-a)	22 and 17·2‡
Van der Kleijn, Guelen, Van Wijk and Baars (1975)	36 (k = 0·02 hour^{-1})
Eadie, Tyrer, Smith and McKauge (1977)	14·5 (k = 0·048 $\pm$ 0·23 hour^{-1})

* value in one subject
† values in two subjects
‡ values on two occasions in one subject

The shorter half-life values obtained by Eadie, Tyrer, Smith and McKauge (1977), and Fig. 11.1, as compared with other authors, may be explained by the former's values being derived from patients chronically dosed with other anticonvulsants. Possibly the other anticonvulsants induced the elimination of clonazepam. Many of the other authors' values quoted above had been derived from otherwise untreated healthy volunteers. Berlin and Dalstrom (1975) found no

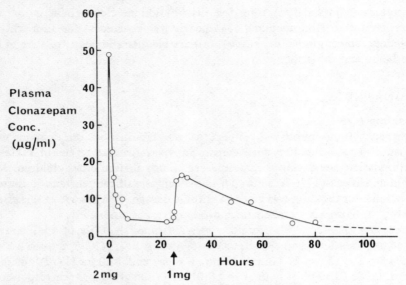

Fig. 11.1 Time-course of plasma clonazepam levels in a patient with epilepsy given two doses of clonazepam 24 hours apart (Eadie, Tyrer, Smith and McKauge, 1978).

evidence that clonazepam induced the enzymatic processes responsible for its own elimination.

Clearance

Diazepam. Values for the clearance of diazepam were $0·0275 \pm 0·0085$ litres kg^{-1} $hour^{-1}$ for premature infants, and $0·1027 \pm 0·0097$ litres kg^{-1} $hour^{-1}$ for 4–8 year old children (Morselli, Mandelli, Tognoni, Principi, Pardi and Sereni, 1974). For mixed populations values were $0·03$ litres kg^{-1} $hour^{-1}$ (Van der Kleijn, Guelen, Van Wijk and Baars, 1975), $26·0 \pm 10·8$ ml/min after the first dose, falling to $18·2 \pm 7·0$ ml/minute after 6 days of therapy (Klotz, Antonin and Bieck, 1976-a; 1976-b), $32·3 \pm 11·0$ ml/minute (Klotz, Antonin, Burgel and Bieck, 1977) and $0·0227$ litres kg^{-1} $hour^{-1}$ (Eatman, Colburn, Boxenbaum, Posmanter, Weinfeld, Ronfeld, Weissman, Moore, Gibaldi and Kaplan, 1977).

Nitrazepam. Iisalo, Kangas and Ruikka (1977) found mean nitrazepam clearance of $4·1 \pm 2·0$ litres $hour^{-1}$ in adults aged 20–38 years and a mean clearance of $4·7 \pm 1·5$ litres $hour^{-1}$ in adults aged 66–89 years. Van der Kleijn, Guelen, Van Wijk and Baars (1975) quoted a similar nitrazepam clearance value of $0·070$ litres kg^{-1} $hour^{-1}$

Clonazepam. Published clearance values include $0·098$ and $0·080$ litres kg^{-1} $hour^{-1}$ in the one subject (Knop, Van der Kleijn and Edmunds, 1975-b) and $0·092 \pm 0·051$ litres kg^{-1} $hour^{-1}$ (Eadie, Tyrer, Smith and McKauge, 1977).

Per cent excreted unchanged

Diazepam. Kaplan, Jack, Alexander and Weinfeld (1973) found that less than $0·05$ per cent of a diazepam dose was excreted unchanged in urine. In 5 subjects whose bile ducts were being drained Klotz, Antonin and Bieck (1976-b) found only $0·3$–$0·4$ per cent of a diazepam dose was excreted unchanged in bile.

Nitrazepam. No data are available.

Clonazepam. Kaplan, Alexander, Jack, Puglisi, De Silva, Lee and Weinfeld (1974) found only about 0·2 per cent of a clonazepam dose was excreted unchanged in urine. Sjo, Hvidberg, Naestoft and Lund (1975) quoted a figure of 0·1–1·4 per cent for this parameter, and Hvidberg and Sjo (1975) a figure of 2 per cent.

Thus both diazepam and clonazepam are eliminated chiefly by biotransformation.

Biotransformation pattern

Diazepam. This substance undergoes a number of chemical alterations in the liver (Jori, Prestini and Pugliatti, 1969). The metabolic pathway is set out in Fig. 11·2. The 13 week fetal human liver is capable of metabolising the drug

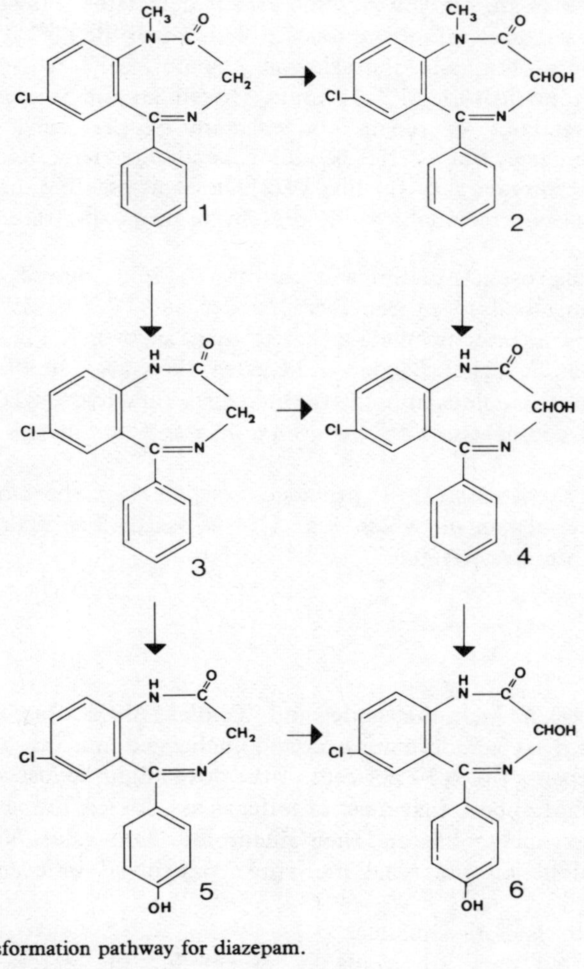

Fig. 11.2 Biotransformation pathway for diazepam.
1. diazepam
2. 3-hydroxydiazepam (temazepam)
3. N-desmethyldiazepam (nordiazepam)
4. oxazepam
5 and 6. 5-(p-hydroxyphenyl) metabolites

(Ackermann and Richter, 1977). The human renal cortex also has a small capacity for biotransforming diazepam (Ackermann, Richter and Sage, 1976). The main product of biotransformation of diazepam is the biologically active desmethyl-diazepam, i.e. nordiazepam (Marcucci, Guaitani, Kvetina, Mussini and Garratini, 1968). In man it was said to first appear in plasma 24 to 36 hours after an initial dose of diazepam (de Silva, Koechlin and Bader, 1966; Foster and Frings, 1970). However, more recent reports suggest that nordiazepam appears in plasma within 30 minutes of diazepam administration in adults (Kaplan, Jack, Alexander and Weinfeld, 1973), within one hour in children, but only after 4 hours in premature infants (Morselli, Mandelli, Tognoni, Principi, Pardi and Sereni, 1974). The hydroxylated derivatives of diazepam are conjugated with glucuronic acid and then, like most glucuronides, are probably fairly rapidly excreted. Thus their plasma levels in man are very low, though usually detectable (Zingales, 1973). The metabolite temazepam is rapidly eliminated with a half-life of 7·25 to 8·25 hours (Fuccella, Bolcioni, Tamassia, Ferrario and Tognoni, 1977) while oxazepam also has a relatively short half-life of 3–21 hours (Greenblatt and Shader, 1974). When the diazepam metabolite oxazepam is given orally, 95 per cent is excreted as its glucuronide conjugate, but a series of minor metabolites have also been detected (Sisenwine, Tio, Shrader and Ruelius, 1972). It seems possible that similar as yet not identified minor metabolites are present in urine in trace amounts after diazepam dosage.

Nitrazepam. Bartosek, Mussini and Garratini (1969) showed that in the rat nitrazepam is metabolised by the liver. Rieder and Wendt (1971) provided a scheme outlining nitrazepam metabolism in man, on which Fig. 11.3 is based. Randall, Schallek, Scheckel, Bagdon and Rieder (1966) also identified the 7-amino and 7-acetamido metabolites in human urine. Again, the hydroxylated metabolites are likely to be conjugated with glucuronic acid and eliminated rapidly via the kidneys.

Clonazepam. Eschenhof (1973) provided a scheme for the biotransformation pathways of clonazepam on which Fig. 11.4 is based. The main metabolite in plasma is the 7-amino derivative.

Excretion

Diazepam. Kaplan, Jack, Alexander and Weinfeld (1973) found that less than 0·5 per cent of a diazepam dose was excreted unchanged in urine, and 2·5 to 9 per cent as nordiazepam. Up to 10 per cent of the dose might be lost in faeces. From their data it would appear that most of a diazepam dose is probably excreted in urine as 3-hydroxy metabolites and their glucuronide conjugates. No work appears to have been done on the renal mechanisms involved in excretion of these substances.

Nitrazepam No data are available.

Clonazepam. No data are available, except for the percentages excreted unchanged given above, and the finding of Sjo, Hvidberg, Naestoft and Lund (1975) that, in the steady state, some 5 to 20 per cent of a clonazepam dose appears in urine as the 7-amino and 7-acetamido-metabolites.

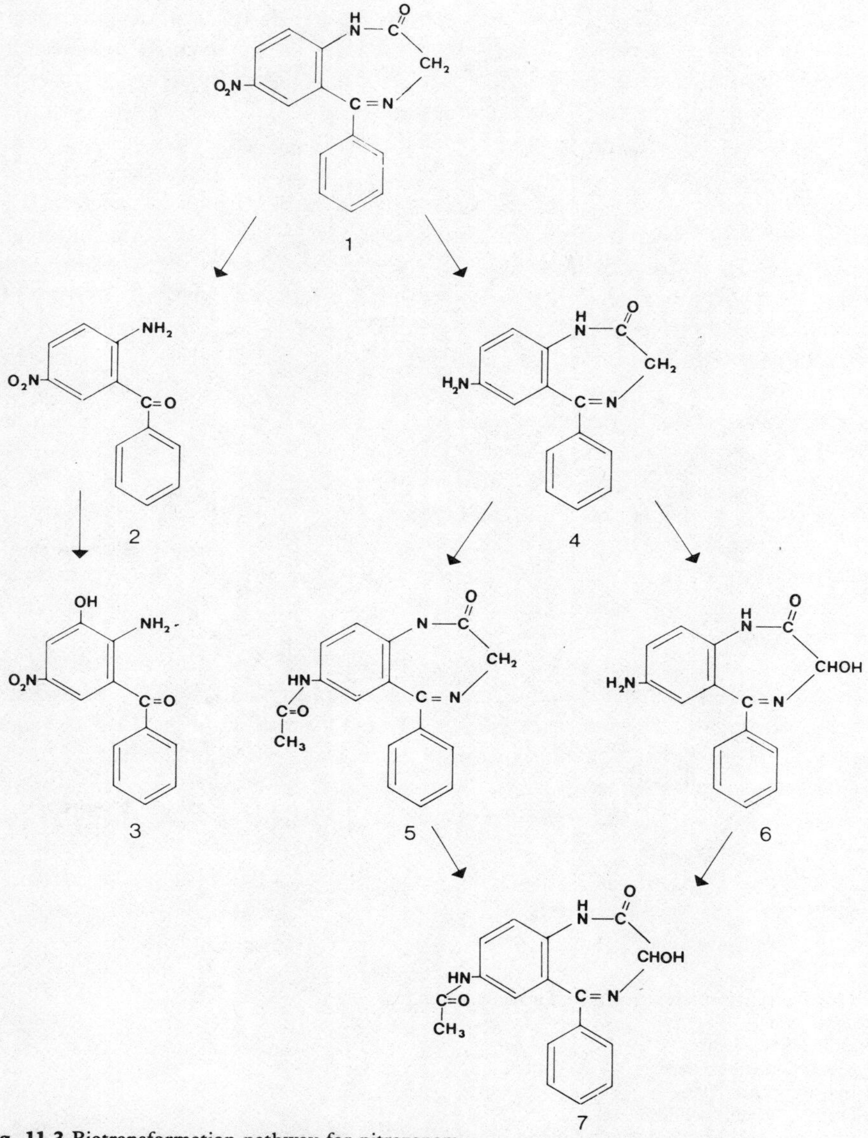

Fig. 11.3 Biotransformation pathway for nitrazepam.
1. nitrazepam
2 and 3. benzophenone metabolites
4. 7-aminonitrazepam
5. 7-acetamidonitrazepam
6 and 7. 3-hydroxyderivatives of 4 and 5 respectively.

CLINICAL PHARMACOKINETICS

Time-Course of Plasma Drug Levels

Single dose

   Diazepam. Peak plasma diazepam levels occur about 1 hour after a single oral

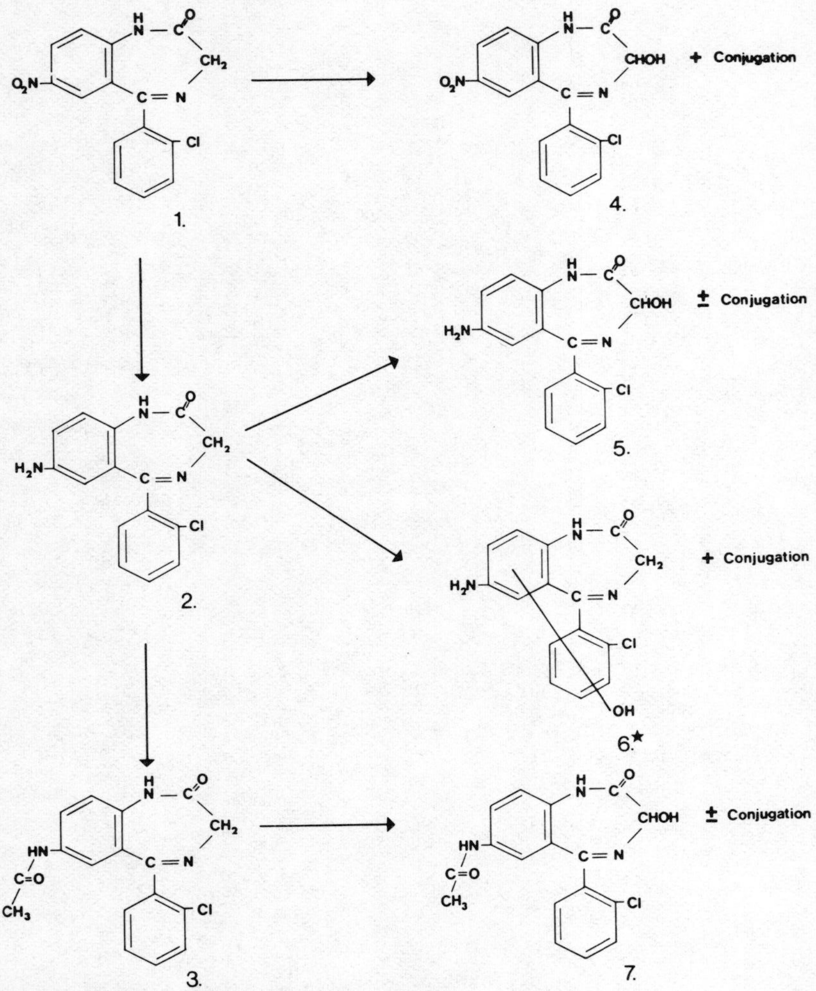

Fig. 11.4 Biotransformation pathway for clonazepam
1. clonazepam
2. 7-aminoclonzaepam
3. 7-acetamidoclonazepam
4. 3-hydroxyclonazepam
5. 3-hydroxy-7-aminoclonazepam
6. phenolic metabolite of 7-aminoclonazepam (it is not known which benzene ring is hydroxylated)
7. 3-hydroxy-7-acetamidoclonazepam

dose of the drug. Levels then decline monoexponentially, with a half-life of some 1 to 2 days. After intramuscular or rectal administration peak plasma diazepam level occurs more slowly (see above). Recent data suggest that nordiazepam may appear in plasma within 1 hour of diazepam administration. Levels of this substance decline more slowly than levels of diazepam itself.

Nitrazepam. After oral dosage, plasma nitrazepam levels peak within 2 hours and then decline with a terminal half-life of about 1 day in younger subjects, and rather longer in older subjects.

Clonazepam. After oral administration, plasma clonazepam levels reach a peak within 3 hours and then decline with a terminal half-life of about 24–36 hours.

Repeated dosage

Diazepam. With repeated dosage, plasma diazepam levels reach steady-state values after the lapse of about 7 days (Hillestad, Hansen and Melson, 1974; Kaplan, Jack, Alexander and Weinfeld, 1973) or 8 days (Gamble, Dundee and Gray, 1976). Available pharmacokinetic data suggest that it would take about twice as long for a steady-state to occur for plasma nordiazepam levels. However, Eatman, Colburn, Boxembaum, Posmanter, Weinfeld, Ronfeld, Weissman, Moore, Gibaldi and Kaplan (1977) quoted a figure of 5–8 days for the time to achieve a steady state for nordiazepam. Zingales (1973) found that plasma levels of diazepam and its metabolites took several weeks to reach a plateau, when diazepam was taken regularly in constant daily dosage. In a few patients plasma drug levels continued to rise for many months. However Kanto, Iisalo, Lehtinen and Salminen (1974) found that after 6 weeks of diazepam therapy plasma levels of both the parent substance and nor-diazepam began to decline.

Steady state plasma nor-diazepam levels are reported to be similar to simultaneous plasma diazepam levels (De Silva, Schwartz, Stefanovik, Kaplan and D'Arconte, 1964; Kaplan, Jack, Alexander and Weinfeld, 1973). However steady-state plasma nor-diazepam levels have also been reported to be 70 per cent (Bond, Hailey and Lader, 1977), about 1/2–1/3 (Gamble, Dundee and Gray, 1976) or 1/5 (Klotz, Antonin and Bieck, 1976-b) of simultaneous plasma diazepam levels. Oxazepam and 3-hydroxydiazepam levels are about 5–10 per cent of plasma diazepam levels (Zingales, 1973).

Despite the relatively slow elimination of diazepam and nor-diazepam, the rapid absorption of diazepam after oral administration suggests that there might be appreciable inter-dose fluctuation in steady state plasma levels of drug and metabolite. In 4 subjects given 10 mg diazepam once a day Kaplan, Jack, Alexander and Weinfeld (1973) showed fluctuations of plasma diazepam levels through a threefold range during the dosage interval.

Nitrazepam. Iisalo, Kangas and Ruikka (1977) found that nitrazepam plasma levels attained steady state values after 3·5 days of therapy in 21 to 38 year old healthy adults, and after 7·5 days in aged patients.

Rieder and Wendt (1971) showed that, with a regular evening 5 mg nitrazepam dose, plasma nitrazepam levels became steady in three days, at an average value of 38·6 ng/ml. The total plasma levels of its two main metabolites, the 7-amino and 7-acetamido derivatives, were similar to those of the parent nitrazepam.

Clonazepam. Elimination rate data suggest that the steady state for clonazepam would usually apply after 5–8 days of regular dosage. In the steady state De Silva, Puglisi and Munno (1974) could not find measurable plasma levels of the 7-amino and 7-acetamido metabolites when clonazepam levels were 20 to 49 ng/ml. However Sjo, Hvidberg, Naestoft and Lund (1975) found that, in the steady state, plasma levels of clonazepam and its metabolites were in a 1:3 to a 3:1 ratio in different subjects. The rapid absorption of clonazepam after oral administration, despite its fairly slow elimination, makes it likely that there will be significant fluctuation in steady-state plasma levels across a 12 or 24 hour dosage interval.

Correlations of plasma drug concentrations and clinical effects

Diazepam. Apparently on a basis of clinical impression, Agurell, Berlin, Ferngren and Hellstrom (1975) proposed that 150–200 ng/ml was the threshold for an anticonvulsant effect of diazepam. Booker and Celesia (1973) had set 600 ng/ml as the threshold diazepam concentration to suppress paroxysmal activity in the human EEG. This value was obtained after intravenous injection of the drug and it may have been determined before final blood to brain distributional ratios had time to apply. The surface EEG shows increased β activity once plasma diazepam levels exceed 100 ng/ml (Fink, Irwin, Weinfeld, Schwartz and Conney, 1975). Bond, Hailey and Lader (1977) stated that no relation has been shown to exist between plasma benzodiazepine level and measured relief of anxiety, but Dasberg, Van der Kleijn, Guelen and Van Praag (1974) claimed that plasma diazepam levels above 400 ng/ml and plasma nordiazepam levels above 300 ng/ml were associated with relief of anxiety and other psychiatric symptoms.

Winek (1976) regarded plasma diazepam levels of 5000–2000 ng/ml as toxic, and levels above 50 000 ng/ml as lethal.

Nitrazepam. We have been unable to find published data on the correlation between plasma levels of this drug and its anticonvulsant effects.

Clonazepam. Huang, McLeod, Sampson and Hensley (1973) obtained some evidence that plasma clonazepam levels above 15 ng/ml tended to correlate with protection against myoclonic seizures. Levels above 30 ng/ml offered protection against other types of epileptic seizure. In a later publication these authors (Huang, McLeod, Sampson and Hensley, 1974) found that plasma clonazepam levels around 25–30 ng/ml had an anticonvulsant effect. Plasma clonazepam levels of 13–72 ng/ml were associated with improved control of epilepsy in 8 of 10 children (Dreifuss, Penry, Rose, Kupferberg, Dyken and Sato, 1975). Naestoft, Lund, Larsen and Hvidberg, (1973) could not determine any correlation between plasma clonazepam level and anticonvulsant effect. We have seen clonazepam control absence seizures at plasma drug levels in the range 20–30 ng/ml, but also fail to control temporal lobe seizures at levels around 200 ng/ml. The drug has not yet been in use long enough, and has been used too often in cases refactory to all other anticonvulsants, for a reliable therapeutic range of plasma levels in epilepsy to have been worked out.

Plasma level—dose correlations in treated populations

Diazepam. Regular oral diazepam doses of 30 mg per day produced maximum plasma diazepam levels of 500–1000 ng/ml (Foster and Frings, 1970). Daily doses of 20–25 mg taken for five days yielded plasma diazepam levels of 160–400 ng/ml and plasma desmethyldiazepam (nordiazepam) levels of 118–410 ng/ml (De Silva, Schwartz, Stetanovik, Kaplan and D'Arconte, 1964). Zingales (1973) found daily oral diazepam doses of 10 mg produced an average plasma diazepam level of 231 ng/ml, and an average desmethyldiazepam level of 0·269 ng/ml in patients taking the drug over periods between 2 days and 2 years. A 20 mg dose led to average levels of 310 ng/ml and 430 ng/ml respectively.

The effects of age, sex and pregnancy on the relation between diazepam level and drug dose are not known.

Nitrazepam. No data are available.

Clonazepam. Steady-state plasma clonazepam levels are linearly related to drug dose (Huang, McLeod, Sampson and Hensley, 1974; Rose, Penry and Dreifuss, 1974; Sjo, Hvidberg, Naestoft and Lund, 1975; Eadie, Tyrer, Smith and McKauge, 1977—Fig. 11.5). The effect of age, sex and pregnancy on this relationship are not known.

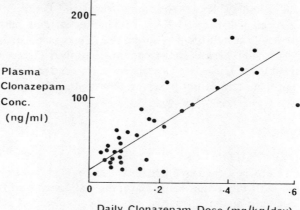

Fig. 11.5 Relation between steady-state plasma clonazepam levels and drug dose in 35 patients (Eadie, Tyrer, Smith and McKauge, 1977).

Plasma level—dose correlations in treated individuals

Diazepam. No data are available.

Nitrazepam. Not data are available.

Clonazepam. In individuals given dose increments to try to attain control of epilepsy, steady-state plasma drug levels appear directly proportionate to drug dose (Eadie, 1976; Fig. 11.6).

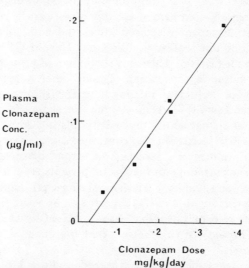

Fig. 11.6 Linear relation between steady-state plasma clonazepam levels and clonazepam dose in a woman who was given increasing clonazepam doses at intervals in an attempt to control her epilepsy (Eadie, 1976).

Effects of disease

Diazepam. Sjoholm, Kober, Odar-Cederlof and Borga (1976) showed that uraemic plasma had a decreased capacity to bind diazepam. Andreasen, Hendel, Griesen and Hvidberg (1976) showed that diazepam half-life was prolonged to a mean of 164 hours in patients with hepatic cirrhosis when compared with normal controls ($T_{\frac{1}{2}} = 32 \cdot 1$ hours). Klotz, Antonin, Brügel and Bieck (1977) found that diazepam had a mean half-life of $99 \cdot 2 \pm 23 \cdot 3$ hours in their patients with liver disease, compared with a half-life of $46 \cdot 6 \pm 14 \cdot 2$ hours in normals; nordiazepam half-life was $108 \cdot 2 \pm 40 \cdot 03$ hours in the patients with liver disease and $50 \cdot 9 \pm 6 \cdot 2$ hours in normal subjects. Diazepam clearance was reduced in cases of liver disease, but the V_d of diazepam and of nordiazepam was unaltered.

INTERACTIONS

PHARMACODYNAMIC INTERACTIONS

Combining one or other of the three benzoidiazepines here considered with other benzodiazepines, with other non-benzodiazepine sedatives or with alcohol, may produce additional anti-anxiety, sedative and anti-convulsant effects. However, it has not been established that these phenomena represent genuine pharmacodynamic interactions. The possibility of pharmacokinetic interactions has not been excluded.

PHARMACOKINETIC INTERACTIONS

Benzodiazepines affecting other substances

Diazepam. Bratlid and Langslet (1973) found that sodium benzoate, which is present in certain parenteral diazepam preparations, could displace bilirubin from plasma albumin, though diazepam itself did not displace bilirubin. Schussler (1971) showed that diazepam displaced thyroxine and triiodothyronine from thyroxine binding globulin. Saldanha, Bird and Havard (1971) considered that diazepam decreased the levels of dialysable thyroxine, of protein bound iodine and of 'free' thyroxine iodine in the plasma of man. They suggested that the drug depressed the release of thyroid stimulating hormone from the pituitary. However Clark, Hall and Ormstow (1971) claimed that diazepam did not reduce protein bound iodine levels or change serum thyroid stimulating hormone concentrations. Argülles and Rosner (1975) showed that continued use of diazepam was associated with raised plasma testosterone levels. Concurrent diazepam therapy caused plasma phenytoin concentrations to rise in the patients studied by Vajda, Prineas and Lovell (1971), and Rogers, Haslam, Longstreth and Lietman (1977). However Richens and Houghton (1975) reported an opposite finding, and showed that the elimination rate of phenytoin was increased in their patients. Orme, Breckenridge and Brooks (1972) showed that diazepam did not alter plasma warfarin concentrations.

Nitrazepam. Concurrent therapy with nitrazepam did not alter plasma warfarin concentrations (Orme, Breckenridge and Brooks, 1972), or tricyclic antidepressant concentrations (Silverman and Braithwaite, 1973).

Clonazepam. The seemingly contradictory finding for the effects of clonazepam on plasma phenytoin levels are discussed on page 92 (see Fig. 11.7). The drug is said to cause raised plasma primidone levels (Windorfer and Sauer, 1977). However Nanda, Johnson, Keogh, Lambie and Melville (1977) found that clonazepam had no effect on plasma phenobarbitone or primidone levels, and Johanessen, Strandjord and Munthe-Kaas (1977) reported that it did not alter plasma phenobarbitone and carbamazepine levels. The data of Fig. 7.19 suggest that clonazepam may not always be without effect on plasma carbamazepine levels.

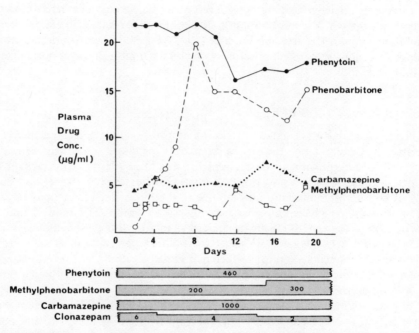

Fig. 11.7 In the majority of patients studied personally, plasma phenytoin levels have tended to fall when clonazepam was added to phenytoin therapy. However, in the patient illustrated, despite constant doses of phenytoin, methylphenobarbitone and carbamazepine, plasma phenytoin and phenobarbitone levels fell when clonazepam dose was reduced.

Other substances affecting benzodiazepines

Diazepam. Ethyl alcohol reduced the plasma protein binding of diazepam from $98 \cdot 5 \pm 0 \cdot 4$ per cent to $97 \cdot 8 \pm 1 \cdot 2$ per cent (Theiessen, Sellers, Denbeigh and Dolman, 1976). Hayes, Pablo, Radomski and Palmer (1977) found higher peak plasma diazepam levels when the drug was taken with alcohol than with water. This suggested that alcohol might enhance the rate of absorption of diazepam. Linnoila, Otterstrom and Anttila (1974) showed that alcohol did not affect serum diazepam levels, but Sellman, Kanto, Raijola and Pekkarinen (1975) found that chronic alcoholics eliminated diazepam faster than control subjects.

Kanto, Philajamaki and Iisalo (1974) showed that halothane anaesthesia in children decreased the plasma clearance of diazepam.

Nitrazepam. No data are available.

Clonazepam. Phenytoin therapy decreased plasma clonazepam levels in 5 patients out of 5 (Hvidberg and Sjo, 1975). Phenobarbitone had a similar effect (Nanda, Johnson, Keogh, Lambie and Melville, 1977).

TOXICITY

LOCAL EFFECTS

The three benzodiazepines here considered rarely cause any local irritation of the alimentary tract when given by mouth. Reactions at parenteral injection sites are uncommon, though Hegarty and Dundee (1977) reported a significant incidence of painless thrombosis at injection sites 7 to 10 days after intravenous diazepam administration.

DOSE-DEPENDENT EFFECTS

The benzodiazepines have sedative actions and nitrazepam is marketed chiefly as a hypnotic. Understandably the drugs frequently produce some drowsiness and feelings of dysequilibrium in doses used for treating epilepsy. Clonazepam may produce drowsiness, ataxia and aggressiveness (Bladin, 1973; Edwards and Eadie, 1973). A considerable measure of tolerance to these sedative effects may develop, particularly if benzodiazepine doses are increased gradually (Elain, Lund and Melsen, 1973). The risk of diazepam toxicity is increased if plasma albumin levels are low (Greenblatt and Koch-Weser, 1974). Nitrazepam may produce increased salivary and bronchial secretion (Millichap and Ortiz, 1966), as may clonazepam. Serious toxic effects. except from gross overdosage, seem exceedingly rare in benzodiazepine therapy.

If chronic therapy with diazepam (Vyas and Carney, 1975) or clonazepam (Edwards, 1974) is ceased abruptly, withdrawal fitting may occur. In the case of clonazepam, status epilepticus has been reported in these circumstances (Edwards, 1974).

IDIOSYNCRATIC EFFECTS

Hypersensitivity rashes occasionally complicate benzodiazepine use. Parenteral diazepam may occasionally cause hypotension and depressed respiration, possibly because of the action of its solvent, propylene glycol (Louis, Kutt and McDowell, 1967).

EFFECTS ON THE FETUS AND NEONATE

Aarskog (1975) and Saxén and Saxén (1975) independently obtained evidence that maternal diazepam intake in the first 3 months of pregnancy was associated with an increased risk of oral clefts in the offspring. Otherwise there is no evidence that the benzodiazepines are dysmorphogenic in humans.

PREPARATIONS AVAILABLE

These include:

Diazepam. *Tablets:* 2 mg; 5 mg
                 Syrup: 2 mg per 5 ml
                 Ampoules: 10 mg per 2 ml
Nitrazepam. *Tablets:* 5 mg
Clonazepam. *Tablets:* 0·5 mg; 2 mg
                 Ampoules: 1 mg

REFERENCES

Aarskog, D. (1975) Association between maternal intake of diazepam and oral clefts. *Lancet*, ii, 921.

Ackermann, E. & Richter, K. (1977) Diazepam metabolism in human foetal and adult liver. *Europ. J. clin. Pharmacol.*, 11, 43–49.

Ackermann, E., Richter, K. & Sage, S. (1976) Diazepam metabolism in human cortex kidney microsomes. *Biochem. Pharmacol.*, 25, 1557–1560.

Agurell, S., Berlin, A., Ferngren, H. & Hellstrom, B. (1975), Plasma levels of diazepam after parenteral and rectal administration in children. *Epilepsia* (Amst.), 16, 277–283.

Andreasen, P. B., Hendel, J., Greisen, G. & Hvidberg, E. F. (1976) Pharmacokinetics of diazepam in disordered liver function. *Europ. J. clin. Pharmacol.*, 10, 115–120.

Archer, G. A. & Sternbach, L. H. (1968) The chemistry of benzodiazepines. *Chem. Rev.*, 68, 747–784.

Argüelles, A. E. & Rosner, J. (1975) Diazepam and plasma-testosterone levels. *Lancet*, 2, 607.

Bartosek, I., Mussini, E. & Garattini, S. (1969) Reduction of nitrazepam by rat liver. *Biochem. Pharmacol.*, 18, 2263–2264.

Berlin, A. & Dahlström, H. (1975) Pharmacokinetics of the anticonvulsant drug clonazepam evaluated from single oral and intravenous doses and by repeated oral administration. *Europ. J. Clin. Pharmacol.*, 9, 155–159.

Bianchi, C., Beani, L. & Bertelli, A. (1975) Effects of some anti epileptic drugs on brain acetylcholine. *Neuropharmacology*, 14, 327–332.

Bladin, P. F. (1973) The use of clonazepam as an anticonvulsant-clinical evaluation. *Med. J. Australia*, 1, 683–688.

Blum, J. E., Haefely, W., Jaffre, M., Polc, P. & Scharer, K. (1973) Parmakologie und Toxicologie des Antiepileptikums Clonazepam. *Arzniem.-Forsch.*, 23, 377–389.

Bond, A. J., Hailey, D. M. & Lader, M. H. (1977) Plasma concentrations of benzodiazepines. *Brit. J. clin. Pharmacol.*, 4, 51–56.

Booker, H. E. & Celesia, G. G. (1973) Serum concentrations of diazepam in subjects with epilepsy. *Arch. Neurol. (Chicago)*, 29, 191–194.

Boyer, P. A. Jnr. (1966) Anticonvulsant properties of benzodiazepines. A review. *Dis. Nerv. Syst.*, 27, 35–42.

Brandt, R. (1976) Passage of diazepam into breast milk. *Arzneim.-Forsch.*, 26, 454–457.

Bratlid, D. & Langslet, A. (1973) Displacement of albumin-bound bilirubin by injectable diazepam preapartions *in vitro*. *Acta Paediat. Scand.*, 62, 510–512.

Breimer, D. D., Bracht, H. & De Boer, A. G. (1977) Plasma level profile of nitrazepam (Mogadon[R]) following oral administration. *Brit. J. Clin. Pharmacol.*, 4, 709–711.

Camerman, A. & Camerman, N. (1970) Diphenylhydantoin and diazepam: molecular structure similarities and steric basic of anticonvulsant activity. *Science*, 168, 1457–1458.

Cartlidge, N. E. F., Hudgson, P. & Weightman, D. (1974) A comparison of baclofen and diazepam in the treatment of spasticity. *J. Neurol. Sci.*, 23, 17–24.

Celesia, G. G., Booker, H. E. & Sato, S. (1973) Effects of diazepam on experimentally induced cortical epilepsy and their correlation with drug concentration. *Electroenceph. Clin. Neurophysiol.*, 34, 727.

Celesia, G. G., Booker, H. E. & Sato, S. (1974) Brain and serum concentrations of diazepam in experimental epilepsy. *Epilepsia* (Amst.), 15, 417–425.

Cendrowski, W. & Sobczyk, W. (1977) Clonazepam baclofen and placebo in the treatment of spasticity. *Europ. Neurol.*, 16, 257–262.

Chandra, B. (1976) The use of clonazepam in the treatment of tic douloureux (a preliminary report). *Proc. Aust. Assoc. Neurol.*, 13, 119–122.

Chou, D. T. & Wang, S. C. (1977) Unit activity of amygdala and hippocampol neurons: effects of morphine and benzodiazepines. Brain Res. (Ast.), 126, 427–440.

Clark, F., Hall, R. & Ormiston, B. J. (1971) Diazepam and tests of thyroid function. Brit. Med. J., ii, 585–586.

Conchie, A. F. & Lowis, G. R. (1973) Diazepam suppositories in prolonged convulsions. Brit. Med. J., iii, 457–458.

Consolo, S., Ladinsky, H., Peri, G. & Garattini, S. (1974) Effect of diazepam on mouse whole brain and brain area acetylcholine and choline levels. Europ. J. Pharmacol., 27, 266–268.

Court, J. E. & Kase, C. S. (1976) Treatment of tic douloureux with a new anticonvulsant (clonazepam). J. Neurol. Neurosurg. Psychiat., 39, 297–299.

Coutinho, C. B., Cheripko, J. A. & Carbone, J. J. (1970) Correlation between the duration of the anticonvulsant activity of diazepam and its physiological disposition in mice. Biochem. Pharmacol., 19, 363–379.

Curtis, D. R., Game, C. J. A. & Lodge, D. (1976) Benzodiazepine and central glycine receptors. Brit. J. Pharmacol., 56, 307–311.

Curtis, D. R., Lodge, D., Johnston, G. A. R. & Brand, S. J. (1976) Central actions of benzodiazepines. Brain Res. (Amst.), 118, 344–347.

Dalton, C., Crowley, H. J., Sheppard, H. & Schallek, W. (1974) Regional cyclic nucleotide phosphodiesterase activity in cat central nervous system: effects of benzodiazepines. Proc. Soc. Exp. Biol. Med. (N.Y.), 145, 407–410.

Dasberg, H. H., Van der Kleijn, E., Guelen, P. J. R. & Van Praag, H. M. (1974) Plasma concentrations of diazepam and of its metabolite N-desmethyldiazepam in relation to anxiolytic effect. Clin. Pharmacol. Therap., 15, 473–483,

De Silva, J. A. F., D'Arconte, L. & Kaplan, J. (1964) The determination of blood levels and the placental transfer of diazepam in humans. Curr. Ther. Res., 6, 115–121.

De Silva, J. A. F., Koechlin, B. A. & Bader, G. (1966) Blood level distribution patterns of diazepam and its major metabolite in man. J. Pharm. Sci., 55, 692–702.

De Silva, J. A. F., Puglisi, C. V. & Munno, N. (1974) Determination of clonazepam and flunitrazepam in blood and urine by electron-capture GLC. J. Pharm. Sci., 63, 520–527.

De Silva, J. A. F., Schwartz, M. A., Stefanovik, V., Kaplan, J. and D'Arconte, L. (1964) Determination of diazepam (Valium) in blood by gas-liquid chromatography. Anal. Chem., 36, 2099–2105.

Dominic, J. A., Sinha, A. K. & Barchas, J. D. (1975) Effect of benzodiazepine compounds on brain amine metabolism. Europ. J. Pharmacol., 32, 124–127.

Dreifuss, F. E., Penry, J. K., Rose, S. W., Kupferberg, H. H., Dyken P. & Sato, S. (1975) Serum clonazepam concentrations in children with absence seizures. Neurology (Minneap.), 25, 255–258.

Eadie, M. J. (1976) Plasma level monitoring of anticonvulsants. Clin. Pharmacokinetics, 1, 52–66.

Eadie, M. J., Tyrer, J. H., Smith, G. A. & McKauge, L. (1977) Pharmacokinetics of drugs used for petit mal absence epilepsy. Clin. Exptl. Neurol., 14, 172–183.

Eatman, F. B., Colburn, W. A., Boxenbaum, H. G., Posmanter, H. N., Weinfeld, R. E., Ronfeld, R., Weissman, L., Moore, J. D., Gibaldi, M. & Kaplan, S. A. (1977) Pharmacokinetics of diazepam following multiple-dose oral administration to healthy human subjects. J. Pharmacokinetics Biopharmaceutics., 5, 481–494.

Edwards, V. E. (1974) Side effects of clonazepam therapy. Proc. Aust. Assoc. Neurol., 11, 199–202.

Edwards, V. E. & Eadie, M. J. (1973) Clonazepam—a clinical study of its effectiveness as an anticonvulsant. Proc. Aust. Assoc., Neurol., 10, 61–66.

Euan, M., Lund, M. & Melsen, S. (1973) The rate of dosage increase in clonazepam (Ro 5 4023). Epilepsia (Amst.), 14, 79–80.

Erkkola, R., & Kanto, J. (1972) Diazepam and breast feeding. Lancet, i, 1235–1236.

Erkkola, R., Kanto, J. & Sellman, R. (1974) Diazepam in early human pregnancy. Acta Obst. Gynac. Scand., 53, 135–138.

Eschenhof, V. E. (1973) Untersuchungen über das Schickoal des anticonvulsivums clonazepam in organismus der ratte des hundes und des menchen. Arznein.-Forsch., 23, 390–400.

Fazio, C., Manfredi, M. & Piccinelli, A. (1975) Treatment of epileptic seizures with clonazepam. A reappraisal. Arch. Neurol. (Chic.), 32, 304–307.

Fennessy, R. R. & Lee, J. R. (1972) The effect of benzodiazepines on brain amines of the mouse. Arch. Int. Pharmacodyn., 197, 37–44.

Fink, M., Irwin, P., Weinfeld, R. E., Schwartz, M. A. & Conney, A. H. (1975) Blood levels and electroencephalographic effects of diazepam and bromazepam. Clin. Pharmacol. Therap., 20, 184–191.

Foster, L. B. & Frings, C. S. (1970) Determination of diazepam (Valium) concentrations in serum by gas liquid chromatography. Clin. Chem., 16, 177–179.

BENZODIAZEPINE ANTICONVULSANTS 259

Fuccella, L. M., Bolcioni, G., Tamassia, V., Ferrario, L. & Tognoni, G. (1977) Human pharmacokinetics and bioavailability of temazepam administered in soft gelatine capsules. *Europ. J. clin. Pharmacol.*, **12**, 383–386.

Fuxe, K., Agnati, L. & Bolme, P. (1975) The possible evolvement of GABA mechanisms in the action of benzodiazepines on central catecholamine neurons. *Psychopharmacol. Bull.*, **11**, 55–56.

Gamble, J. A. S., Dundee, J. W. & Gray, R. C. (1976) Plasma diazepam concentrations following prolonged administration. *Brit. J. Anaesth.*, **48**, 1087–1090.

Gastaut, H., Catier, J., Dravet, C. & Roger, J. (1970) Exceptional anticonvulsive properties of a new benzodiazepine. *Epilepsy. Mod. Probl. Pharmacopsychiat.*, **4**, 261–269.

Gastaut, H., Courjon, J., Poiré, R. & Weber, M. (1971) Treatment of status epilepticus with a new benzodiazepine more active than diazepam. *Epilepsia* (Amst.), **12**, 197–214.

Gilbert, J. C. & Wyllie, M. G. (1976) Effects of anticonvulsant drugs on the ATPase activities of synaptosomes and their components. *Brit. J. Pharmacol.*, **56**, 49–57.

Giles, H. H., Zium, D. H., Frecker, R. C., Macleod, S. M. & Sellers, E. M. (1977) Saliva and plasma concentrations of diazepam after a single oral dose. *Brit. J. clin. Pharmacol.*, **4**, 711–712.

Guinta, F., Ottino, C. A., Rossi, G. F. & Tercero, E. (1970) Experimental study of the action of a new benzodiazepine derivative (Ro 5-4023). *Riv. Neurol.*, **11**, 213–223.

Goldberg, M. A. & Dorman, J. D. (1976) Intention myoclonus: successful treatment with clonazepam. *Neurology* (Minneap.), **26**, 24–26.

Govoni, S., Fresia, P., Spano, P. F. & Trabucchi, M. (1976) Effect of desmethyldiazepam and chlordesmethyldiazepam on 3′, 5′ cyclic guanosine monophosphate levels in rat cerebellum. *Psychopharmacology*, **50**, 241–244.

Greenblatt, D. J., & Koch-Weser, J. (1974) Clinical toxicity of chlordiazepoxide and diazepam in relation to serum albumin concentration: a report from the Boston Collaborative Drug Surveillance Program. *Europe. J. clin. Pharmacol.*, **7**, 259–262.

Greenblatt, D. J. & Shader, R. I. (1974) *Benzodiazepines in Clinical Practice*. New York: Raven Press.

Hayes, S. L., Pablo, G., Radomski, T. & Palmer, R. F. (1977) Ethanol and oral diazepam absorption. *New Eng. J. Med.*, **296**, 186–189.

Hegarty, J. E. & Dundee, J. W. (1977) Sequelae after intravenous injection of three benzodiazepines—diazepam, lorazepam and flunitrazepam. *Brit. Med. J.*, ii, 1384–1385.

Hillestad, L., Hansen, T. & Melsom, H. (1974) Diazepam metabolism in normal man. II Serum concentration and clinical effect after oral administration and cumulation. *Clin. Pharmacol. Therap.*, **16**, 485–489.

Hillestad, L., Hansen, T., Melsom, H. & Driveness, A. (1974) Diazepam metabolism in normal man. I Serum concentrations and clinical effects after intravenous, intramuscular and oral administration. *Clin. Pharmacol. Therap.*, **16**, 479–484.

Huang, C. Y., McLeod, J. G., Sampson, D. & Hensley, W. J. (1973) Clonazepam in the treatment of epilepsy. *Proc. Aust. Assoc. Neurol.*, **10**, 67–74.

Huang, C. Y., McLeod, J. G., Sampson, D., & Hensley, W. J. (1974) Clonazepam in the treatment of epilepsy. *M. J. Australia*, **2**, 5–8.

Hvidberg, E. F. & Sjo, O. (1975) Clinical pharmacokinetic experiences with clonazepam, in *Clinical pharmacology of antiepileptic drugs* ed. Schneider, H., Janz, D., Gardner-Thorpe, C., Meinardi, H., & Sherwin, A. L. Berlin. Springer. 242–246.

Idaenpaeaen Hiekkilae, J. E., Taska, R. J., Allen, H. A. & Schoolar, J. C. (1971) Autoradiographic study of the fate of diazepam C_{14} in the monkey brain. *Arch. Int. Pharmacodyn.*, **194**, 68–77.

Iisalo, E., Kangas, L. & Ruikka, I. (1977) Pharmacokinetics of nitrazepam in young volunteers and aged patients. *Brit. J. clin. Pharmacol.*, **4**, 646 P–647 P.

Jenner, P., Chadwick, D., Reynolds, E. H. & Marsden, C. D. (1975) Altered 5HT metabolism with clonazepam, diazepam and diphenylhydantoin. *J. Pharm. Pharmacol.*, **27**, 707–710.

Johanessen, S. I., Strandjord, R. E. & Munthe-Kaas, A. W. (1977) Lack of effect of clonazepam on serum levels of diphenylhydantoin, phenobarbital and carbamazepine. *Acta neurol. Scandinav.*, **55**, 506–512.

Jori, A., Prestini, P. E. & Pugliatti, C. (1969) Effect of diazepam and chlordiazepoxide on the metabolism of other drugs. *J. Pharm. Pharmacol.*, **21**, 387–390.

Kangas, L., Kanto, J. & Erkkola, R. (1977) Transfer of nitrazepam across the human placenta. *Europ. J. clin. Pharmacol.*, **12**, 355–357.

Kangas, L., Kanto, J. & Siirtola, T. (1974) Cerebro-spinal fluid concentrations and serum protein binding of diazepam and N-demethyldiazepam. *Acta Pharmacol.* (Kbh), **35**, Suppl. 1 (No. 48).

Kanto, J., Iisalo, E., Lehtinen, V., & Salminen, J. (1974) The concentration of diazepam and its metabolites in the plasma after an acute and chronic administration. *Psychopharmacologica (Berlin)*, **36**, 123–131.

Kanto, J., Kangas, L., & Siirtola, T. (1975) Cerebro-spinal fluid concentrations of diazepam and its metabolites in man. *Acta Pharmacol. (Kbh)*, **36**, 328–334.

Kanto, J. H., Pihlatamaki, K. K. & Iisalo, E.U. M. (1974) Concentrations of diazepam in adipose tissue of children. *Brit. J. Anaesth.*, **46**, 168.

Kaplan, S. A., Alexander, K., Jack, M. L., Puglisi, C. V., De Silva, J. A. F., Lee, T. L. & Weinfeld, R. A. (1974) Pharmacokinetic profiles of clonazepam in dog and humans and of flunitrazepam in dog. *J. Pharm. Sci.*, **63**, 527–532.

Kaplan, S. A., Jack, M. L., Alexander, K. & Weinfeld, R. E. (1973) Pharmacokinetic profile of diazepam in man following single intravenous and oral and chronic oral administration. *J. Phar. Sci.*, **62**, 1789–1796.

Klotz, U., Antonin, K-H. and Bieck, P. R. (1976-a), Pharmacokinetics and plasma binding of diazepam in man, dog, rabbit, guinea pig and rat. *J. Pharmacol. exp. Therap.*, **199**, 67–73.

Klotz, U., Antonin, K. H. & Bieck, P. R. (1976-b), Comparison of the pharmacokinetics of diazepam after single and subchronic doses. *Europ. J. clin. Pharmacol.*, **10**, 121–126.

Klotz, U., Antonin, K. H., Brügel, H. & Bieck, P. R. (1977) Disposition of diazepam and its major metabolite desmethyldiazepam in patients with liver disease. *Clin. Pharmacol. Therap.*, **21**, 430–436.

Knop, H. J., Van der Kleijn, E. & Edmunds, L. C. (1975-a) The determination of clonazepam in plasma by gas-liquid chromatography. *Pharmaceutisch Weekblad.*, **110**, 297–309.

Knop, H. J., Van der Kleijn, E. & Edmunds, L. C. (1975-b) Pharmacokinetics of clonazepam in man and laboratory animals, in *Clinical pharmacology of antiepileptic drugs* ed. Schneider, H., Janz, D., Gardner-Thorpe, C., Meinardi, H. & Sherwin, A. L. Berlin. Springer. 247–259.

Korttila, K., Mattila, M. J. & Linnoila, M. (1975) Saturation of tissues with N-desmethyldiazepam as a cause for elevated serum levels of this metabolite after repeated administration of diazepam. *Acta pharmacol. et toxicol.*, **36**, 190–192.

Linnoila, M., Otterstrom, S. & Anttila, M. (1974), Serum chlordiazepoxide diazepam and thioridazine concentrations after the simultaneous ingestion of alcohol or placebo drink. *Ann. Clin. Res.* (Helsinki), **6**, 4–6.

Loescher, W. & Frey, H. H. (1977) Effect of convulsant and anticonvulsant agents on level and metabolism of γ-aminobutyric acid in mouse brain. *Nauyn Schmied. Arch. Phar.*, **296**, 263–269.

Louis, S., Kutt, H. & McDowell, F. (1967) The cardiocirculatory changes caused by intravenous Dilantin[R] and its solvent. *Am. Heart. J.*, **174**, 523–529.

Mahon, W. A., Inaba, T., Umeda, T., Tsutsumi, E. & Stone, R. (1976) Biliary elimination of diazepam in man. *Clin. Pharmacol. Therap.*, **19**, 443–450.

Mandelli, M., Morselli, P. L., Nordio, S., Parki, G., Sereni, F. & Tognoni, G. (1975) Placental transfer of diazepam and its disposition in the newborn infant. *Clin. Pharm. Therap.*, **17**, 564–572.

Mao, C. C., Guidotti, A. & Costa, E. (1975) Evidence for an involvement of GABA in the mediation of the cerebellar cGMP decrease and the anticonvulsant action of diazepam. *Nauyn-Schmied. Arch. Pharm.*, **289**, 369–378.

Marcucci, C., Guaitani, A., Kvetina, J., Mussini, E. & Garattini, S. (1968) Species difference in diazepam metabolism and anticonvulsant effect. *Europ. J. Pharmacol.*, **4**, 467–470.

Millichap, J. G. & Ortiz, W. R. (1966) Nitrazepam in myoclonic epilepsies. *Amer. J. Dis. Child.*, **112**, 242–248.

Morselli, P. L., Mandelli, M., Tognoni, G., Principi, N., Pardi, G. & Sereni, F. (1974) Drug interaction in the human fetus and in the new born infant. in Morselli, P. L., Garattini, S. & Cohen, S. N. *Drug Interactions*. New York. Raven Press. 259–270.

Morselli, P. L., Principi, N., Tognoni, G., Reali, E., Belvedere, G., Standen, S. M., & Sereni, F. (1973) Diazepam elimination in premature and full term infants and children. *J. Perinat. Med.*, **1**, 133–141.

Müller, W. & Wollert, U. (1973) Characterization of the binding of benzodiazepines to human serum albumin. *Naunyn. Schmied. Arch. Pharm.*, **280**, 229–237.

Müller, W. E., & Wollert, U. (1976) Interaction of benzodiazepine derivatives with bovine serum albumin. I. Gel filtration studies. *Biochem. Pharmacol.*, **25**, 141–145.

Naestoft, J., Lund, M., Larsen, N. E., & Hvidberg, E. (1973) Assay and pharmacokinetics of clonazepam in humans. *Acta Neurol. Scandinav.*, **49**, 103–108.

Nanda, R. N., Johnson, R. H., Keogh, H. J., Lambie, D. G. & Melville, I. D. (1977), Treatment of epilepsy with clonazepam and its effect on other anticonvulsants. *J. Neurol. Neurosurg. Psychiat.*, **40**, 538–543.

Olsen, R. W., Lamar, E. E. & Bayless, J. D. (1977) Calcium-induced release of γ-aminobutyric acid from synaptosomes: effects of tranquilliser drugs. *J. Neurochem.*, **28**, 299–305.

Orme, M., Breckenridge, A. & Brooks, R. V. (1972), Interactions of benzodiazepines with warfarin. *Brit. Med. J.*, **iii**, 611–614.

Ostrovskaya, R. U. & Molodavkin, G. M. (1977) The GABAergic mechanism of the effects of diazepam on cortical neurons. *Bull. Exp. Biol. Med.*, **82**, 1343–1346.

Ostravskaya, R. U., Molodavkin, G. M., Porfireva, R. P. & Zubovskaya, A. M. (1975). Mechanism of the anticonvulsant action of diazepam. *Bull. Exp. Biol. Med.*, **79**, 270–273.

Petsche, H. (1972) Demonstration of cortical point of application of the benzodiazepine derivative clonazepam (Ro 5-4023). *E.E.G.*, *E.M.G.*, **3**, 145–153.

Pieri, L. & Haefely, W. (1976) The effect of diphenylhydantoin, diazepam and clonazepam on the activity of Purkinje cells in the rat cerebellum. *Nauyn-Schmied. Arch. Pharm.*, **296**, 1–4.

Pieris, J. B., Boralessa, H. & Lionel, N. D. W. (1976) Clonazepam in the treatment of choreiform activity. *Med. J. Australia*, **1**, 225–227.

Polc, P. & Haefely, W. (1976) Effects of two benzodiazepines, phenobarbitone and baclofen on synaptic transmission in the cat cuneate nucleus. *Nauyn Schmied. Arch. Pharm.*, **294**, 121–131.

Raabe, W. & Gumnit, R. J. (1977) Anticonvulsant action of diazepam: increase of cortical postsynaptic inhibition. *Epilepsia* (Amst.), **18**, 117–120.

Racine, R. J., Livingstone, K. & Joaquin, A. (1975) Effects of procaine HCl, diazepam and diphenylhydantoin on cortical and subcortical structures in rats. *Electroenceph. clin. Neurophysiol.*, **38**, 355–365.

Randall, L. O., Schallek, W., Scheckel, C., Bagdon, R. E. & Rieder, J. (1965) Zur Pharmakologie von Mogadon Einem Schlafmittel mit neuartigem Wirkungsmechanismus. *Schweiz. med. Wschr.*, **95**, 334–337.

Richens, A. & Houghton, G. W. (1975) Effect of drug therapy on the metabolism of phenytoin, in *Clinical pharmacology of anti-epileptic drugs* ed. Schneider, H., Janz, D., Gardner-Thorpe, G., Meinardi, H. & Sherwin, A. L. Berlin. Springer. 87–95.

Rieder, J. (1965) Methoden zur Bestimmung von 1,3-Dihydro-7-nitro,5-phenyl-2H-1,4-benzodiazepine-2-on-und seined Hauptmetaboliten im biologischen Proben und Ergebrisse von Versuchen uber die Pharmakokinatik and den Metabolismus dieser substanz bei Mensch und Ratte. *Arzneim.-Forsch.*, **15**, 1134–1148.

Rieder, J. (1973) Plasma levels and derived pharmacokinetic parameters of unchanged nitrazepam in man. *Arzneim.-Forsch.*, **23**, 212–218.

Rieder, J. & Wendt, G. (1971) Pharmacokinetics and metabolism of the hypnotic nitrazepam. *Symposium of Benzodiazepines*, Milan 1.11.71 to 4.11.71.

Rogers, H. J., Haslam, R. A., Longstreth, J. & Lietman, P. S. (1977) Phenytoin intoxication during concurrent diazepam therapy. *J. Neurol., Neurosurg. Psychiat.*, **40**, 890–895.

Rose, S. W., Penry, J. K. & Dreifuss, F. E. (1974) Serum clonazepam concentrations in children with absence seizures. *Neurology (Minneap.)*, **24**, 386.

Saldanha, V. J., Bird, R. & Havard, C. W. H. (1971) Effect of diazepam (Valium) on dialysable thyroxine. *Postgrad. Med. J.*, **47**, 326–328.

Saxén, I. & Saxén, L. (1975) Association between maternal intake of diazepam and oral clefts. *Lancet.*, **iii**, 498.

Schussler, G. C. (1971) Diazepam competes for thyroxine binding sites. *J. Pharmacol. exp. Therap.* **178**, 204–209.

Schwartz, D. E., Koechlin, B. A., Postma, E., Palmer, S. & Krol, G. (1965) Metabolites of diazepam in rat, dog and man. *J. Pharmacol. exp. Therap.*, **149**, 423–435.

Sellman, R., Kanto, J., Raijola, E. & Pekkarinen, A. (1975) Induction effect of diazepam on its own metabolism. *Acta. Pharmacol. (Kbh)*, **37**, 345–351.

Silverman, G. & Braithwaite, R. A. (1973) Benzodiazepines and tricyclic anti-depressant plasma levels. *Brit. Med. J.*, **iii**, 18–20.

Sisenwine, S. F., Tio, C. O., Shrader, S. R. & Ruelis, H. W. (1972) The biotransformation of oxazepam (7-chloro-1,3-dihydro-3-hydroxy-5-phenyl-2H-1,4-benzodiazepin-2-one) in man, miniature swine and rat. *Arzneim.-Forsch.*, **22**, 682–687.

Sjo, O., Hvidberg, E. F., Naestoft, J. & Lund, M. (1975) Pharmacokinetics and side-effects of clonazepam and its 7-amino-metabolite in man. *Europ. J. clin. Pharmacol.*, **8**, 249–254.

Sjoholm, I., Kober, A., Odar-Cederlof, I. & Borga, O. (1976) Protein binding of drugs in uremic and normal serum: the role of endogenous binding inhibitors. *Biochem. Pharmacol.*, **25**, 1205–1213.

Stark, L. G., Killam, K. F. & Killam, E. K. (1970) The anticonvulsant effects of phenobarbital, diphenylhydantoin and two benzodiazepines in the baboon, Papio papio. *J. Pharmacol. exp. Therap.*, **173**, 125–132.

Sternbach, L. H., Fryer, R. I., Keller, O., Metlesics, W., Sach, G. & Steiger, N. (1963) Quinazolines and 1–4 Benzodiazepines. X. Nitro-substituted 5-phenyl-1,4-benzodiazepine derivatives. *J. med. pharm. Chem.*, **6**, 261–265.

Sternbach, L. H. & Reeder, E. (1961) Quinzolines and 1,4 benzodiazepines. IV. Transformation of 7-chloro-2 methylamine-5-phenyl-3H-1,4 benzodiazepine 4-oxide. *J. Organic Chem.*, **26**, 4936–4941.

Sturdee, D. W. (1976) Diazepam: routes of administration of rate of absorption. A study of women with pre eclampsia. *Brit. J. Anaesth.*, **48**, 1091–1096.

Swinyard, E. A. & Castellion, A. W. (1966) Anticonvulsant properties of some benzodiazepines. *J. Pharmacol. exp. Therap.*, **151**, 369–375.

Tanaka, A. (1972) Progressive change of behavioral and electroencephalographic responses to daily amygdaloid stimulation in rabbits. *Fukuoka Med. J.*, **62**, 152–164.

Taylor, K. M. & Laverty, R. (1969) The effect of chlordiazepoxide, diazepam and nitrazepam on catecholamine metabolism in regions of the rat brain. *Europ. J. Pharmacol.*, **9**, 296–301.

Thiessen, J. J., Sellers, E. M., Denbeigh, P. & Dolman, I. (1976) Plasma protein binding of diazepam and tolbutamide in chronic alcoholics. *J. Clin. Pharmacol.*, **16**, 345–351.

Tsuchiya, T., Fukushima, H. & Kitagawa, S. (1976) Effect of benzodiazepines on penicillin induced epileptic discharges. *Folia Pharmacol. Jap.*, **72**, 861–877.

Tsutsumi, E., Inada, T., Mahon, W. A. & Kalow, W. (1975) The displacing effect of a fatty acid on the binding of diazepam to human serum albumin. *Biochem. Pharmacol.*, **24**, 1361–1362.

Vajda, F. J. E., Prineas, R. J. & Lovell, R. R. H., (1971) Interaction between phenytoin and benzodiazepines. *Brit. Med. J.*, i, 346.

Van der Kleijn, E. (1969) Kinetics of distribution and metabolism of diazepam in animals and humans. *Arch. int. Pharmacodyn.*, **182**, 433–436.

Van der Kleijn, E. (1971) Pharmacokinetics of distribution and metabolism of ataractic drugs and an evaluation of the site of antianxiety activity. *Proc. N.Y. Acad. Sci.*, **179**, 115–125.

Van der Kleijn, E., Guelen, P. J. M., Van Wijk, C. & Baars, I. (1975) Clinical pharmacokinetics in monitoring chronic medication with anti-epileptic drugs, in *Clinical pharmacology of antiepileptic drugs* ed. Schneider, H., Janz, D., Gardner-Thrope, C., Meinardi, H. and Sherwin, A. L. Berlin. Springer. 11–13.

Van der Kleijn, E., Van Rossum, J. M., Muskens, E. T. J. M. & Rijntjes, N. V. M. (1971) Pharmacokinetics of diazepam in dogs, mice and humans. *Acta. pharmacol. toxicol.*, **29**, suppl. 3. 109–127.

Vyas, I. & Carney, M. W. P. (1975) Diazepam withdrawal fits. *Brit. Med. J.*, iv, 44.

Windorfer, A. Jr. & Sauer, W. (1977) Drug interactions during anticonvulsant therapy in childhood: Diphenylhydantoin, primidone, phenobarbitone, clonazepam, nitrazepam, carbamazepine and dipropylacetate. *Neuropaediatrie*, **8**, 29–41.

Winek, C L. (1976) Tabulation of therapeutic, toxic and lethal concentrations of drugs and chemicals in blood. *Clin. Chem.*, **22**, 832–836.

Young, A. B., Zukin, S. R. & Snyder, S. H. (1974) Interaction of benzodiazepines with central nervous glycine receptors: possible mechanism of action. *Proc. Nat. Acad. Sci. U.S.A.*, **71**, 2246–2250.

Zingales, I. A. (1973) Diazepam metabolism during chronic medication. Unbound fraction in plasma, erythrocytes and urine. *J. Chromatog.*, **75**, 55–78.

Zsilla, G., Cheney, D. L. & Costa, E. (1976) Regional changes in the rate of turnover of acetylcholine in rat brain following diazepam or muscimol. *Naunyn-Schmied. Arch. Pharm.*, **294**, 251–255.

12

Valproic acid

Common proprietary names: Epilim, Depakine, Depakene, Eugenyl
The molecule of valproic acid has been known since 1881. Its anticonvulsant properties were discovered accidentally in France in 1961, while it was being used as a solvent for testing prospective anticonvulsants. The drug was first marketed in Europe, but more recently has become available on a wider basis. Valproate appears particularly useful in the absence and myoclonic seizures of generalized epilepsy, but may have a role in other types of epileptic seizure.

Major reviews of the substance and its uses are available (Simon and Penry, 1975; Pinder, Brogden, Speight and Avery, 1977).

CHEMISTRY

Valproic acid is the trivial name for n-propylpentanoic acid (also called dipropylacetic acid). It is usually prescribed as its sodium salt, which has a molecular weight of 166·198.
Sodium valproate is a hygroscopic white powder which is soluble in polar solvents (e.g. water, ethanol and methanol) but is poorly soluble in solvents of lower polarity (e.g. acetone, chloroform, diethylether, benzene). Its pKa value, as valproic acid, is 4·95.

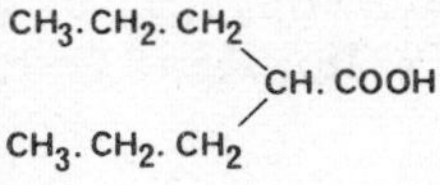

$$CH_3.CH_2.CH_2 \diagdown$$
$$CH.COOH$$
$$CH_3.CH_2.CH_2 \diagup$$

PHARMACODYNAMICS

ACTIONS IN MAN

Anticonvulsant actions
Valproate appears to be a very effective anticonvulsant, when used as sole therapy, in the absence and myoclonic seizures of generalized epilepsy (Jeavons, Clark and Maheshwari, 1977). It is also reported to be an effective anticonvulsant for febrile convulsions in infancy (Cavazzuti, 1975). The drug has been used successfully for the tonic-clonic seizures of generalized epilepsy, and for all varieties of partial epilepsy (Simon and Penry, 1975). In these varieties of epilepsy, however, valproate has nearly always been given in conjunction with other anticonvulsants.

The possible occurrence of pharmacokinetic interactions between valproate and the major anticonvulsants makes it difficult to know the direct effect of valproate in controlling seizures in these circumstances. Valproate has the reputation of being less sedative than the other anticonvulsants in common use (Simon and Penry, 1975).

Other actions

Striatal γ-aminobutyrate levels are reduced in Huntington's chorea. In experimental animals, valproate raises brain γ-aminobutyrate concentrations. However valproate has been used to treat Huntington's chorea, without success (Pearce, Heathfield and Pearce, 1977).

ACTIONS IN ANIMALS

Models of generalized epilepsy

Valproate protects against photic seizures in the baboon Papio papio (Patry and Naquet, 1971) and against audiogenic seizures in mice (Simler, Ciesielski, Maitre, Randrian and Mandel, 1973). The drug also protects against seizures provoked by the following systemically administered chemical convulsants: pentylenetetrazole (Frey and Loscher, 1976), bemegride (Van Duijn and Beckman, 1975) and, to a lesser extent, bicuculline (Frey and Loscher, 1976) and strychnine (Frey and Loscher, 1976).

Although valproate offers some protection against maximum electroshock seizures (Frey and Loscher, 1976) it is more effective against seizures produced by the systemic administration of chemical convulsants.

Models of partial epilepsy

Valproate protects against seizures beginning in an experimentally induced cobalt focus in the hippocampus of cats (Mutani, Doriguzzi, Fariello and Furlan, 1968; Mutani and Fariello, 1969). The drug prevents the development of kindled seizures produced by amygdaloid stimulation in cats (Leviel and Naquet, 1977). However valproate facilitates the development of seizures induced by electrical stimulation of the cat visual cortex (Ito, Hori, Yoshida and Shimizu, 1977).

MECHANISMS OF ACTION

Neuron pools

In cats valproate decreased the frequency of seizure discharges in a cobalt-induced hippocampal focus (Mutani, Dorigussi, Fariello and Furlan, 1968). In this preparation the drug raised the threshold for after-discharge production, and shortened the duration of any after-discharges that developed (Mutani and Fariello, 1969).

Single neurons

Ostrovskaya and Molodavkin (1977) showed that valproate reduced the spontaneous activity of neurons in the sensory and motor cortices of rats.

Biochemical effects

Effects on energy production
Valproate alters biochemical function in the so-called GABA shunt. This action has not yet been shown to alter energy availability in neural tissue.

Effects on inorganic ions
No information is available as to the effects of valproate on the inorganic ions relevant to neuronal function.

Effects on synaptic transmitters
  Gamma-aminobutyrate. This is the only synaptic transmitter about which there is information regarding the effects of valproate. The drug raises brain GABA levels (Godin, Heiner, Mark and Mandel, 1969; Simler, Ciesielski, Maitre, Randrian and Mandel, 1973; Elazar and Gottesfeld, 1975; Simler, Gensburger, Ciesielski and Mandel, 1976). Kupferberg, Lust and Penry (1975) showed that not only did valproate raise cerebellar GABA levels, but that the time course of the raised GABA levels paralleled the time course of the drug's anticonvulsant action. However Anlezark, Horton, Meldrum and Sawaya (1976) found that valproate could protect against audiogenic seizures in mice, even though brain GABA levels were not increased. Valproate produces raised GABA levels chiefly by inhibiting the enzyme succinate semialdehyde dehydrogenase, which degrades GABA. Sawaya, Horton and Meldrum (1975) showed that valproate at the clinically relevant concentration of 10^{-3} M was an efficient inhibitor of this enzyme. The drug also inhibits another enzyme involved in GABA degradation viz. GABA transaminase (Godin, Heiner, Mark and Mandel, 1969; Simler, Ciesielski, Maitre, Randrian and Mandel, 1973) although Fowler, Beckford and John (1975) found that the inhibition was relatively weak. Godin, Heiner, Mark and Mandel (1969) found that valproate was a weak inhibitor of glutamate dehydrogenase.

Effects on folates
No information is available relating to this matter.

Effects on macromolecules
No information is available.

PHARMACOKINETICS

ABSORPTION AND BIOAVAILABILITY

Eadie, Tyrer, Smith and McKauge (1977) calculated that valproate had an absorption rate constant of $1\cdot67 \pm 1\cdot37$ hour^{-1}, corresponding to a mean absorption half-time of $0\cdot42$ hours. Klotz and Antonin (1977) showed that the bioavailability of the drug from tablets was 68–100 per cent and from solution 86–100 per cent while Perucca, Gatti, Frigo and Crema (1978) found the drug in tablets had a 100 ± 10 per cent bioavailability. Peak plasma levels occur relatively early after oral administration e.g. in 1–3 hours (Loiseau, Brachet and Henry, 1975), 3–7 hours (Klotz and Antonin, 1977), within 3·75 hours (Eadie, Tyrer, Smith and

McKauge, 1977) or in 3·7 ± 0·5 hours, after a lag time of 1·3 ± 0·5 hours (Gugler, Schell, Eichelbaum, Froscher and Schulz, 1977). In some countries an enteric coated preparation is available. This produces a slower absorption profile (Van de Mortel and Franck, 1976).

DISTRIBUTION

V_d

Published values for V_d include the following:

0·15 to 0·40	litres kg^{-1}:	Schobben, Van der Kleijn and Gabreels (1975)
0·127 ± 0·040	litres kg^{-1}:	in healthy volunteers ⎱ Richens, Schoular,
0·198 ± 0·029	litres kg^{-1}:	in epileptics ⎰ Ahmad and Jordan (1976)
0·14 ± 0·05	litres kg^{-1}:	Klotz and Antonin (1977)
0·161 ± 0·030	litres kg^{-1}:	in persons over 10 years ⎱ Eadie, Tyrer, Smith
0·363 ± 0·077	litres kg^{-1}:	in young children ⎰ and McKauge (1977)
0·15 ± 0·02	litres kg^{-1}:	Gugler, Schell, Eichelbaum, Froscher and Schulz (1977)
0·147 ± 0·004	litres kg^{-1}:	Perucca, Gatti, Frigo and Crema (1978)
0·175 ± 0.025	litres kg^{-1}:	Perucca, Gatti, Frigo, Crema, Galzetti and Visintini (1978)

These V_d values suggest that the drug is probably distributed through extracellular water. However the statistically significantly higher value found by Eadie, Tyrer, Smith and McKauge (1977) in young children as compared with adolescents and adults, raises the possibility that the drug may have a more extensive distribution in the young.

Plasma protein binding

Jordan, Shillingford and Stead (1976) showed only a slight decrease in the percentage binding of valproate to plasma protein as valproate concentrations were increased from 50 to 200 μg/ml while Gugler and Mueller (1978) found binding decreased once plasma valproate levels exceeded 100 μg/ml. At concentrations of 50–100 μg/ml about 90 per cent of the drug in plasma was bound, but circulating fatty acids competed with valproate for binding sites on albumin. Other figures for the plasma protein binding of the drug are 84 per cent (Meinardi, Van der Kleijn, Meijer and Van Rees, 1975), 85–95 per cent (Espir, Benton, Will, Hayes and Walker, 1975), 80–94 per cent (Klotz and Antonin, 1977), 84–95 per cent (Wulff, Flachs, Würtz-Jorgensen and Gram, 1977), 91·6 ± 2·5 per cent (Gugler and Mueller, 1978), 93·3 per cent (Gugler, Schell, Eichelbaum, Fröscher and Schulz, 1977) and 94·8 ± 0·45 per cent (Loscher, 1978).

Concentrations in body fluids

Apart from plasma, valproate concentration data have been reported in CSF, saliva and milk. Takeda, Goto, Amano and Kukino (1976) found CSF valproate levels were 12 per cent of serum levels. Gugler, Schell, Eichelbaum, Fröscher and Schulz (1977) found that the salivary valproate level was 0·4–4·5 per cent of the plasma level of this substance. Espir, Benton, Will, Hayes and Walker (1976) found a valproate level in milk of 7 μg/ml when the maternal serum level of the drug was 95 μg/ml.

Concentrations in tissues

Autoradiographs illustrating the tissue distribution of valproate in experimental animals were published by Meinardi, Van der Kleijn, Meijer and Van Rees (1975). The drug showed very little accumulation in the central nervous system, though there was some tendency for preferential uptake in the arbor vitae of the cerebellum. Ciesielski, Maitre, Cash and Mandel (1975) found that the drug tended to accumulate in brain regions in direct proportion to the GABA transaminase activity of these regions.

ELIMINATION

Elimination rate

Some of the available figures for the elimination rate constant and/or half-life of valproate are set out below.

k (hour^{-1})	$T_{\frac{1}{2}}$ (hours)	
–	8–10	Loiseau, Brachet and Henry (1975)
–	8–15	Schobben, Van der Kleijn and Gabreels (1975)
0·0860 ± 0·0109	9·00 ± 1·01	in healthy volunteers ⎱ Richens, Scoular
0·01238 ± 0·0107	5·88 ± 0·47	in epileptics ⎰ Ahmad and Jordan (1976)
–	7·4 ± 1·4	Espir, Benton, Will, Hayes, and Walker (1976)
–	24	Takeda, Goto, Amano and Kikino (1976)
0·084 ± 0·022	8·2	Eadie, Tyrer, Smith and McKauge (1977)
0·045 ± 0·007(β)	15·9 ± 2·6	Gugler, Schell, Eichelbaum, Fröscher and Schulz (1977)
0·0549 ± 0·0083	12·8 ± 1·6	Perucca, Gatti, Frigo and Crema (1978)
–	9·0 ± 1·4	Perucca, Gatti, Frigo, Crema, Calzetti and Visintini (1978)

The above authors gave the drug by mouth. Most found a monoexponential decline in plasma drug levels. Klotz and Antonin (1977) gave the drug intravenously and found a bi-exponential decline in plasma drug levels. They obtained an α half-life of 1·0 ± 0·86 hours, and a β half-life value of 12·2 ± 3·7 hours. After giving the drug orally Gugler, Schell, Eichelbaum, Fröscher and Schulz (1977) found a bi-exponential pattern of decline in plasma drug levels, with a β half-life of 15·9 ± 2·6 hours.

Clearance

Published clearance values for valproate include the following:

0·011 to 0·36	litres kg^{-1} hour^{-1}	Schobben, Van der Kleijn and Gabreels (1975)
0·74 ± 0·065	litres hour^{-1}	in healthy volunteers ⎱ Richens, Schoular
1·46 ± 0·18	litres hour^{-1}	in epileptics ⎰ Ahmad and Jourdan (1976)
0·0108 ± 0·0021	litres kg^{-1} hour^{-1}	Espir, Benton, Will, Hayes and Walker (1976)
0·468 ± 0·144	litres hour^{-1}	Klotz and Antonin (1977)
0·018 ± 0·008	litres kg^{-1} hour^{-1}	Eadie, Tyrer, Smith and McKauge (1977)
0·0064 ± 0·0011	litres kg^{-1} hour^{-1}	Gugler, Schell, Eichelbaum, Fröscher and Schulz (1977)
0·008 ± 0·001	litres kg^{-1} hour^{-1}	Perucca, Gatti, Frigo and Crema (1978)
0·014 ± 0·002	litres kg^{-1} hour^{-1}	Perucca, Gatti, Frigo, Crema, Calzetti, and Visintini (1978)

Per cent excreted unchanged

Very little of a valproate dose is excreted unchanged in urine. Schobben, Van der Kleijn and Gabreels (1975) gave a figure of 7 per cent for the percentage excreted unchanged, Gugler, Schell, Eichelbaum, Fröscher and Schulz (1977) a figure of 3·2 per cent (with 21·2 per cent excreted as conjugated metabolites) while Klotz and Antonin (1977) could not measure any unchanged drug in urine. The elimination of the drug is chiefly by means of biotransformation.

Biotransformation pattern

The biotransformation of valproate in man appears to involve both omega oxidation and glucuronide conjugation (Kuhara and Matsumoto, 1974; Ferrandes and Eymard, 1977). The main pathway appears to be as shown (Fig. 12·1).

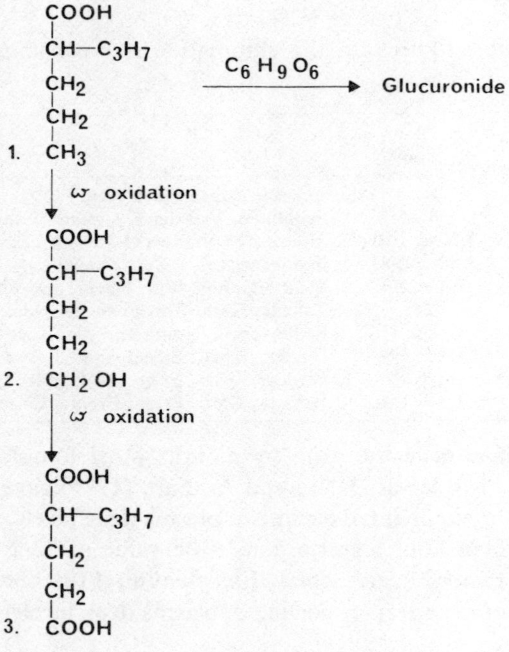

$$
\begin{array}{l}
\text{COOH} \\
\text{CH---C}_3\text{H}_7 \\
\text{CH}_2 \\
\text{CH}_2 \\
1.\quad \text{CH}_3
\end{array}
\xrightarrow{\text{C}_6\text{H}_9\text{O}_6}\ \text{Glucuronide}
$$

ω oxidation

$$
\begin{array}{l}
\text{COOH} \\
\text{CH---C}_3\text{H}_7 \\
\text{CH}_2 \\
\text{CH}_2 \\
2.\quad \text{CH}_2\,\text{OH}
\end{array}
$$

ω oxidation

$$
\begin{array}{l}
\text{COOH} \\
\text{CH---C}_3\text{H}_7 \\
\text{CH}_2 \\
\text{CH}_2 \\
3.\quad \text{COOH}
\end{array}
$$

Fig. 12.1 Valproate biotransformation
1. Valproic acid
2. 2-n-propyl-5-hydroxypentanoic acid
3. 2-n-propylglutaric acid

Schmidt (1977) has obtained evidence in man that propionic acid ($CH_3.CH_2.COOH$) is also a metabolite of valproate.

Excretion

No data are available as to factors influencing the urinary excretion of valproate.

CLINICAL PHARMACOKINETICS

Time course of plasma drug levels

Single doses

Following a single oral dose of valproate, plasma levels rise to their peak after a mean of 2·1 hours from dosage, and then decline mono-exponentially with a mean half-life of 8·2 hours (Eadie, Tyrer, Smith and McKauge, 1977). A typical example of the time course is illustrated in Fig. 12.2.

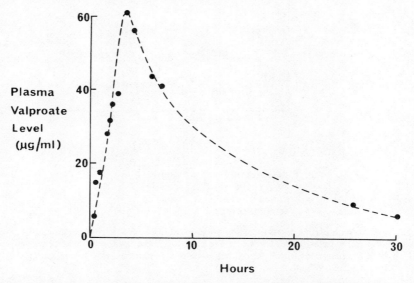

Fig. 12.2 Time course of plasma valproate levels in a subject who took a single dose of 800 mg sodium valproate at the start of the study (Eadie, Tyrer, Smith and McKauge, 1977).

Repeated doses

With repeated doses of valproate, plasma drug levels should achieve steady-state values after 2 days. Because of the relatively rapid absorption and elimination of the drug there is likely to be appreciable fluctuation in plasma valproate level across an 8 hour, or longer, dosage interval (Fig. 12.3).

Authors who attempt to correlate plasma valproate levels with clinical effects or with drug dosages often do not specify the time during the dosage interval at which the levels have been measured. Clearly this is important because of the short half-life of valproate and consequent inter-dosage fluctuation in drug concentrations in plasma.

Correlations of plasma drug concentration and clinical effect

Anticonvulsant effects

Valproate has not been available long enough or used often enough as the sole anticonvulsant for its therapeutic range to have been determined with certainty. Indeed, some have said that plasma levels of the drug do not correlate with clinical

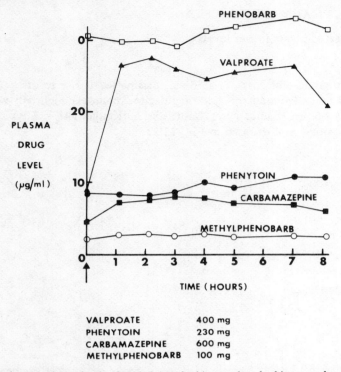

Fig. 12.3 Steady-state plasma levels of methylphenobarbitone, phenobarbitone, carbamazepine, phenytoin and valproate across an 8 hour dosage interval. While the levels of the other drugs show relatively little fluctuation over this period, valproate levels show appreciable changes (Eadie, Tyrer, Smith and McKauge, 1977).

response of epilepsy (Haigh and Forsythe, 1975; Jeavons, Clarke and Maheshwari, 1977; Wulff, Flachs, Würtz-Jorgensen and Gram, 1977). A tentative lower limit to the therapeutic range is 50 μg/ml (Vajda, Morris, Drummer and Bladin, 1976). Schobben Van der Kleijn and Gabreels (1975) proposed a therapeutic range of 50–100 μg/ml, Takeda, Goto, Amano and Kukino (1976) a range of 65–150 μg/ml and Van der Kleijn, Guelen, Van Wijk and Baars (1975) a range of 60–80 μg/ml.

Unwanted effects
Meinardi (1976) stated that valproate levels above 110 μg/ml are usually associated with muscular weakness and tremor. Our limited experience with the drug is not in accord with this view.

Plasma level—dose correlations in treated populations
There has been relatively little systematic study of valproate plasma level-dose correlations, and of the effect of factors such as age, sex and disease on the relationship. However, data such as those of Haigh and Forsythe (1975) indicate that steady state plasma level and dose are linearly related, though there is considerable scatter of plasma level values when plotted against dose (Wulff, Flachs, Würtz-Jorgensen and Gram, 1977).

Plasma level—dose relations in treated individuals
No information on this matter is available.

Effects of disease
Gugler and Mueller (1978) showed that plasma protein binding capacity for valproate is reduced in patients with renal insufficiency.

INTERACTIONS

PHARMACODYNAMIC INTERACTIONS

As yet there are no proven pharmacodynamic interactions between valproate and other drugs. The apparent additive anti-epileptic effect when valproate is added to other anticonvulsants may involve pharmacokinetic interactions (*see below*).

PHARMACOKINETIC INTERACTIONS

Valproate affecting other substances

Plasma protein binding
Patsalos and Lascelles (1977) showed that valproate decreased the plasma protein binding of phenytoin. Jordan, Shillingford and Steed (1976) found that the drug at a concentration of 25 μg/ml decreased the plasma protein binding of phenobarbitone. This drug-displacing effect did not increase as valproate concentrations were increased. These authors also found that valproate concentrations of 100 μg/ml, or more, decreased the plasma protein binding of phenytoin.

Other anticonvulsants
Phenytoin. Vajda, Morris, Drummer and Bladin (1976), Windorfer, Sauer and Gaedeke (1975) and Windorfer and Sauer (1977) all reported that valproate therapy causes a rise in plasma phenytoin levels. However Windorfer and Sauer (1977) indicated that, in the longer term, valproate therapy caused a fall in plasma phenytoin levels. An immediate fall in plasma phenytoin level in one patient when valproate was added to previous anticonvulsant therapy is shown in Fig. 12.4. Vakil, Critchley, Philips, Fahim, Haydock, Cocks and Dyer (1976), Gram, Wulf, Rasmussen, Flachs, Würtz-Jorgensen, Somerbeck and Lohren (1977) and Adams, Luders and Pippenger (1978) also noted this latter effect. Richens, Scoular, Ahmad and Jordan (1976) found no consistent effect of valproate on phenytoin level. The mechanisms of the possible interaction between valproate and phenytoin are not yet worked out. Possibly more than one mechanism is involved.
Phenobarbitone. Schobben, Van der Kleijn and Gabreels (1975), Richens, Scoular, Ahmad and Jordan (1976), Vakil, Critchley, Philips, Fahim, Haydock, Cocks and Dyer (1976), Gram, Wulff, Rasmussen, Flachs, Würtz-Jorgensen, Sommerbeck and Lohren (1977) and Adams, Luder and Pippenger (1978) showed that valproate therapy can cause a substantial rise in plasma phenobarbitone levels. The same effect occurs if the phenobarbitone is derived from the biotransformation of methylphenobarbitone (Fig. 12.5), or primidone (Adams, Luders and Pippenger, 1978).

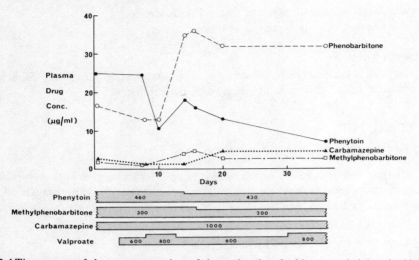

Fig. 12.4 Time courses of plasma concentrations of phenytoin, phenobarbitone, methylphenobarbitone and carbamazepine in a patient to whom valproate was given, commencing on day 3 of the study. Without any change in phenytoin dose, plasma phenytoin levels fell in the week after valproate dosage began. Subsequent changes in the plasma levels of the various drugs are difficult to interpret, because of changes in dosages of the drugs.

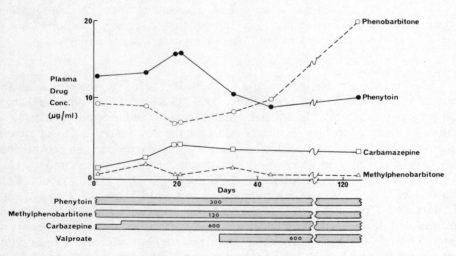

Fig. 12.5 Time courses of plasma levels of phenobarbitone, phenytoin, carbamazepine and methylphenobarbitone in a patient who had taken constant daily doses of methylphenobarbitone, phenytoin and carbamazepine for more than 3 weeks before valproate was added to his therapy. Though there was no subsequent change in the dose of any of the anticonvulsants, plasma phenobarbitone level rose substantially in the weeks after valproate intake began.

Primidone. Windorfer, Sauer and Gaedeke (1975) and Adams, Luders and Pippenger (1978) found that valproate therapy caused a rise in plasma primidone levels, but Windorfer and Sauer (1977) noted the opposite effect.

Other substances affecting valproate
Takeda, Goto, Amano and Kukino (1976) stated that plasma valproate levels were reduced by phenytoin and phenobarbitone, but not by carbamazepine.

TOXICITY

LOCAL EFFECTS AT ADMINISTRATION SITE

Relatively mild and often temporary abdominal discomfort, sometimes with decreased appetite, nausea, vomiting and diarrhoea, occurs in a minority of patients given valproate. These symptoms are rarely severe enough to make cessation of therapy necessary.

DOSE DETERMINED SYSTEMIC EFFECTS

Central nervous system
The true incidence of sedation from valproate is difficult to assess as the drug has usually been given to patients already taking other anticonvulsants. In this case possible pharmacokinetic interactions make the interpretation of apparent side effects of valproate uncertain. Jeavons, Clark and Maheshwari (1977) encountered no sedation in 58 patients given valproate alone. In high dosage the drug can cause tremor and weakness (Meinardi, 1976) and ataxia (Haigh and Forsythe, 1975). However it is possible that pharmacokinetic interactions with other anticonvulsants were involved in the production of these unwanted effects.

Valproate seems capable of producing mental stimulation and excitement in some patients (Haigh and Forsythe, 1975). Again it is possible that these symptoms may represent consequences of a pharmacokinetic interaction with other anticonvulsants which the subjects were taking simultaneously.

Haematological effects
Sutor and Jesdinsky-Buscher (1976) found an increased bleeding time in 8 out of 12 subjects taking valproate. In two of these subjects there was thrombocytopenia. In 6 out of 10 subjects studied, platelet adhesiveness was decreased. Winfield, Benton, Espir and Arthur (1976) also reported thrombocytopenia in one patient, who was taking no drug except valproate. The abnormality disappeared when valproate was ceased. Otherwise, clinical problems related to valproate-induced alterations in platelet function appear rare.

Other unwanted effects
Scalp hair loss, generally of mild degree, has been reported by some workers (Simon and Penry, 1975). Toxicological studies in animals suggest that the drug, given in high dosage, may cause damage to the seminiferous epithelium. These findings have led to concern that the drug might have a similar effect in man (Schedule of Benefits for Medical Practitioners, Commonwealth Department of Health, 1978). As far as we can ascertain, this occurrence has not yet been reported. Diaz and Shields (1978) showed that chronic high dose valproate intake (200 mg/kg) caused a reduction in brain weight in young rats.

IDIOSYNCRATIC EFFECTS

As yet there do not appear to be reports of clear cut idiosyncratic unwanted effects due to valproate.

EFFECTS ON THE FETUS AND NEONATE

The drug is said to have dysmorphogenic effects in animals (Whittle, 1976). There may not yet have been time for its dysmorphogenic potential in humans to become apparent. However Pinder, Brogden, Speight and Avery (1977) cited Whittle as stating that there had been one example of possible dysmorphogenesis reported in humans.

PREPARATIONS AVAILABLE

These include
   Tablets. 200 mg sodium valproate.
   These tablets are individually foil wrapped, because of the hygroscopic nature of the drug.

REFERENCES

Adams, D., J., Luders H. & Pippenger, C. (1978) Sodium valproate in the treatment of intractable seizure disorders: A clinical and electroencephalographic study. *Neurology* (Minneap.), **28**, 152–157.

Anlezark, G., Horton, R. W., Meldrum, B. S. & Sawaya, M. C. B. (1976), Anticonvulsant action of ethanolamine-0-sulphate and di-n-propylacetate and the metabolism of γ-aminobutyric acid (GABA) in mice with audiogenic seizures. *Biochem. Pharmacol.*, **25**, 413–417.

Cavazzuti, G. B. (1975) Prevention of febrile convulsions with dipropylacetate (Depakine). *Epilepsia* (Amst.), **16**, 647–648.

Ciesielski, C., Maitre, M., Cash, C. & Mandel, P. (1975) Regional distribution in brain and effect on cerebral mitochondrial respiration of the anticonvulsive drug n-dipropylacetate. *Biochem. Pharmacol.*, **24**, 1055–1058.

Diaz, J. & Shields, W. D. (1978) Chronic administration of dipropylacetate early in life: effects on brain development and behaviour. *Ann. Neurol.*, **4**, 198.

Eadie, M. J., Tyrer, J. H., Smith, G. A. & McKauge, L. (1977) Pharmacokinetics of drugs used for petit mal absence epilepsy. *Clin. Exptl. Neurol.*, **14**, 172–183.

Elazar, Z. & Gottesfeld, Z. (1975) Effect of drug induced increase of brain GABA levels on penicillin focus. *Experimentia* (Basel), **31**, 676–678.

Espir, M. L. E., Benton, P., Will, E., Hayes, M. J. & Walker, G. (1975) Sodium valproate (Epilim)—some clinical and pharmacological aspects, in *Clinical and pharmacological aspects of sodium valproate (Epilim) in the treatment of epilepsy* ed. Legg, N. J. Tunbridge Wells. M. C. S. Consultants, 145–151.

Ferrandes, B. & Eymark, P. (1977) Metabolism of valproate sodium in rabbit, rat, dog and man. *Epilepsia* (Amst.), **18**, 169–182.

Fowler, L. J., Beckford, J. & John, R. A. (1975) Analysis of the kinetics of the inhibition of rabbit brain γ-aminobutyrate aminotransferase by sodium n-dipropylacetate and some other simple carboxylic acids. *Biochem. Pharmacol.*, **24**, 1267–1270.

Frey, H. H. & Löscher, W. (1976) Di-n-propylacetic acid—profile of anticonvulsant activity in mice. *Arzneim.-Forsch.*, **26**, 299–301.

Godin, Y., Heiner, L., Mark, J. & Mandel, P. (1969) Effect of dipropylacetate an anticonvulsive compound on GABA metabolism. *J. Neurochem.*, **16**, 869–873.

Gram, L., Wulff, K., Rasmussen, K. E., Flachs, H., Würtz-Jorgensen, A., Sommerbeck, K. W. & Lohren, V. (1977) Valproate sodium: a controlled clinical trial including monitoring of drug levels.

Epilepsia (Amst.), **18**, 141–148.

Gugler, R. & Mueller, G. (1978) Plasma protein binding of valproic acid in healthy subjects and in patients with renal disease. *Brit. J. clin. Pharmacol.*, **5**, 441–446.

Gugler, R., Schell, A., Eichelbaum, A., Fröscher, W. & Schulz, H-U. (1977) Disposition of valproic acid in man. *Europ. J. clin. Pharmacol.*, **12**, 125–132.

Haigh, D. & Forsythe, W. I. (1975) The treatment of childhood epilepsy with sodium valproate. *Develop. Med. Child. Neurol.*, **17**, 743–748.

Ito, T., Hori, M., Yoshida, K. & Shimizu, M. (1977) Effect of anticonvulsants on cortical focal seizures in cats. *Epilepsia (Amst.)*, **18**, 63–71.

Jeavons, P. M., Clark, J. E. & Maheshwari, M. C. (1977) Treatment of generalised epilepsies of childhood and adolescence with sodium valproate ('Epilim'). *Develop. Med. Child. Neurol.*, **19**, 9–25.

Jordan, B. J., Shillingford, J. S. & Steed, K. P. (1976) Preliminary observations of the protein-binding and enzyme-inducing properties of sodium valproate (Epilim), in *Clinical and Pharmacological aspects of sodium valproate (Epilim) in the treatment of epilepsy* ed. Legg, N. J. Tunbridge Wells. M. C. S. Consultants, 112–116.

Klotz, U. & Antonin, K. H. (1977) Pharmacokinetics and bioavailability of sodium valproate. *Clin. Pharmacol. Therap.*, **21**, 736–743.

Kuhara, T. & Matsumoto, J. (1974) Metabolism of branch medium chain length fatty acid. I—Omega oxidation of sodium dipropylacetate in rats. *Biomed. Mass Spectrometry*, **1**, 291–294.

Kupferberg, H. J., Lust, W. D. & Penry, J. K. (1975) Anticonvulsant activity of dipropylacetic acid (DPA) in relation to GABA and cGMP brain levels in mice. *Fed. Proc.*, **34**, 283.

Leviel, V. & Naquet, R. (1977) A study of the action of valproic acid on the kindling effect. *Epilepsia* (Amst.), **18**, 229–234.

Loiseau, P. Brachet, A. & Henry, P. (1975) Concentration of dipropylacetate in plasma. *Epilepsia* (Amst.), **16**, 609–615.

Loscher, W. (1978) Serum protein binding and pharmacokinetics of valproate in man, dog, rat and mouse. *J. Pharmacol. exp. Therap.*, **204**, 255–261.

Meinardi, H. (1976) Discussion, in *Clinical and Pharmacological Aspects of Sodium Valproate (Epilim) in the Treatment of Epilepsy* ed. Legg, N. J. Tunbridge Wells. M. C. S. Consultants, 48.

Meinardi, H., Van der Kleijn, E., Meijer, J. W. A. & Van Rees, H. (1975) Absorption and distribution of antiepileptic drugs. *Epilepsia* (Amst.), **16**, 353–365.

Mutani, R., Doriguzzi, T., Fariello, R. & Furlan, P. M. (1968) Arizone antiepilettica del sale di sodio dell'acido n-dipropilacetico. Studio experimentale sul gatto. *Riv. Patol. Nerv. Ment.*, **89**, 24–33.

Mutani, R. & Fariello, R. (1969) Effetti dell'acido n-dipropylacetico (Depakine) sull-attivita del focus epilettiogeno corticale da cobalto. *Riv. Patol. Ner. Ment.*, **90**, 40–49.

Ostrovskaya, R. U. & Molodavkin, G. M. (1977) The GABAergic mechanism of the effects of diazepam on cortical neurons. *Bull. Exp. Biol. Med.*, **82**, 1343–1346.

Patry, G. & Naquet, R. (1971) Action de l'acide dipropylacétique chez le Papio papio photosensible. *Canad. J. Physiol. Pharmacol.*, **49**, 568–572.

Patsalos, P. N. & Lascelles, P. T. (1977) *In vitro* hydroxylation of diphenylhydantoin and its inhibition by other commonly used anticonvulsant drugs. *Biochem. Pharmacol.*, **26**, 1929–1933.

Perucca, E., Gatti, G., Frigo, G. M. & Crema. A. (1978) Pharmacokinetics of valproic acid after oral and intravenous administration. *Brit. J. clin. Pharmacol.*, **5**, 313–318.

Perucca, E., Gatti, G., Frigo, G. M., Crema, A., Calzetti, S. & Visintini, D. (1978) Disposition of sodium valproate in epileptic patients. *Brit. J. clin. Pharmacol.*, **5**, 495–499.

Pinder, R. M., Brogden, R. N., Speight, T. M. & Avery, G. S. (1977) Sodium valproate: a review of its pharmacological properties and therapeutic efficacy in epilepsy. *Drugs*, **13**, 81–123.

Richens, A., Scoular, I. T., Ahmad, S. & Jordan, B. J. (1976) Pharmacokinetics and efficacy of Epilim in patients receiving long-term therapy with other anticonvulsants, in *Clinical and pharmacological aspects of sodium valproate (Epilim) in the treatment of epilepsy* ed. Legg, N. J., Tunbridge Wells. M.C.S. Consultants. 78–88.

Sawaya, M. C. B., Horton, R. W. & Meldrum, B. S. (1975) Effects of anticonvulsant drugs on the cerebral enzymes metabolizing GABA. *Epilepsia* (Amst.), **16**, 649–655.

Schmid, R. D. (1977) Propionic acid and dipropylacetic acid in the urine of patients treated with dipropylacetic acid. *Clin. Chim. Acta*, **74**, 39–42.

Schobben, E., Van der Kleijn, E. & Gabreels, F. J. M. (1975) Pharmacokinetics of di-N-propylacetate in epileptic patients. *Europ. J. clin. Pharmacol.*, **8**, 97–105.

Simler, S., Ciesielski, L, Maitre, M., Randrian, H. & Mandel, P. (1973) Effect of sodium-n-dipropylacetate on audiogenic seizures and brain γ-aminobutyric acid. *Biochem. Pharmacol.*, **22**, 1701–1708.

Simler, S., Gensburger, C., Ciesielski, L. & Mandel, P. (1976) Effets du N-dipropylacetate de sodium sur le taux de GABA de certaines zones du cerveaux de la souris. *C. R. Seances Soc. Biol. Ses. Fil.*,

170, 1285–1288.

Simon, D. & Penry, J. K. (1975) Sodium di-n-propylacetate (DPA) in the treatment of epilepsy. A review. *Epilepsia* (Amst.), **16**, 549–573.

Sutor, A. H. & Jesdinsky-Buscher, C. (1976) The effect of dipropylacetate (Ergenyl) upon haemostasis during anticonvulsant therapy. *Fortschr. der Medizin.*, **94**, 411–414.

Takeka, A., Goto, H., Amano, Y. & Kukino, K. (1976) A study on serum and cerebrospinal fluid levels of sodium valproate (DPA), a new antiepileptic drug. *Brain Develop.*, **8**, 401–408.

Vajda, F., Morris, P., Drummer, O. & Bladin, P. (1976) Studies on sodium valproate—a new anticonvulsant, in *Clinical and pharmacological aspects of sodium valproate (Epilim) in the treatment of epilepsy* ed. Legg, N. J., Tunbridge Wells. M.C.S. Consultants. 92–100.

Vakil, S. D., Critchley, E. M. R., Philips, J. C., Fahim, Y., Haydock, C., Cocks, A. & Dyer, T. (1976) The effect of sodium valproate (Epilim) on phenytoin and phenobarbitone blood levels, in *Clinical and pharmacological aspects of sodium valproate (Epilim) in the treatment of epilepsy* ed. Legg, N. J., Tunbridge Wells. M.C.S. Consultants. 75–77.

Van de Morel, I. & Franck, G. (1976) Etude pharmacocinétique du di-n-propylacétate de sodium sous ses formes ordinaire et retard. *Acta Neurol. Belg.*, **76**, 165–172.

Van der Kleijn, E., Guelen, P. J. M., Van Wijk, C. & Baars, I. (1975) Clinical pharmacokinetics in monitoring chronic medication with anti-epileptic drugs, in *Clinical pharmacology of antiepileptic drugs* ed. Schneider, H., Janz, D., Gardner-Thorpe, C., Meinardi, H. & Sherwin, A. L. Berlin. Springer. 11–33.

Van Duijn, H. & Beckman, M. K. F. (1975) Dipropylacetic acid (Depakine) in experimental epilepsy in the alert cat. *Epilepsia* (Amst.), **16**, 83–90.

Whittle, B. A. (1976) Pre-clinical teratological studies on sodium valproate (Epilim) and other anticonvulsants, in *Clinical and pharmacological aspects of sodium valproate (Epilim) in the treatment of epilepsy* ed. Legg, N. J. Tunbridge Wells. M. C. S. Consultants. 105–110.

Windorfer, A. Jr. & Sauer, W. (1977) Drug interactions during anticonvulsant therapy in childhood: Diphenylhydantoin, primidone, phenobarbitone, clonazepam, nitrazepam, carbamazepine and dipropylacetate. *Neuropediatrie*, **8**, 29–41.

Windorfer, A., Sauer, W. & Gaedeke, R. (1975) Elevation of diphenylhydantoin and primidone serum concentrations by addition of dipropylacetate, a new anticonvulsant drug. *Acta Paediat. Scand.*, **64**, 771–772.

Winfield, D. A., Benton, P., Espir, M. L. E. & Arthur, L. J. H. (1976) Sodium valproate and thrombocytopenia. *Brit. Med. J.*, **ii**, 981.

Wulff, K., Flachs, H., Wurtz-Jorgensen, A. & Gram, L. (1977) Clinical pharmacological aspects of valproate sodium. *Epilepsia* (Amst.), **18**, 149–157.

13

Sulthiame

Common proprietary name: Ospolot
This substance, which can be regarded as a sulphonamide derivative, lacks antibacterial activity. It has found a place as an anticonvulsant, particularly in temporal lobe epilepsy (Sutherland and Bowman, 1963). However, there is an increasing impression that it is not a very effective antiepileptic drug (Green, Troupin, Halpern, Friel and Kanarek, 1974).

CHEMISTRY

Sulthiame (tetrahydro-2-p-sulphamoylphenl-l, 2-thiazine 1,1-dioxide) is a white crystalline substance with a molecular weight of 290·37. It is an acid which dissolves in aqueous alkaline solution but is poorly soluble in water or ethanol.

PHARMACODYNAMICS

ACTIONS IN MAN

Sulthiame at first appeared to be a reasonably effective anticonvulsant in partial epilepsy of temporal lobe origin (Sutherland and Bowman, 1963; Liu, 1966). Subsequently there were reports that sulthiame was also a useful anticonvulsant for myoclonic seizures (Ingram and Ratcliffe, 1963; Lerman and Nussbaum, 1975). In such studies the drug had often been given in combination with other anticonvulsants. When the effect of sulthiame in raising plasma phenytoin levels became known (p. 91) the question arose as to what extent sulthiame was an anticonvulsant in its own right. Green, Troupin, Halpern, Friel and Kanarek (1974) demonstrated that it was a less efficient anticonvulsant than phenytoin in the same patients, when each drug was used alone.

ACTIONS IN ANIMALS

Wirth, Hoffmeister, Friebel and Sommer (1960) found that sulthiame protected rats and mice against pentylenetetrazole-induced seizures and against maximum electroshock seizures. It was ineffective against strychnine-provoked seizures.

MECHANISMS OF ACTION

Biochemical
Biochemically sulthiame is a carbonic anhydrase inhibitor. However it is only about 1/16 as potent as acetazolamide, another carbonic anhydrase inhibitor which has sometimes been used as an adjuvant in the treatment of epilepsy (Wirth, Hoffmeister and Sommer, 1961). Both acetazolamide and sulthiame produce peripheral paraesthesiae as side effects. Unlike acetazolamide, sulthiame is not a diuretic. It is possible that sulthiame exerts its anticonvulsant effect by producing an intracellular acidosis, which diminishes Na^+ entry into cells. Geets and Pinon (1971) found that successful therapeutic results with sulthiame correlated with a lowering of plasma pH. Gray and Rauh (1967) found that noradrenaline was required for carbonic anhydrase inhibitors to exert anticonvulsant effects.

Spector (1972) showed that sulthiame, at concentrations similar to those found in patients treated with the drug, reduced oxygen consumption in a rat microsome-synaptosome preparation. This effect was reversed by noradrenaline or by formyl-tetrahydrofolic acid. Therefore it is conceivable that sulthiame may act in part by limiting the energy available for the excessive activity of epileptic discharging.

PHARMACOKINETICS

Very little pharmacokinetic data for humans are available.

ABSORPTION AND BIOAVAILABILITY

Studies in rats showed that isotopically labelled sulthiame was well absorbed from the gut (Duhm, Maul, Medenwald, Patzchke and Wegner, 1963). Over 90 per cent of the dose is said to absorb in man (Diamond and Levy, 1963).

DISTRIBUTION

In rats Duhm, Maul, Medenwald, Patzchke and Wagner (1963) found that sulthiame concentrations in brains were similar to those in serum. However sulthiame tended to be more concentrated in tissues, including red blood cells, than it was in serum. There is no direct evidence available that sulthiame is bound to plasma protein. However the data of Hooper, Sutherland, Bochner, Tyrer and Eadie (1973), which showed that sulthiame to some extent displaced phenytoin from serum albumin, raise the possibility that sulthiame in plasma may be partly bound to plasma protein.

ELIMINATION

In man Diamond and Levy (1963) found that a total of 60–70 per cent of a sulthiame dose was excreted unchanged in urine, with about 25–50 per cent being present in urine as a metabolite. Duhm, Maul, Medenwald, Patzchke and Wagner (1963) identified the sulthiame metabolite as a hydroxylated derivative devoid of anticonvulsant activity. Olesen (1968) found 32 per cent of a sulthiame dose in man was excreted in urine unchanged in 24 hours.

CLINICAL PHARMACOKINETICS

Olesen (1968) found plasma sulthiame levels of 0·5 to 12·5 μg/ml in patients taking sulthiame doses of between 200 and 1000 mg per day, with a mean plasma level of 4·0 μg/ml. These figures give an indication of the order of magnitude of plasma sulthiame levels likely to be encountered in practice. Sufficient data are not available to define a 'therapeutic' or 'toxic' range of plasma sulthiame concentrations.

INTERACTIONS

PHARMACODYNAMIC INTERACTIONS

No proven pharmacodynamic interactions involving sulthiame have been traced.

PHARMACOKINETIC INTERACTIONS

Reports that other drugs influence plasma sulthiame concentrations are not available. There have been several reports that sulthiame therapy increases plasma phenytoin concentrations (Hansen, Kristensen and Skovsted, 1968; Hoglmeier and Wenzel, 1969; Olesen and Jensen, 1969). This matter is more fully documented on page 91. Morselli, Rizzo and Garattini (1970) found that, when sulthiame was given to rats already receiving phenytoin, brain concentrations of phenytoin rose though there was no alteration in plasma phenytoin levels.

TOXICITY

LOCAL EFFECTS

Orally-administered sulthiame may cause some local alimentary irritation with gastric distress and nausea.

DOSE-RELATED SYSTEMIC EFFECTS

In many patients once a sufficient dose of sulthiame is given two troublesome side-effects often appear. These are hyperpnoea with dyspnoea, and paraesthesiae of the extremities (Sutherland and Bowman, 1963). These symptoms can be relieved by dosage reduction. Sometimes they do not develop again when the dose is slowly increased beyond the threshold at which the symptoms had appeared previously. Patients sometimes find these symptoms intolerable so that their occurrence may limit sulthiame dosage.

IDIOSYNCRATIC EFFECTS

In some patients sulthiame may produce headache, drowsiness, ataxia and anorexia, and occasionally mental changes (e.g. hallucinations). Transient catatonia has been reported (Mykyta, 1968). Increased salivation has been noted in occasional patients. There have been other reports of probably idiosyncratic type side-effects (e.g. acute renal tubular necrosis, as described by Aviram, Czaczkes and Rosenmann, 1965).

EFFECTS ON THE FETUS AND NEONATE

No reports of dysmorphogenesis due to sulthiame have been traced. However, this lack of information may only reflect the fact that the drug is not widely used at the present time.

PREPARATIONS AVAILABLE

These include:

Tablets: 50 mg; 200 mg.

REFERENCES

Aviram, A., Czaczkes, J. W. & Rosenmann, E. (1965) Acute renal failure associated with sulthiame. *Lancet*, **i**, 818.

Diamond, S. & Levy, L. (1963) Metabolic studies on a new anti-epileptic drug, Riker 594. *Current Therapeutic Research*, **5**, 325–330.

Duhm, B., Maul, W., Medenwald, H., Patzchke, K. & Wegner, L-A. (1963) Tierexperimentelle untersuchungen mit ^{35}S-markiertem N-(4'-sulfamylphenyl)-butansultam-(1,4). *Z. Naturforsch.*, **18**, 475–492.

Geets, W. & Pinon, A. (1971) L'action métabolique et anti-épileptique de 'Ospolot'. *Acta Neurol. Belg.*, **71**, 164–172.

Gray, W. D. & Rauh, C. E. (1967) The anticonvulsant action of inhibitors of carbonic anhydrase; relation to endogenous amines in brain. *J. Pharmacol. exp. Therap.*, **155**, 127–134.

Green, J. R., Troupin, A. S., Halpern, L. M., Friel, P. & Kanarek, P. (1974) Sulthiame: evaluation as an anticonvulsant. *Epilepsia* (Amst.), **15**, 329–349.

Hansen, J. M., Kristensen, M. & Skovsted, L. (1968) Sulthiame (Ospolot) as inhibitor of diphenylhydantoin metabolism. *Epilepsia* (Amst.), **9**, 17–22.

Hogmeier, H. & Wenzel, U. (1969) Zerebellarer Dauerschaden durch vorübergehende Hydantoinüberdosierung. *Deutsche Med. Wochenschrift.*, **94**, 1330–1332.

Hooper, W. D., Sutherland, J. M., Bochner, F., Tyrer, J. H. & Eadie, M. J. (1973) The effect of certain drugs on the plasma protein binding of diphenylhydantoin. *Aust. N.Z. J. Med.*, **3**, 377–381.

Ingram, T. T. S. & Ratcliffe, S. G. (1963) Clinical trail of Ospolot in epilepsy. *Develop. Med. Child. Neurol.*, **5**, 313–315.

Lerman, P. & Nussbaum, E. (1975) The use of sulthiame in myoclonic epilepsy of childhood and adolescence. *Acta Neurol. Scandinav. Suppl.*, **60**, 7–12.

Liu, M. C. (1966) Clinical experience with sulthiame (Ospolot). *Brit. J. Psychiat.*, **112**, 621–628.

Morselli, P. L., Rizzo, M. & Garattini, S. (1970) Effect of sulthiame on blood and brain levels of diphenylhydantoin in the rat. *Biochem. Pharmacol.*, **19**, 1846–1847.

Mykyta, G. J. (1968) A case of sulthiame overdosage. *M. J. Australia*, **2**, 118–119.

Olesen, O. V. (1968) Determination of Sultiam (Ospolot) in serum and urine by thin-layer chromatography: serum levels and urinary output in patients under long term treatment. *Acta Pharmacol. et Toxicol.*, **26**, 22–28.

Olesen O. V. & Jensen, O. N. (1969) Drug-interaction between sulthiame (Ospolot (R)) and phenytoin in the treatment of epilepsy. *Danish Med. Bull.*, **16**, 154–158.

Spector, R. G. (1972) The influence of anticonvulsant drugs on formyl tetrahydrofolic acid stimulation of rat brain respiration *in vitro*. *Biochem. Pharmacol.*, **21**, 3198–3201.

Sutherland, J. M. & Bowman, D. A. (1963) Sulthiame (Ospolot) in the treatment of temporal lobe epilepsy. *M. J. Australia*, **2**, 532–533.

Wirth, W., Hoffmeister, F., Friebel, H. & Sommer, S. (1960) Zur Pharmakologie des N-(4-Sulfamylphenyl)-butansultam-(1–4)'. *Dtsch. Med. Wschr.*, **85**, 2195–2199.

Wirth, N., Hoffmeister, F. & Sommer, S. (1961) The pharmacology of Ospolot[R]. *Ger. Med. Mon.* **6**, 309–312.

14

Chlormethiazole

Common proprietary names: Hemineurin, Heminevrin

Recently there has been interest in using chlormethiazole intravenously as an anticonvulsant for status epilepticus (Bentley and Mellick, 1975; Harvey, Higenbottam and Loh, 1975). The drug has too great a dependence potential (McLean, 1975) and is too rapidly eliminated to be suitable for use as an orally administered maintenance anticonvulsant.

CHEMISTRY

Chlormethiazole (clomethiazole: 5-(2-chloroethyl)-4-methylthiazole) is an oily viscous liquid with a molecular weight of 161·66. It is a base with a pKa of 3·2.

The drug is often given as its methanesulphonate. This is a water-soluble colourless crystalline material which is strongly acid in solution.

PHARMACODYNAMICS

ACTIONS IN MAN

Chlormethiazole is a rapidly-acting sedative and hypnotic. Given intravenously it often controls convulsive status epilepticus. It is also used to control delerium tremens (Sattes, 1966).

ACTIONS IN ANIMALS

The animal pharmacology of the drug was reviewed by Lechat (1966). Chlormethiazole protects against generalized epilepsy induced by systemically administered chemical convulsants (pentylenetetrazole, bemegride, 2-aminopyridine and isoniazid, but not strychnine). It also protects against maximum electroshock seizures. The drug has hypnotic effects in animals, and inhibits their respiratory, thermoregulatory and vomiting centres.

MECHANISMS OF ACTION

Microelectrode studies showed that chlormethiazole inhibited strychnine-induced paroxysmal activity in guinea pig cerebral cortex (Nystrom, Riihimaki, Riihimaki and Vainio, 1974). The drug may inhibit Na^+ uptake into cerebral tissue after electrical stimulation (Wallgren, Nikander, Boguslawsky and Linkola, 1947). The manufacturer's literature suggests that chlormethiazole has its anticonvulsant effect at central nervous system glycine receptors.

The structure of the molecule of chlormethiazole resembles that of half the molecule of thiamine. However, chlormethiazole will not relieve the manifestations of thiamine deficiency.

PHARMACOKINETICS

The investigations of Moore, Triggs, Shanks and Thomas (1975) and Nation, Learoyd, Barber and Triggs (1976) provide pharmacokinetic information about the drug. Moore, Robertson, Smyth, Thomas and Vine (1975) elucidated its metabolic pathways.

ABSORPTION AND BIOAVAILABILITY

Chlormethiazole is said to absorb rapidly and completely after it is given orally to experimental animals. In man the bioavailability is only 15 per cent. This is not due to poor absorption but to extensive first-pass biotransformation.

DISTRIBUTION

The apparent V_d of the drug is 5.4 litres kg^{-1}, suggesting substantial tissue binding. Approximately 70 per cent of the drug in plasma is bound to plasma proteins in the young, and 60 per cent in the aged (Nation, Vine, Triggs and Learoyd, 1977). Svedin (1966-a) published whole body autoradiographs illustrating the distribution of the drug in mice. In these animals drug levels were higher in the blood than in the tissues, except for the adrenals and kidneys, where radioactivity levels were high.

ELIMINATION

In young subjects the β phase half-life is 4.05 ± 0.60 hours, while in the elderly it averages 8.49 hours. In the young the clearance is 1.378 ± 0.244 litres kg^{-1} $hour^{-1}$, which is close to the value of hepatic blood flow. In the healthy aged, the plasma clearance is even higher than in the young (Nation, Learoyd, Barber and Triggs, 1976). Less than 5 per cent of a chlormethiazole dose is excreted unchanged in urine. The known biotransformation pathways are shown in Fig. 14.1. However, even when all known metabolites in urine are measured, over 80 per cent of a chlormethiazole dose is still not accounted for.

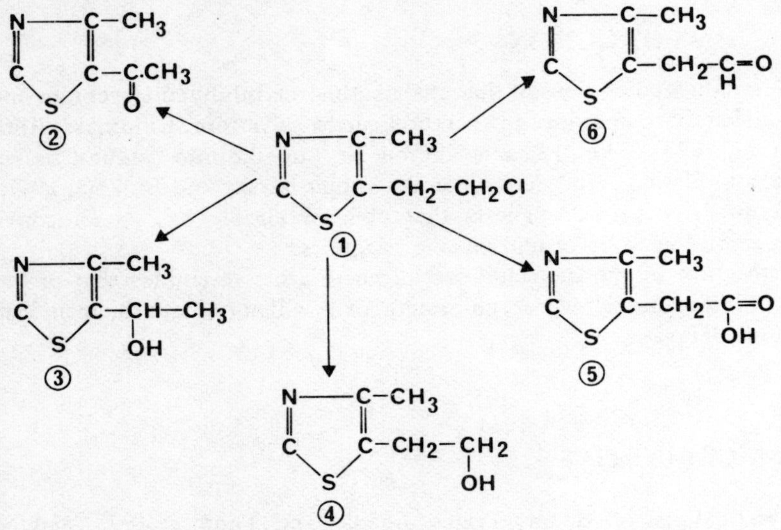

Fig. 14.1 Biotransformation pathways of chlormethiazole (after Moore, Robertson, Smythe, Thomas and Vine, 1975).
1. chlormethiazole
2. 5-acetyl-4-methylthiazole
3. 5-(1-hydroxyethyl)-4-methylthiazole
4. 5-(2-hydroxyethyl)-4-methylthiazole
5. thiazolacetic acid
6. 4-methyl-5-thiazoleacetaldehyde

CLINICAL PHARMACOKINETICS

There have been no published attempts to correlate plasma chlormethiazole levels with anticonvulsant effect.

INTERACTIONS

Chlormethiazole might be expected to interact additively with other hypnotics and sedatives. However no work on its interactions appears to have been published.

TOXICITY

LOCAL EFFECTS

Irritative phenomena at the infusion site are uncommon, when the drug is given intravenously.

DOSE-DEPENDENT EFFECTS

According to Svedin (1966-b) the unwanted effects of the drug include annoying tingling in the nose, sneezing, conjunctival injection and bronchorrhoea. Drowsiness, slurred speech, nystagmus and hiccup may occur, with increasing depression of consciousness if the dose is increased further. Intravenous doses of the drug may cause tachycardia without change in blood pressure or cardiac output. There is a risk of haemolysis if solutions more concentrated than 0·8 per cent are given intravenously.

Chlormethiazole has the potential to produce dependence if given for more than a few days (Lundquist, 1966; McLean, 1975).

IDIOSYNCRATIC EFFECTS

Rarely the drug causes erythema and uricaria (Sattes, 1966). Khan (1976) recorded an instance in which the drug provoked the acute onset of a painful itchy rash.

EFFECTS ON THE FETUS AND NEONATE

In experimental animals the drug does not appear to cause dysmorphogenesis (Lechat, 1966).

PREPARATIONS AVAILABLE

These include

Chlormethiazole: 192·0 mg (of the base) in capsules
Chlormethiazole ethanedisulphonate: 0·8 per cent solution, 500 mls.

REFERENCES

Bentley, G. & Mellick, R. (1975) Chlormethiazole in status epilepticus: three cases. *M. J. Australia*, 1, 537–538.

Harvey, P. K. P., Higenbottam, T. W. & Loh, L. (1975) Chlormethiazole in treatment of status epilepticus. *Brit. Med. J.*, ii, 603–605.

Khan, A. A. (1976) Severe allergic reaction to chlormethiazole. *Brit. Med. J.*, ii, 1105.

Lechat, P. (1966) Toxicological and pharmacological properties of clomethiazole. *Acta Psychiat. Scandinav.*, 42, Suppl., 192, 15–22.

Lundquist, G. (1966)The risk of dependence on chlormethiazole. *Acta. Psychiat. Scandinav.*, 42, Suppl. 192, 203–207.

McLean, D. D. (1975), Hemineurin danger. *M. J. Australia*, 2, 725.

Moore, R. G., Robertson, A. V., Smyth, M. P., Thomas, J. & Vine, J. (1975) Metabolism and urinary excretion of chlormethiazole in humans. *Xenobiotica* 5, 687–696.

Moore, R. G., Triggs, E. J., Shanks, C. A. & Thomas, J. (1975) Pharmacokinetics of chlormethiazole in humans. *Europ. J. clin. Pharmacol.*, 8, 353–357.

Nation, R. L., Learoyd, B., Barber, J. & Triggs, E. J. (1976) The pharmacokinetics of chlormethiazole following intravenous administration in the aged. *Europ. J. clin. Pharmacol.*, 10, 407–415.

Nation, R. L., Vine, J., Triggs, E. J. & Learoyd, B. (1977) Plasma levels of chlormethiazole and two metabolites after oral administration to young and aged human subjects. *Europ. J. clin. Pharmacol.*, 12, 137–145.

Nystrom, S. H. M., Riihimaki, E. J., Riihimaki, M. & Vainio, J. (1974) Action of chlormethiazole on seizure activity in strychnine-induced experimental epilepsy in guinea-pigs. *I.R.C.S. Res. Neurobiol. Neurophysiol. Pharmacol.* 2, 1236.

Sattes, H. (1966) Treatment of delerium tremens with chlormethiazole. *Acta Psychiat. Scandinav.* 42, Suppl., 192, 139–143.

Svedin, C. D. (1966-a) Tissue distribution of chlormethiazole and compatibility with ethanol and certain drugs. *Acta Psychiat. Scandinav.*, **42**, (Suppl. 192) 27–34.

Svedin, C. O. (1966-b) Side effects of chlormethiazole therapy. *Acta Psychiat. Scandinav. Suppl.*, **192**, 199–201.

Wallgren, H., Nikander, P., Boguslawsky, P. V. & Linkola, J. (1947) Effects of ethanol, tert-butanol, and chlormethiazole on net movements of sodium and potassium in electrically stimulated cerebral tissue. *Acta Physiol. Scand.*, **91**, 83–93.

PART III

The use of anticonvulsants

15

The classification of epilepsy

In the chapter on the Principles of Anticonvulsant Therapy (Chapter 5) the types of drug useful in particular forms of human epilepsy were correlated with an abbreviated version of the classification of epileptic seizures produced by the International League Against Epilepsy (Gastaut, 1969). This classification is becoming increasingly adopted throughout the world. The classification is based on the site of origin and pattern of spread of epileptic activity. It is systematic and logically consistent, though it may have to undergo modification as knowledge of epileptogenesis increases. Once mastered, the classification is generally more satisfactory than older classifications. The International League's Classification has abandoned old and familiar terms where these may lead to possible ambiguity. Certain words long hallowed by use have disappeared, perhaps the most notable being *petit mal*. To some people, *petit mal* was a particular form of hereditary epilepsy occurring in a particular age group, associated with a specific EEG appearance and having a special therapeutic requirement. To others, *petit mal* referred to any epilepsy less severe than *grand mal*. Once the words *petit mal* were replaced by the term 'absence', the words *grand mal* became potentially misleading and were replaced by the descriptive term 'tonic-clonic seizure'.

The International League's Classification (1969) divides epileptic seizures (not patients with epilepsy) into four major groups, as follows:

1. generalized seizures
2. partial seizures
3. unilateral seizures
4. unclassifiable seizures (due to inadequate data)

GENERALIZED SEIZURES

In these seizures an epileptic discharge suddenly activates the cerebrum widely, or diffusely. Such generalized seizures are not quite the same as Penfield and Jasper's (1954) original concept of 'centrencephalic' epilepsy. In that type of epilepsy the epileptic discharge was believed to originate in certain areas of the mesencephalic and diencephalic grey matter, the so-called 'centrencephalic integrating system', which projects widely to the hemispheres. Such centrencephalic discharges were conceived as spreading to activate the whole of both hemispheres simultaneously. Thus the resultant seizures appeared to involve the whole cerebrum from the outset. Such centrencephalic seizures, often hereditary, are a common type of generalized epilepsy, though it is now thought that they may result from a sudden loss of meso-diencephalic control of the cortex. It also appears that widespread cerebral pathological processes of various kinds (e.g. hypoxic damage), and metabolic disturbances (e.g. uraemia) may alter function in cortico-diencephalic (and perhaps cortico-mesencephalic) circuits to produce widespread discharges in the cortex. In the surface EEG and in their clinical effects these discharges also appear generalized from the outset, though their origin may be outside the centrencephalic system. Thus they may arise in the orbital surface of a frontal lobe. The matter is well discussed by Gloor (1969), who proposed the term 'generalized cortico-reticular epilepsies' for all these varieties of generalized epilepsy.

There are a number of subdivisions of generalized epilepsy. The principal types are listed below:

1. **Absences:** (*petit mal* seizures in the limited sense of that term). These are the classic manifestation of centrencephalic epilepsy. Absences are usually of hereditary origin and consist of sudden transient lapses of consciousness. They often begin in the 4 to 10 year age group, occur frequently, and are commonly associated with generalized bursts of bilaterally symmetrical 3 Hz spike and wave activity in the surface EEG. Typical absences, as defined above, are comparatively rare. Such absences occurred in only 2·3 per cent of the patients attending Livingstone's epilepsy clinic (Livingstone, 1972). Absences comprised only 9·1 per cent of the 76·3 per cent of classifiable cases in the series of 6000 epileptic patients collected by Gastaut, Gastaut, Goncalves e Silva and Sanchez (1976).

2. **Myoclonic and akinetic attacks:** (the other two elements of the old '*petit mal* triad' which accounted for 4·4 per cent of the classifiable cases in the series of Gastaut, Gastaut, Goncalves e Silva and Sanchez, 1976). These consist of momentary lapses of consciousness with either brief, bilateral clonic jerking of face, limbs and/or trunk ('minor motor' epilepsy to some paediatricians) or with sudden loss of postural tone, in some instances causing a 'drop' attack. They may be hereditary and are then usually associated with the typical 3 Hz spike and wave surface EEG discharges of *petit mal* absences. More often they are of acquired origin (due to metabolic disorders or widespread cerebral abnormality). They are then associated in the surface EEG with generalized discharges, often of spike and wave, or polyspike and wave form, at 2–5 Hz.

3. **Tonic, clonic and tonic-clonic (grand mal) seizures,** which comprised 28·4 per cent of classifiable cases in the series of Gastaut, Gastaut, Goncalves e Silva and Sanchez (1976). These seizures consist of bilateral tonic spasms and/or clonic jerks involving the head, the limbs on both sides and the trunk. The onset of these motor events is associated with sudden loss of consciousness. Such seizures may occur in persons who have, or who have had, absences or myoclonic or akinetic seizures, or they may occur as the sole manifestation of epilepsy. They may be of hereditary or acquired origin. If hereditary, they tend to be associated with generalized 3 Hz spike and wave disturbances in the interseizure surface EEG. If acquired, the interseizure EEG characteristically shows 'atypical' (2–5 Hz) spike and wave activity. However other forms of bilateral paroxysmal discharge may occur. The older the patient, the less likely is his EEG to show characteristic appearances.

Generalized epilepsy accounted for 37·7 per cent of the classifiable cases in the series of Gastaut, Gastaut, Goncalves e Silva and Sanchez (1976). Individual patients may have more than one subvariety of generalized epilepsy.

PARTIAL SEIZURES

This pattern of seizure, formerly called focal epilepsy, probably is the most common type of epilepsy (Tower, 1957). Partial epilepsy comprised 62·3 per cent of the classifiable 76·3 per cent of cases in the series of Gastaut, Gastaut, Goncalves e Silva and Sanchez (1976). Partial epilepsy is always due to local structural pathological changes in the brain. These changes are almost always acquired, but rarely may be hereditary. There is clinical, and/or surface EEG evidence that partial epileptic discharges begin locally in some region of the brain (other than those structures which are primarily involved in the initiation of generalized epilepsy). The clinical expression of partial epilepsy is determined by the site of origin and direction and extent of spread of the epileptic discharge. In the past, partial epilepsy was often subdivided in terms of the site of origin of the discharges (e.g. temporal lobe epilepsy). The International League's Classification subdivides partial epilepsy in terms of its pattern of clinical symptomatology, as follows:

a. with elementary symptomatology, consisting of
   (i) motor symptoms
   (ii) special sensory or somato-sensory symptoms
   (iii) autonomic symptoms
   (iv) compound forms
b. with complex symptomatology (partial complex seizures)
   (i) with impaired consciousness only
   (ii) with cognitive symptomatology
   (iii) with affective symptomatology
   (iv) with psychosensory symptomatology
   (v) with psychomotor symptomatology
   (vi) compound forms
c. partial seizures, secondarily generalized.

The discharge in any partial seizure may spread sufficiently to activate those structures or circuits involved in initiating generalized epilepsy. If so a secondarily generalized seizure (with loss of consciousness and bilateral motor events) may be grafted onto the primary partial seizure. If the primary partial seizure is subclinical, as it may be, only the secondarily generalized seizure may appear clinically. However the surface EEG at the onset of the seizure, and between seizures, often shows the focal origin of the discharges. It is this EEG appearance which differentiates (perhaps artificially) such secondarily generalized epilepsy from certain forms of acquired but primarily generalized epilepsy. (Such acquired primarily generalized epilepsy is sometimes confusingly called 'secondary generalized epilepsy'.) In these latter form of generalized epilepsy, as mentioned above, a focal disturbance in certain cortico-diencephalic circuits produces an extremely rapid generalization of paroxysmal activity, without there being clear evidence of the local origin of the discharge in the interictal or seizure surface EEG. However, in this type of generalized epilepsy evidence of the primary local site of seizure origin may be obtained from depth electrode studies.

UNILATERAL SEIZURES

These are comparatively uncommon and are usually due to acquired pathological abnormalities in the brains of young children. The epileptic discharge seems to activate one whole hemisphere simultaneously. The surface EEG may show widespread unilateral or sometimes bilateral discharges, perhaps with varying or consistent unilateral preponderance.

UNCLASSIFIABLE SEIZURES

Despite the best efforts of the clinician, it is sometimes impossible to classify a patient's epileptic seizures. Such was the case in 23·7 per cent of the 6000 patients collected by Gastaut, Gastaut, Goncalves e Silva and Sanchez (1967).

REFERENCES

Gastaut, H. (1969) Clinical and electroencephalographical classification of epileptic seizures. *Epilepsia*, (Amst.), **10**, Suppl: 2.

Gastaut, H., Gaustaut, J. L., Goncalves e Silva, G. E. & Sanchez, G. R. F. (1976) Relative frequency of different types of epilepsy: a study employing the classification of the International League against Epilepsy. *Epilepsia*, (Amst.), **16**, 457–461.

Gloor, P. (1969) Neurophysiological bases of generalized seizures termed centrencephalic, in *The physiopathogenesis of the epilepsies* ed. Gaustaut, H., Jasper, H., Bancaud, J. & Waltregny, A. Springfield: Charles C. Thomas, 209–236.

Livingstone, S. (1972) *Comprehensive Management of Epilepsy in Infancy, Childhood and Adolescence*. Springfield. Charles C. Thomas.

Penfield, W. & Jasper, H. (1954) *Epilepsy and the Functional Anatomy of the Human Brain*. Boston: Little, Brown & Co.

Tower, D. B. (1957) The status of the medical treatment of seizures, in *Modern trends in neurology*—2nd series ed. Williams, D. London: Butterworth & Co. Ltd., 317–337.

16

Treatment of various types of epilepsy

It should be noted that, in what follows, it is the drug therapy of the patient's seizures which is discussed, rather than the total management of the person with epilepsy. The whole broad question of the social management of patients with epilepsy, and of their families, and the smaller question of the role of surgery in epilepsy, are outside the scope of this book. Here attention is concentrated on developing and applying a rational scheme of drug treatment for epilepsy. However the voluminous literature relating to drug treatment is not reviewed in detail. The earlier literature on this matter was summarized by Coatsworth (1971).

THE INTERVAL TREATMENT OF EPILEPSY

The questions that should have been asked before prescribing anticonvulsant therapy have been set out in Chapter 5. In summary, it should have been determined whether:

1. the patient's attacks are epileptic;
2. there is a treatable cerebral or extracerebral (e.g. metabolic) disorder which is responsible for the epilepsy;
3. there is a removable or reversible factor which aggravates the epilepsy or precipitates individual attacks, and
4. the epilepsy, if left untreated, is likely to recur.

Once these matters have been determined and treatment appears indicated, oral anticonvulsant therapy should be prescribed. The drug selected depends on the patient's pattern, or patterns, of seizure. The choice of an appropriate anticonvulsant for treating particular forms of epileptic seizure is set out in Table 16.1. The most effective drugs for treating particular types of seizures are listed in the appropriate columns. However drugs often have a degree of activity against the type of epilepsy considered in the adjacent columns. Hereditary and acquired varieties of myoclonic seizure may tend to require different therapy unless the newer anticonvulsants clonazepam and valproate are used. Consequently myoclonic seizures are further subdivided in the classification, whereas other varieties of epileptic seizure are not.

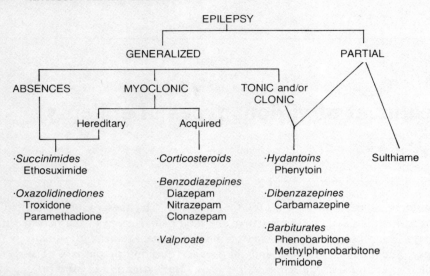

Table 16.1 Correlation of types of epilepsy with appropriate anticonvulsant drugs.

ABSENCES (*Petit mal*)

Ethosuximide

It seems generally agreed at the present time that ethosuximide is the treatment of choice for *petit mal* absences. The drug is more effective and less toxic than the oxazolidinediones (Schmidt and Wilder, 1968; Livingstone, 1972). The more recently introduced clonazepam and sodium valproate have not yet found their definitive places in treating absence seizures. Both appear effective. *Petit mal* absences (as defined in Chapter 15) rarely occur in very young children. Therefore it should not often be necessary to prescribe ethosuximide except in capsule form, though syrup preparations are available.

Ethosuximide is rapidly absorbed from the alimentary tract and has a half-life in children of approximately 30 hours (Buchanan, Fernandez and Kinkel, 1969). Therefore the drug need not be given more than once a day to produce reasonably stable steady-state plasma levels over the course of a dosage interval (Buchanan and Smith, 1971). In children it will take about 7 days after therapy commences for ethosuximide to attain approximate steady-state plasma levels and to exert its maximal effect. Plasma ethosuximide concentrations of 40–80 μg/ml or 40–120 μg/ml (Sherwin and Robb, 1972; Penry, Porter and Dreifuss, 1972) appear to offer optimal protection against *petit mal* absences. However, the present authors have treated patients who required ethosuximide levels up to 180 μg/ml to obtain control of this type of epilepsy. These ethosuximide levels were tolerated without clinical toxicity. A total daily oral ethosuximide dose of 25–35 mg/kg gives the average patient a plasma ethosuximide concentration of 60–80 μg/ml. Pharmacokinetic considerations might suggest that one should prescribe oral ethosuximide in a single oral daily dose of 30 mg/kg once the diagnosis of *petit mal* absence epilepsy is made. If a rapid onset of maximal action is required one might use a single loading dose of perhaps twice the daily maintenance dose. Thereafter the usual maintenance dose should be given each day. Unless the clinical situation indicates the need for earlier action, ethosuximide dosages should not be increased more often than once a week. Such a dosage policy allows the effects of steady-state ethosuximide concentrations to be ascertained before dosages are changed.

Absence epilepsy is probably the easiest of all varieties of epilepsy to treat on a basis of clinical judgement. The individual attacks are brief and only minimally disturb the sufferer. The attacks usually occur several or many times each day and tend to cease during the second decade of life. One can use the clinical response of the patient to ethosuximide treatment to assess the efficacy of therapy quite quickly. It is rarely calamitous if further attacks occur while dosages are being adjusted. (With forms of epilepsy in which individual attacks are more severe, but usually less frequent, one nearly always has to wait much longer to know if therapy is effective, whilst further attacks are a greater disadvantage for the patient.) Rarely would it be imperative to obtain very rapid control of *petit mal* absences. Perhaps the only circumstance is so-called *petit mal* status (for which intravenous benzodiazepine therapy is usually effective–see below). Therefore in treating *petit mal* absences with oral ethosuximide it has usually proved satisfactory to adjust dosages on clinical grounds, without needing to monitor plasma drug levels. Therapy might begin with 250 mg of the drug twice daily for a 5 or 6 year old, or 250 mg t.d.s. for a 10 year old. At weekly intervals the dose may be increased by 250 mg daily until the absences cease, or until side effects preclude further dosage increase. In the first weeks of such a regime a few patients may experience alimentary distress after ethosuximide doses. This symptom tends to lessen with time and can be relieved by the concurrent use of antacids. Apart from this complaint, side effects from ethosuximide (Chapter 9) are comparatively uncommon. However the patient should be asked about their presence. Otherwise the earliest manifestations of serious toxicity may not be detected.

The above empirical approach to ethosuximide dosage usually means that the child will receive less than 25 mg/kg/day of ethosuximide initially. Such a dosage is likely to lead to plasma ethosuximide levels in the lower part of the therapeutic range, but these levels may suffice to control absence seizures. If not, ethosuximide dose should be increased. When ethosuximide doses in individual patients are increased, and particularly when plasma ethosuximide levels are used as a guide to therapy, it should be remembered that steady-state plasma ethosuximide level tends to rise out of proportion to dose increase, particularly within and above the therapeutic range (Fig. 9.7). Once a satisfactory daily dose is achieved, one can consider whether to have the child take the whole dose once a day. It is convenient for patients not to have to take ethosuximide three or more times a day. Particularly in children, mid-day doses tend to be omitted, whether accidentally or deliberately. However, especially for a large child, who may for instance weigh 50 kg and require ethosuximide in a dose of 30 to 40 mg/kg each day, a single dose of 6 or 8 ethosuximide (250 mg) capsules once every day may be unacceptable. Here divided doses may be more realistic, even though once-daily ethosuximide dosage may be all that is necessary on pharmacokinetic grounds. In practice, twice daily ethosuximide administration as a routine may be preferable for most patients. Patients seem to manage to remember morning and evening doses of anticonvulsant drugs more easily, possibly because these doses are nearly always taken in the home. If one dose out of two is omitted there is likely to be less fall in plasma and brain level of drug than if the whole day's (single) dose is missed. At least in relation to phenytoin Terrence and Alberts (1978) showed that compliance decreased if the drug was prescribed more often than twice a day.

Another practical matter arises in connection with ethosuximide therapy. The oxazolidinediones (e.g. troxidone) when used for *petit mal* absences, appear to decrease the threshold for major convulsions (Schmidt and Wilder, 1968). There is also suspicion that, if ethosuximide is prescribed for patients whose only form of epilepsy is *petit mal* absences, a few may develop major tonic-clonic fits within a short time (Lorentz de Haas and Kuilman, 1964). However, some authors have stated that they have not encountered this complication (Heathfield and Jewesbury, 1964). In any event, one in two or one in three persons with absences might be expected to ultimately develop major fits (Rodin, 1968). Therefore, it may be argued whether ethosuximide really precipitates major epilepsy, or whether the latter develops purely as a temporal coincidence in a predisposed person. However the coincidence may occur occasionally, and if it does it is not easy to justify to irate parents why treatment has apparently made a child's epilepsy 'worse', i.e. more severe. Consequently, many neurologists make a practice of prescribing an anticonvulsant effective against generalized tonic-clonic seizures (e.g. a hydantoin or barbiturate) together with ethosuximide, even when such major epilepsy has not yet occurred in the patient with *petit mal* absences. If this policy is followed it would seem prudent to prescribe the major anticonvulsant first, and to ensure that its dose is potentially adequate (preferably assessed by plasma level measurements), before ethosuximide is added. If the two drugs are prescribed simultaneously from the outset, and idiosyncratic type side effects occur, it may be difficult to know which drug is responsible.

As mentioned above, there often appears little need to measure plasma ethosuximide levels in the clinical situation. Sherwin, Robb and Lechter (1973) found the measurements a help clinically, in that they thereby detected patients who were not taking their prescribed ethosuximide dosage. This may be the main advantage that the estimations offer in many circumstances. To treat *petit mal* absences all that may be needed in many instances is to prescribe a major anticonvulsant and adjust to its dose to provide an adequate plasma (and brain) drug concentration, as explained later; then oral ethosuximide is commenced once or twice daily, beginning with the nearest convenient dosage multiple of 250 mg (the capsule size) that permits a daily intake of no more than 20–25 mg/kg body weight. Thereafter, recognizing that ethosuximide has a half-life of 30 to 60 hours and that the initial dose will sometimes be inadequate, 250 mg dosage increments are made each 7 to 10 days till the absences cease or side effects prevent further dosage increase. It should be realized that the elimination of ethosuximide, and the response to the drug, vary so much in different patients that the upper limit of dose should be determined solely by the patients' response, and not by some notion of the upper limit of a therapeutic range of plasma drug concentrations.

If *petit mal* absences are controlled, ethosuximide therapy is usually continued in full dosage into the teenage years. By this stage the absences tend to cease spontaneously, even if not previously fully controlled (Livingstone, 1972). Then, particularly if the EEG no longer shows the characteristic discharges, the ethosuximide may be withdrawn. It is customary to do this gradually over several months (Livingstone, 1972). However, we know of no proof that such a protracted withdrawal is necessary. There is an appreciable risk of generalized tonic-clonic fits occurring, even after *petit mal* absences have ceased. It is therefore prudent to continue the anticonvulsant prescribed to prevent tonic-clonic epilepsy for at least three years after the ethosuximide is withdrawn. This is a situation in which it may be possible to prevent the later development of a form of severe epilepsy to which a patient is predisposed. In fact it may be the prevention of severe epilepsy years later, rather than the slight risk of precipitating an immediate tonic-clonic fit, which justifies the prescription of a major anticonvulsant together with ethosuximide from the outset of therapy. If ethosuximide in maximum tolerated dosage fails to control *petit mal* absences, or if it cannot be tolerated, other anticonvulsants should be tried. Clonazepam or sodium valproate (both considered below) are the best therapeutic alternatives, but there are other possibilities.

Other succinimides
When ethosuximide cannot be tolerated its congeners methsuximide or phensuximide may still be tolerated. However they often prove relatively ineffective. Further, if a potential serious side effect of idiosyncratic type has been produced by ethosuximide it probably is safer to avoid the other succinimides. When the latter are used their dosages are adjusted on clinical grounds, as for ethosuximide. While both drugs have much shorter half-lives than ethosuximide (Kinkel, 1971), they produce slowly eliminated active metabolites. Therefore these drugs should need to be given only once a day to maintain reasonably steady plasma and brain concentrations of anticonvulsant substances.

Oxazolidinediones
The oxazolidinediones, troxidione and paramethadione, are now largely superseded drugs, used as adjuncts to ethosuximide therapy, or as replacements if ethosuximide, clonazepam and valproate cannot be tolerated. Both these oxazolidinediones are less effective than ethosuximide, and both have potentially serious, even dangerous, side effects (e.g. aplastic anaemia, nephrotic syndrome). In addition, both oxazolidinediones may produce distressing glare phenomena. These may be more intolerable than *petit mal* absences for some patients.

For both drugs, dosages can be adjusted on clinical grounds, as are ethosuximide dosages, and for the same reasons. Again it probably is wise to prescribe a major anticonvulsant before the 'dione' is given, for the reasons indicated above. The half-life of dimethadione, the major (biologically active) metabolite of troxidione, is so long that it would seem reasonable to give troxidione once daily, and to adjust dosages no more often than at fortnightly intervals. The troxidione dose that controls absences may be about 60 mg/kg/day. Renal and haemopoietic function should be checked by appropriate laboratory tests, particularly during the first few months of therapy with these agents, and the patient questioned about possible side effects. If the oxazolidinediones prove effective they should be continued in full dosage, and withdrawn as recommended for ethosuximide after the patient's epilepsy has been controlled for a sufficient period.

Other drugs

If *petit mal* absences fail to respond to the above agents (and also clonazepam and valproate, which are discussed below) the carbonic anhydrase inhibitor acetazolamide may be tried, particularly in cases where the attacks are worsened by overbreathing. Acetazolamide seems to offer no more than minor benefits and Livingstone (1972) has found that it practically never produces sustained control of epilepsy. Benzodiazepines other than clonazepam (e.g. diazepam) may be successful at times in absence epilepsy (Geller and Christoff, 1971).

MYOCLONIC AND AKINETIC SEIZURES

It is convenient to discuss the therapy of infantile myoclonic seizures of hypsarrhythmic type (infantile spasms, salaam seizures or West's syndrome) separately from the remaining types of myoclonic attack.

HYPSARRHYTHMIA

In this variety of myoclonic epilepsy, which occurs between the ages of 6 months and 3 years, it is necessary to treat the condition successfully within a few weeks of its onset if permanent mental retardation is to be avoided (Rodin, 1968). All too often the significance of the story of an infant with a series of clustered, sudden flexion jerks of the trunk, with extension of the limbs, is not appreciated for many days or weeks. The diagnosis may then be made too late to prevent intellectual impairment, even though the epileptic component of the disorder may still be controlled by therapy.

ACTH, tetracosactrin and corticosteroids

Whether the hypsarrhythmia is idiopathic, as it is in perhaps 50 per cent of cases (Bower and Jeavons, 1959), or related to detectable pathological change in the brain, the treatment of first choice is ACTH, tetracosactrin, cortisone or synthetic glucocorticoids. The mode of action of these agents in hypsarrhythmia is unknown. If the seizures respond, they usually do so within a few days of commencing treatment. Concurrently there is then a degree of impovement in the associated mental impairment. ACTH, tetracosactrin and steroids are the only known treatments which may, if given in the first few weeks of the disorder, reverse the intellectual retardation associated with hypsarrhythmia. They also control the epileptic element. Certain benzodiazepines and other anticonvulsants may exert a degree of control over the myoclonic jerks only (see below). It has been suggested that ACTH is more effective than steroids in treating hypsarrhythmia (Finne, 1963). However Jeavons and Bowers (1964) in their review found no real evidence that this was so and steroids are now recommended also (Schmidt and Wilder, 1968). One has occasionally seen substantial doses of prednisone fail to control the spasms of hypsarrhythmia in an infant whose attacks were promptly terminated by ACTH. This might suggest that ACTH sometimes may be superior to steroids in treating hypsarrhythmia, a conclusion with which Livingstone (1972) would appear to agree. However recent doubts about the bioavailability of certain glucocorticoid preparations (Sugita and Niebergall, 1973) raise the possibility that a portion of the steroid doses may not have absorbed in some instances, even though a potentially adequate dose was prescribed.

The average infant with hypsarrhythmia may be given ACTH by daily intramuscular injection in a dose of 20 I.U. (or tetracosactrin in a dose of 0·5 mg second daily) immediately the diagnosis is made. If there is no response in a fortnight the ACTH dose should be increased to 30 or 40 I.U. daily for another fortnight (or the tetracosactrin dose increased correspondingly). If there has still been no response by this stage it is unlikely that continued ACTH or tetracosactrin will prove of use. Logically it may then be worth trying synthetic glucocorticoids (e.g. prednisone or prednisolone 30 mg per day, in divided doses). The ACTH may have failed to produce a sufficient adrenal response, though the use of a steroid itself still may be effective. It would appear that, when ACTH fails, a successful outcome is unlikely. De Negri, Lamedica and Ravera (1973) considered that plasma cortisol levels in excess of 40 μg/100 ml were needed to benefit hypsarrhythmia, and that better results were attained at levels of 80 μg/100 ml.

Little is known as to the minimal effective steroid or ACTH dose for hypsarrhythmia, or the optimal dosage interval. Hypsarrhythmia is an intellect-threatening emergency. It must be treated vigorously and the response to treatment judged on clinical and EEG grounds. An unnecessarily high dose of therapy is preferable to underdosage. It is remarkable how often nursing staff fail to observe the individual spasms in a child with hypsarrhythmia. This failure may lead to an erroneous belief that the hypsarrhythmia is controlled a few days after ACTH therapy is begun in hospital. The mother's report that her infant's attacks have ceased is usually more reliable. However such a report should be confirmed by finding that the hypsarrhythmic discharges have cleared from the EEG before ACTH therapy is suspended. Generally hypsarrhythmia should be treated with ACTH for at least 7 days after the disorder is controlled clinically and electroencephalographically. If this is done, relapse is rare after cessation of therapy. Any relapse usually responds to a second, longer, course of treatment.

If hypsarrhythmia fails to respond to ACTH or steroid therapy given in high dosage for a month or more it would seem that the prognosis for cure of the disorder is indeed poor. The child is likely to have residual permanent mental retardation. Although the myoclonic spasms probably will cease after several months or more, other forms of epilepsy are likely to occur later, if they are not already present. Other authors would seem to agree with this prognosis (Jeavons and Bower, 1964). When the hypsarrhythmia cannot be cured it may still be possible to control the myoclonic element to some extent with the forms of therapy ordinarily used for myoclonic epilepsy in older age groups (e.g. clonazepam, nitrazepam or valproate).

Pyridoxine

It should be mentioned that rare forms of hypsarrhythmia appear to be due to pyridoxine deficiency (Cochrane, 1959, cited by Jeavons and Bower, 1964; French, Grueter, Druckman and O'Brien, 1965). Therefore it may be reasonable to prescribe this relatively inexpensive and apparently inocuous substance in all infants with hypsarrhythmia without waiting to establish a diagnosis of pyridoxine deficiency by biochemical means (as described by French, Grueter, Druckman and O'Brien, 1965).

OTHER MYOCLONIC AND AKINETIC EPILEPSIES

Some varieties of myoclonic seizure in the post-hypsarrhythmic age group are of hereditary origin. These are not associated with detectable pathological change in the brain and show interseizure EEG appearances similar to those seen in typical *petit mal* absences. More often myoclonic and akinetic seizures are due to detectable pathological changes in the brain or to chemical abnormalities affecting the brain. Rarely the pathological changes may be of hereditary origin, as in the Unverricht-Lundborg syndrome of myoclonus epilepsy, where there are Lafora inclusion bodies (Seitelberger, 1968). In these acquired myoclonic epilepsies of childhood, adolescence and adult life the interseizure EEG differs from the typical generalized 3 Hz spike and wave appearance of the hereditary variety of myoclonic epilepsy. Instead, the EEG tends to show generalized multiple spike and wave discharges, or spike and wave discharges at frequencies above or below 3 Hz, though in the frequency range 2–5 Hz. On the whole, the older the patient, the less likely clear cut spike-wave discharges are in the surface EEG. Further, the older the patient when the attacks begin the more responsive to treatment the disorder is likely to be.

HEREDITARY MYOCLONIC EPILEPSY

Ethosuximide

In the hereditary types of myoclonic epilepsy (without associated cerebral structural changes) ethosuximide may be used as for *petit mal* absences. If it fails, the attacks may be treated with the agents used for acquired myoclonic epilepsy.

ACQUIRED MYOCLONIC EPILEPSY IN CHILDHOOD

Myoclonic seizures of acquired type in childhood (the Lennox-Gastaut syndrome) are generally regarded as being among the more difficult forms of epilepsy to control, unless the underlying cause is a reversible metabolic disorder (e.g. renal failure). Nitrazepam was for a time regarded as the drug of choice for myoclonic attacks (Lance, 1968). However, many clinicians would now prefer either valproate or clonazepam. Corticotrophin is not useful (Tudor, Milea and Stoica, 1974).

Valproate

Sodium valproate is hygroscopic. It is marketed as individually foil-wrapped tablets, each containing 200 mg active substance (300 mg in some countries). The initial dose for a 10–20 kg child might be 100 mg b.d., or for a larger child 100 mg t.d.s. The unused half-tablets from each dose may have to be discarded. Valproate has a relatively short half-life (about 8 hours) and is fairly rapidly absorbed. Plasma valproate levels therefore show appreciable fluctuation over a single 8 hour, or longer, dosage interval (Fig. 12.3). So long as plasma valproate levels remain above the therapeutic threshold at all times, this fluctuation in plasma drug levels is unlikely to affect control of epilepsy adversely. However, excessive fluctuation in plasma valproate levels increases the risk of both overdosage and underdosage effects. To reduce this risk it seems reasonable to suggest that valproate should be given two, or preferably three, times a day. Wulff, Flachs, Würtz-Jorgensen and Gram (1977) stated that the drug should be given at least four times a day. The short half-life of valproate means that steady-state conditions should apply by 48 hours after a dosage change. Consequently dosages can be increased as often as every 2 or 3 days, if the clinical situation indicates it, without risk of delayed-onset overdosage manifestations.

In practice, valproate dosage may be increased as necessary till epilepsy is controlled or until unwanted effects of the therapy preclude further dosage increase. The timing of the doses, and of the increases in dose, should be determined by the considerations discussed above. The effective dose often lies between 400 and 2000 mg per day. At the present time measurements of plasma valproate levels do not provide a particularly helpful guide to treatment. There may be several reasons for this. Firstly, myoclonic seizures in children usually occur frequently. Therefore it is usually easy to determine clinically whether therapy is adequate, and to act accordingly. Secondly, the therapeutic range of plasma valproate levels (50–100 μg/ml) is not well established and therefore is not a secure guide to therapy. Thirdly, alterations in plasma valproate level from one measurement to the next may not necessarily indicate that valproate dosage should be revised. Unless immediately predosage (i.e. minimal) plasma drug levels have been measured on all occasions, differences in level may be due merely to differences in the timing of the measurements relative to the time of drug intake.

If valproate is given to patients already taking other anticonvulsants, it is wise to measure the plasma levels of the other drugs, particularly if apparent unwanted effects of the valproate occur. Interactions between valproate and other anticonvulsants, especially phenobarbitone and phenytoin (see pp. 178, 93 and 269) can lead to substantial alterations in the plasma levels of these drugs, necessitating changes in their dosages.

Valproate appears to be an effective drug for myoclonic epilepsy (and for *petit mal* absences). Its unwanted effects usually are not severe. In particular drowsiness (excluding that due to pharmacokinetic interactions with phenobarbitone) is not often troublesome. Reservations about regarding valproate as the drug of first choice for myoclonic epilepsy stem chiefly from concern that the drug-induced testicular damage which sometimes occurs in experimental animals might also prove to occur in man. Until this possibility can be excluded, it may be prudent to prefer clonazepam in this type of epilepsy.

Clonazepam

Clonazepam has a half-life of approximately 24 hours. Even though it is fairly rapidly absorbed its plasma levels are unlikely to fluctuate through an unacceptably wide range if it is taken twice a day, or more often. Plasma level fluctuations might not be excessive even with once-daily dosage, so long as the individual's therapeutic threshold plasma level is exceeded throughout the 24 hours. Steady-state conditions should apply by 5 days after a dosage change. These pharmacokinetic considerations suggest that clonazepam should be given twice daily. Therapy should begin in low dosage (e.g. 0·5 mg b.d. for a 10–20 kg child, 1 mg b.d. for a 50 kg or heavier individual). Dosage should be increased every 5 days, as necessary to control epilepsy. Sometimes the initial dose may have to be reduced, because it has produced excessive drowsiness. It often proves wise to use initial clonazepam doses well below the expected therapeutic doses. Although the drug produces drowsiness, tolerance to this symptom often develops fairly rapidly. If the clonazepam dose can be kept below the threshold for this symptom, and increased at 5 to 7 day intervals, it may often be possible to achieve a therapeutic effect without the patient having any problem from unwanted effects of treatment. If the initial dose is too high, or dose increments are too frequent or too large, the patient may be unwilling to persevere with the drug because it has made him too drowsy and irritable. Occasional patients become quite aggressive when taking clonazepam.

Plasma clonazepam levels do not appear a very helpful guide to either therapeutic or adverse effects of the drug. Dosage adjustments are best made on clinical grounds, though plasma level measurements can serve as an indication of patient compliance, and can show whether levels in the tentative therapeutic range of 25–75 ng/ml have been attained. Patients may tolerate, and obtain benefit from, much higher plasma clonazepam levels, provided doses have been increased gradually. The upper limit of clonazepam dose should be determined by the occurrence of sufficiently troublesome adverse effects of the drug, and not by achieving some arbitrary plasma drug level.

If clonazepam therapy is to be ceased, the drug should not be stopped abruptly, because of the danger of withdrawal fits or status epilepticus.

Nitrazepam

The pharmacokinetic data of Rieder (1973) suggest that nitrazepam need not be given more often than twice daily (possibly once daily would be sufficient) to maintain reasonably constant steady-state plasma drug concentrations. However the nitrazepam concentration that gives optimal protection against myoclonic seizures is unknown. At the present time nitrazepam dosages must be worked out by trial and error in each individual. The drug's half-life (about 24 hours) suggests that nitrazepam dosage could be increased every 5 to 7 days without undue risk of exceeding the minimum effective dose for the individual. Dosage increases should be made until the myoclonic attacks cease or until side effects (mostly drowsiness) preclude further dosage increase. The initial dosage and the dosage increments are usually 2·5 mg daily for smaller children and 5 mg daily for larger children and for adults.

Diazepam

Oral diazepam may be used for myoclonic seizures in the unlikely event that other benzodiazepines cannot be tolerated. Diazepam is often less effective than nitrazepam for this disorder (Lance, 1968). It tends to produce intolerable drowsiness before an adequate long-term anticonvulsant effect occurs. The plasma half-lives of diazepam (1–2 days) and its biologically active desmethyl metabolite (2–4 days) are long enough to suggest that diazepam need be given only once each day to keep plasma level fluctuations of drug and metabolite within acceptable limits. No guidelines are yet available as to the correlation of plasma diazepam or nordiazepam concentrations with protection against myoclonic seizures. Therefore dosage adjustments should be made on clinical grounds. However one should not increase dosages too frequently (e.g. not more often than once a fortnight) to allow a steady-state to occur after each dose change. Thus unnecessarily high dosages are avoided. A representative initial dose for younger children might be 2 to 4 mg daily, with a correspondingly larger dose for older children and adults (e.g. 5 to 10 mg daily). The usual dose increment would be 2 mg or 5 mg daily.

The benzodiazepines and valproate, singly or in combination, may fail to control myoclonic epilepsy of acquired origin in childhood. It then may be worth trying anticonvulsants from the succinimide or oxazolidinedione families alone, or in combination with the benzodiazepines or valproate. In particular, ethosuximide, in doses sufficient to produce plasma levels in the range 100–150 μg/ml, or higher, may occasionally be useful.

In resistant myoclonic epilepsy in younger children the ketogenic diet (Livingstone, 1972) is likely to have its best effects, and may be worth trying. The diet can be made more palatable by using medium chain triglycerides as the source of ketone bodies (Huttenlocker, Wilbourn and Sigmore, 1971). If myoclonic epilepsy remains uncontrolled, major tonic-clonic fits may develop. These require treatment in their own right. If myoclonic seizures are completely controlled the full dose of the effective anticonvulsant agent, or agents, should be continued for 3 or 4 years before a dosage reduction is attempted.

MYOCLONIC EPILEPSY IN ADOLESCENCE AND ADULT LIFE

Except when due to progressive brain disease, myoclonic epilepsy in adolescence and adult life is usually milder than the disorder in childhood. It responds to the same drugs, used in higher initial doses, though not necessarily in higher final doses. However the barbiturate anticonvulsants and carbamazepine may also be useful. There is a not uncommon type of epilepsy with pre-breakfast myoclonic attacks which occurs in the second decade of life. This disorder often does not present clinically until a major seizure ensues. Barbiturate anticonvulsants are usually efficacious for this disorder, and their pharmacokinetic properties make them convenient to employ.

ALL OTHER VARIETIES OF EPILEPSY

This category comprises the majority of all instances of epilepsy. It includes all cases of partial epilepsy, and all tonic-clonic fits, whether part of primary generalized epilepsy or due to the secondary generalization of partial epilepsy, and all unilateral seizures. For all these varieties of epilepsy the effective anticonvulsants for interval treatment are the hydantoins, the barbiturates, carbamazepine, probably clonazepam and perhaps valproate and sulthiame. In these varieties of epilepsy the problem of organizing therapy is rather different from that in *petit mal* absences and in myoclonic seizures. In the latter types of epilepsy the individual seizures are brief and, apart from myoclonic 'drop' attacks, are generally mild in their effects. Further, the individual seizures are frequent. Therefore it usually does not take long for a given anticonvulsant dosage to be proved adequate or inadequate. Thus therapy can be adjusted on clinical grounds relatively easily and quickly. By way of contrast, in the types of epilepsy now to be discussed, the individual seizures generally are less frequent, and sometimes are quite infrequent. However these seizures may be very much more severe and disrupting for the sufferer's life. Consequently it is often more difficult to adjust therapy for these epilepsies on purely clinical grounds, yet at the same time it is more important to control the seizures quickly. Here the monitoring of plasma anticonvulsant concentrations is particularly useful.

Drugs of the hydantoin and barbiturate families, and carbamazepine, are used as the primary anticonvulsants for these types of epilepsy. Clonazepam has not yet found its place as the sole drug to be used. Sulthiame is usually employed as a secondary anticonvulsant in combination with hydantoins, barbiturates or carbamazepine (Sutherland and Bowman, 1963). Nevertheless, sulthiame may well be an anticonvulsant in its own right, particularly for partial epilepsy. However in many patients side effects prevent adequate sulthiame dosage. Valproate has not had time to establish itself as a sole anticonvulsant in the types of epilepsy now considered. It appears to reinforce the effects of hydantoin and barbiturate anticonvulsants. However this reinforcement may involve pharmacokinetic interactions between the drugs so that similar results might have been achieved by adjusting the dose of the primary drug. Overall there may be little to choose between phenytoin, phenobarbitone, methylphenobarbitone, primidone and carbamazepine as the initial anticonvulsant for the types of epilepsy here considered. Carbamazepine now has been in use long enough to prove itself the equal of the older drugs in these circumstances. Some might prefer one of the barbiturates on the grounds that such drugs are less likely than phenytoin to produce serious side effects. However barbiturates cause much more chronic mental dullness and irritability than does phenytoin. Carbamazepine occupies an intermediate position between phenytoin and the barbiturates in relation to patterns of unwanted effects. This might commend it in the eyes of some. Serious phenytoin side effects are relatively rare if its dosage is managed carefully. The majority of patients taking phenytoin feel more 'normal' than do the majority who take barbiturate anticonvulsants. The pharmacokinetics of phenytoin are more thoroughly understood than those of other anticonvulsants. Therefore many would regard phenytoin as the drug of first choice for the types of epilepsy now under consideration.

Phenytoin

Initial dosage
In partial epilepsy, seizures may be individually minor but sometimes occur quite frequently. However, in many instances tonic-clonic epileptic seizures occur only at intervals of weeks or months. Consequently there may be considerable delay in obtaining control of epilepsy where dosage adjustments are made purely on clinical grounds. This delay may reduce the chances of obtaining final seizure control, and possibly cure of the epilepsy (Rodin, 1968). Statistically, when phenytoin is used, plasma drug concentrations of 10–20 μg/ml correlate with the best chance of controlling epilepsy with minimal risk of side effects due to overdosage (Kutt and McDowell, 1968). Therefore it is logical to try to attain plasma phenytoin concentrations in this range soon after phenytoin therapy is commenced. The data of Fig. 16.1 indicate that in persons 14 years of age and over, a daily oral phenytoin

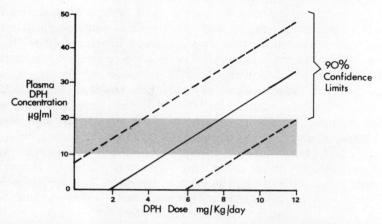

Fig. 16.1 Regression for steady-state plasma phenytoin (DPH) level on phenytoin dose in 97 adults. The therapeutic range and 90 per cent confidence limits for predicting plasma phenytoin level from drug dose are shown.

dose of 4–5 mg/kg offers an approximate 50 per cent probability of achieving a steady-state plasma phenytoin level over 10 μg/ml. There is only a 5 per cent probability of producing a level in excess of 22 μg/ml, and thus possible side effects from overdosage. For children below 11 years of age (this group behaves differently from adults in respect to their elimination of phenytoin) a daily dose of 4–5 mg/kg offers a 50 per cent probability of a steady-state phenytoin level over 6·5 μg/ml. There is a 5 per cent probability of a level exceeding 23 μg/ml, with a risk of overdosage effects (Fig. 16.2). In this age group to obtain a 50 per cent chance of producing plasma phenytoin levels over 10 μg/ml a minimum dose of 7·5 mg/kg/day would be needed. A dose of 7·5 mg/kg/day would be associated with a 10 per cent risk of producing plasma levels over 23 μg/ml, a possibility which might be regarded with disquiet. If the initial daily phenytoin dose, calculated on the basis of 4–5 mg/kg for adults, and 7–8 mg/kg for children is prescribed, there

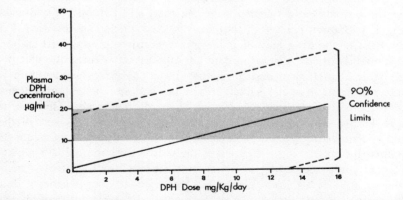

Fig. 16.2 Regression for steady-state plasma phenytoin (DPH) level on phenytoin dose in 120 children. The therapeutic range and 90 per cent confidence belt for predicting plasma phenytoin level from drug dose are shown.

would be a moderate chance of the patient being protected against his epilepsy within a week of commencing therapy. By this time, drug concentrations in the body would have had time to reach a steady state, yet there would be little risk of serious overdosage. In practice, it is often not possible to prescribe the exact dosage suggested by the 4–5 or 7–8 mg/kg/day formulae. Except for suspensions, which can be inconvenient and may deliver dosages imprecisely if not used carefully, oral phenytoin is available in 30, 50 or 100 mg dosage units. The drug must be prescribed in terms of these units. Because of its comparatively slow elimination from the body, an extra 100 mg of phenytoin taken second daily appears to keep plasma drug levels fairly steady at the approximate concentration that would be expected from an extra 50 mg of the drug taken daily. Similarly, an extra 30 mg second daily proves equivalent to an extra 15 mg daily. The correlation between steady-state plasma phenytoin level and dose increment in the individual patient is not linear (Figs. 6.21 and 6.22). Therefore if one aims to achieve a phenytoin plasma level of 10–20 μg/ml and has to alter a patient's phenytoin dose even slightly (to prescribe the drug in a commercially available preparation) this can rather substantially reduce the chances of the patient being correctly dosed. In nearly all circumstances it is preferable to underdose the patient initially rather than to overdose him. A reasonable working rule is to prescribe an initial phenytoin dose of 4–5 mg/kg daily for patients of all ages, and to reduce this dose if necessary to permit the drug's being supplied as a commercially available preparation. There is no need to give phenytoin more often than once a day to maintain plasma levels (Loeser, 1961; Buchanan, Kinkel, Goulet and Smith, 1972; Vajda, Merory and Bladin, 1975). However, for the reasons given when discussing the use of ethosuximide, it may be preferable in practice to prescribe the drug twice daily. From the outset of therapy the patient should organize a routine such as the following for taking his treatment. Once a week he should put out each day's treatment for the next 7 days into a separate container marked with the name of the day on which that container will be used. Once each day (e.g. on going to bed) he should check the containers and ensure that the previous 24 hours' therapy has been taken. If not, the omitted drugs should be taken there and then. The knowledge that phenytoin need not be taken at frequent intervals and exact times during the day (and night) can relieve patients, and parents, of a considerable burden. If maximum phenytoin action is required quickly (in less than 4 days) a loading dose of the drug may be given intravenously. As explained earlier (page 55) this method of administration is rather cumbersome. Intramuscular injection of phenytoin is inefficient and unreliable (page 72). An oral phenytoin loading dose (10 mg/kg for an adult) is likely to produce a plasma phenytoin concentration in the region of 10 μg/ml within 12 hours of its administration. This dose may be given in several stages over 1–2 hours or longer, to reduce the risk of the drug causing gastric irritation and vomiting. Plasma phenytoin levels can then be maintained by prescribing the expected daily dose (averaging 2–2·5 mg/kg twice daily for an adult), beginning 12 hours after the loading dose.

Although initial phenytoin therapy as recommended above carries little risk of overdosage, this possibility should not be ignored. Each patient (and his relatives, if possible) should be warned of potential side effects of the drug, especially ataxia and skin rashes, and of their attendant dangers. It may be prudent for the patient to limit his activities for several days after the introduction of therapy with any anticonvulsant and also after any subsequent dosage change. Unless there is urgency it may be convenient to make dosage changes just prior to a weekend. Thus business responsibilities and car driving may be restricted with lessened inconvenience. Sporting activities may also be curtailed at this time, if considered necessary.

Follow up

The patient's condition should be reviewed 7 to 10 days after phenytoin therapy is initiated. This is important because there is much individual variation in the plasma phenytoin levels achieved with any given daily dosage of the drug. The doses recommended above are likely to produce satisfactory plasma phenytoin levels in only about 50 per cent of patients. Also, by the expiry of 7 to 10 days many of the potential idiosyncratic side effects of phenytoin will have had time to appear. Overdosage manifestations, if they have occurred, will not have been present too long, yet steady-state tissue drug concentrations will apply. At this stage plasma phenytoin concentration should be measured, if possible, and then any necessary dosage adjustment made. If attacks of epilepsy are still occurring after the drug has been taken for at least a week, the dosage should be increased unless the plasma level is already in the toxic range (e.g. over 25 μg/ml), or unless unwanted effects are already present. If, as is so often the case, the natural history of the epilepsy is such that attacks usually occur only at intervals of weeks, or months, the absence of attacks during the first 7 to 10 days of therapy does not necessarily mean that the epilepsy is controlled. In this circumstance, if the plasma phenytoin concentration is below 10 μg/ml, the dose should be increased, as discussed below. If facilities for measuring phenytoin levels are unavailable one may wait and see if the dose proves adequate as time passes. Alternatively one may increase the dose cautiously till nystagmus appears. This sign usually appears before ataxia occurs. Nystagmus usually, but unfortunately not always, occurs when the plasma phenytoin level is a little above 20 μg/ml. A slight dosage reduction is then likely to achieve a plasma phenytoin level in the therapeutic range of 10–20 μg/ml. Phenytoin doses should not be altered more often than once a week or the full effect of one dose change may not have appeared before the dose is altered again.

Dosage adjustment

Some 50 per cent of patients taking phenytoin may require dosage adjustment after their initial plasma phenytoin level measurement. In adjusting phenytoin dosages it is essential to be aware of the shape of the curve relating plasma drug level to dose change in the individual (Fig. 6.22). If this is not appreciated and it is assumed that the relation between dose change and plasma level change is linear, dosage adjustments made when the plasma level is above 6–9 μg/ml will almost certainly produce changes in the plasma level of the drug well in excess of those desired. In order to help the clinician adjust patients' phenytoin doses to achieve plasma levels in the desired range, a set of figures (Figs. 16.3, 16.4 and 16.5) is included. These figures show the likely effects of phenytoin dosage increments of 30, 50 and 100 mg per day on plasma phenytoin concentrations in the average 70 kg patient,

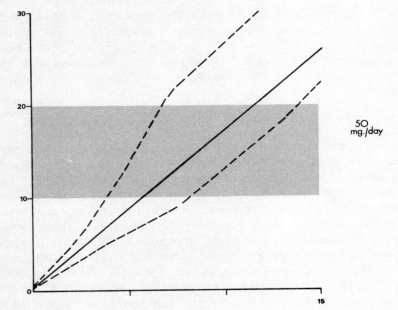

Fig. 16.3

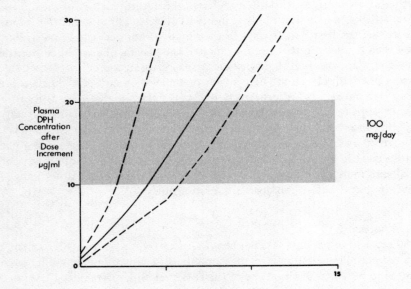

Fig. 16.4

and in patients near the extremes of the ranges of response of plasma phenytoin level to dosage change.

If phenytoin dose has been altered, the plasma level of the drug should be measured again in another 7 to 10 days to ensure that the dosage change has had its desired effect. If not, a further dosage adjustment may be made, guided by data

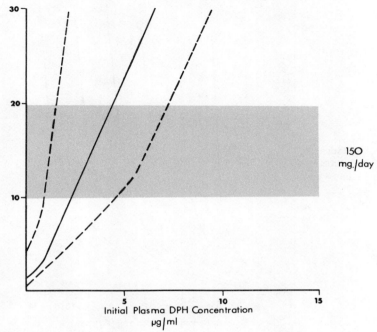

Fig. 16.5

Figs. 16.3, 16.4 and 16.5. These figures show respectively the calculated effects of 50, 100 and 150 mg daily phenytoin dose increments on plasma phenytoin levels in a 70 kg man. The calculated average vaules are shown on solid lines, and the calculated range of values likely to be found is enclosed by the broken lines.

such as the set of curves shown in Fig. 16.6. The effect of this further adjustment may be confirmed by another estimation of plasma phenytoin concentration a week or more after the most recent dose alteration.

There have been other more refined attempts to guide the clinician in adjusting phenytoin dosage. Richens and Dunlop (1975) and Richens (1975) produced a nomogram based on mean population Michaelis-Menten elimination parameters of the drug. There have been reports that this nomogram was not always a satisfactory predictor of the effects of dosage changes on plasma drug levels (Lund and Alvan, 1975). The problem may be that the nomogram was derived from too small a range of K_m and V_{max} values.

An intrinsically more accurate method was described by Ludden, Hawkins, Allen and Hoffman (1976). This required two accurate steady-state plasma phenytoin measurements at different drug doses in each patient. From the data an Eadie-Hofstee plot was constructed for each patient, and V_{max} and K_m were read from the plot. From these values the effects of a dose change on plasma phenytoin level in the individual could be calculated with reasonable accuracy, utilising the formula

$$\text{Concentration} = \frac{\text{Dose} \cdot K_m}{(V_{max} - \text{Dose})}$$

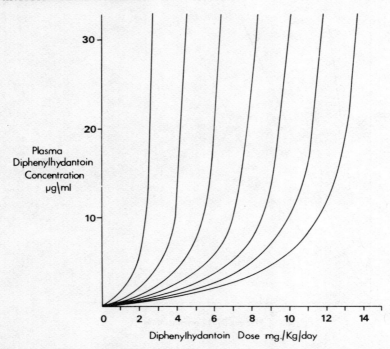

Fig. 16.6 Theoretical curves for predicting the effects of phenytoin dosage changes on plasma phenytoin concentrations in individual patients.

However, by the time phenytoin doses have been changed to permit two steady-state plasma phenytoin levels at different doses to be obtained, one may have already achieved a plasma phenytoin level in the therapeutic range in the majority of patients. Therefore, by the time one is in a position to be able to use this technique to manipulate drug levels in a patient, this patient often needs no further dosage change. Another method of using individual Michaelis-Menten parameters for the same purpose was described by Mullen (1978).

If a patient's plasma phenytoin level appears disproportionately low in relation to his dose it may be prudent to suspect that he is not taking his full prescribed dose, even if he denies omitting some doses of the drug. This possibility should be borne in mind in making further dosage adjustments.

Should epilepsy still occur when plasma phenytoin levels are in the therapeutic range, it still may be possible to control the seizures by giving more drug. However at this stage even small increases in drug dose are likely to produce considerable increases in plasma phenytoin level and in biological effects. Some patients may feel perfectly well with plasma phenytoin levels of 20 to 30 μg/ml, and their epilepsy may be controlled or improved. However it should be realized that these patients are in a potentially brittle pharmacokinetic and therapeutic situation. Their phenytoin elimination capacity is virtually saturated. Anything which alters the drug's elimination slightly (e.g. liver disease, administration of certain other drugs for intercurrent illness or variation in alcohol intake) may suffice to precipitate phenytoin intoxication.

Long-term management

If a phenytoin dose is found which completely controls a patient's epilepsy, and produces no serious side effects (see page 98) that dose should be continued till the patient has had no epilepsy for 3 or 4 years or longer. Then withdrawal of therapy can be considered, particularly if the EEG has shown clearing of epileptiform activity. It is customary to withdraw phenytoin slowly, over weeks or months (Livingstone, 1972). Some patients in these circumstances may prefer to continue taking their anticonvulsants indefinitely because of the feeling of security this engenders. There would seem no logical reason for not respecting this attitude if the phenytoin dose is properly adjusted and careful assessment shows that no unwanted effects are present.

Prescribing phenytoin as described above is tantamount to suggesting that the drug usually should be used in or near its maximum tolerated dose. No doubt some would argue that it is preferable to use the drug in its minimal effective dose. However, trying to find a minimal effective dose in a patient subjects him to an increased risk of further epilepsy while the desired minimal dose is sought. The more epileptic seizures that have occurred in a person, the less the chance of finding any anticonvulsant dose that will be effective for him (Rodin, 1968). Therefore a vigorous approach to phenytoin therapy seems preferable, with dosages guided by clinical judgement in conjunction with plasma phenytoin concentration measurements. Without the latter, to be therapeutically vigorous may present some hazard for the patient.

Measurement of plasma phenytoin concentrations should when possible be carried out in the following circumstances:

1. 7 to 10 days after therapy is initiated.
2. 7 to 10 days after any change in phenytoin dosage.
3. 7 to 10 days after the dose of any other drug (whether used for epilepsy or for intercurrent illness) is changed.
4. whenever symptoms appear which could be phenytoin side effects.
5. at 6 to 12 monthly intervals during a course of therapy. This serves to encourage the patient to take his drugs. Non-compliance is a major problem in managing epilepsy (Lund, Jorgensen and Kuhl, 1964; Gibberd, Dunne, Handley and Hazleman, 1970). Such measurements are also a protection against the insidious development of overdosage, which may be obvious to the patient and the clinician only in retrospect.
6. whenever epilepsy escapes from control.

When phenytoin estimations are done after some months of therapy it may be wise to measure serum folate and calcium levels also. If a patient has uraemia, liver disease or a disorder known to alter plasma proteins, or if he is taking multiple drugs which may alter the plasma protein binding of phenytoin, it may be wise to measure phenytoin concentration in plasma water or in saliva. These levels may provide a more reliable index of the biological effect of the drug than does the phenytoin level in whole plasma. For these fluids the 'therapeutic' range is probably about $1 \cdot 5$–$2 \cdot 8$ μg/ml (Fig. 6.2).

If phenytoin cannot be tolerated it should be replaced by another anticonvulsant. Should phenytoin fail to control epilepsy in its maximum tolerated dosage, a second anticonvulsant may be added to the highest phenytoin dose that can be comfortably tolerated. In these circumstances a barbiturate type anticonvulsant or carbamazepine should probably be used next. The other hydantoin anticonvulsants are either too potentially toxic (methoin) or too relatively ineffective (ethotoin) to warrant consideration apart from the most exceptional circumstance.

Barbiturate anticonvulsants

The principal anticonvulsants in this group are phenobarbitone, methylphenobarbitone and primidone (desoxyphenobarbitone). It seems fair to say that there is as yet no published proof that either methylphenobarbitone or primidone is superior to phenobarbitone as an anticonvulsant, when dosages are taken to their limits of tolerance or adjusted till all drugs give similar plasma phenobarbitone concentrations. Olesen and Dam (1967) provided evidence supporting this view in respect to phenobarbitone and primidone though Pippenger (personal communication) has recently obtained evidence to the contrary. Because of the simultaneous presence of biologically active metabolites, the pharmacokinetic situation is more complex to interpret when methylphenobarbitone or primidone is used than when phenobarbitone itself is given. Therefore, in the interests of simplicity, it might be argued that phenobarbitone should be the preferred barbiturate anticonvulsant. However, there are also arguments that methylphenobarbitone should be the preferred drug. Changes in methylphenobarbitone dose in the individual have more easily predicted effects on plasma phenobarbitone levels, and biological actions, than do changes in phenobarbitone dose. Methylphenobarbitone dosage units are more appropriately sized than are those of phenobarbitone, and methylphenobarbitone lacks the occasional tendency of primidone to produce extreme drowsiness with the first dose. It would seem irrational to combine two or more barbiturate-type anticonvulsants. If the first had really been taken to its limit of tolerance, overdosage type side effects should occur if the drugs were combined, since in effect more phenobarbitone would have been supplied.

Phenobarbitone

Oral phenobarbitone need be given only once a day to adults, and perhaps twice a day to children, to maintain steady-state plasma levels of the drug with relatively little interdosage fluctuation (Butler, Makaffee and Waddell, 1954; Faero, Kastrup, Lykkegaard Nielsen, Melchior and Thorn, 1972). Reasons have been given above for preferring the practice of twice daily anticonvulsant administration for all the more commonly used anticonvulsants in all age groups. This preference is determined both by convenience and by pharmacokinetic considerations. Steady-state conditions are likely to apply after 2 to 3 weeks of phenobarbitone therapy in constant dosage. Plasma phenobarbitone levels in the range 10–30 μg/ml are likely to be associated with an optimal anticonvulsant effect. There is said to be a reasonable chance of obtaining these levels in one to two weeks with regular phenobarbitone doses of approximately 2·5 mg/kg/day (Buchthal and Lennox-Buchthal, 1972). The data of Fig. 8·4 and 16.7 suggest that different age groups require different daily phenobarbitone doses to attain a mean mid-therapeutic range plasma phenobarbitone level of 20 μg/ml. For persons under 4 years, between 4 and 14 years, between 15 and 40 years, and over 40 years, the mean daily

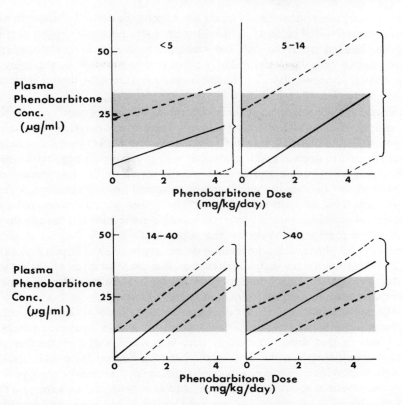

Fig. 16.7 Regressions for steady-state plasma phenobarbitone level on phenobarbitone dose, together with 90 per cent confidence limits for predicting the plasma level from the dose, in persons of various ages. The therapeutic range is shaded (Eadie, Lander, Hooper and Tyrer, 1976). This information may be used as a guide for determining potentially adequate phenobarbitone doses in persons of various ages.

doses required are respectively, 4·7, 3·1, 2·2 and 1·7 mg/kg. Such data indicate that a 70 kg young adult would require about 150 mg of the drug daily, whereas in the past the conventional phenobarbitone dose was 30 mg t.d.s. The above figures may be used as a basis for prescribing initial doses. If doses of this magnitude are used from the outset, an appreciable number of patients will be troubled by drowsiness and some will insist on ceasing treatment. If doses of about half this size are used at first, and increased after 1 to 2 weeks of therapy, steady-state conditions will be attained more slowly. However, tolerance to the sedative effects of the drug will have had time to develop and fewer patients will be troubled by drowsiness. More will finally be able to tolerate full dosage of the drug.

In adjusting phenobarbitone dosage it should be realized that the relation between plasma drug level and dose in the individual is curvilinear (Fig. 8.8). The second of two successive dose increments of equal size will produce a relatively greater increase in plasma phenobarbitone level than the first. The patient may easily become intoxicated as doses are increased. He may then refuse to continue therapy with the drug. Sufficient data are not yet available to permit firm guidance on how to manipulate phenobarbitone dosage to produce desired changes in plasma drug level in individual patients. It would seem a safe policy to suggest that doses should be changed by about half the amount one would have expected if one assumed plasma drug level was directly proportionate to dose in the individual. Subsequent steady-state plasma phenobarbitone measurement should indicate the need for any further dosage change.

It is important not to adjust phenobarbitone doses too frequently (probably not more often than once in 3 weeks) because it takes a comparatively long time to attain a steady-state plasma level after a dosage change. Unless the clinical response suggests otherwise, one's initial aim should be to prescribe a phenobarbitone dose regime which will provide steady-state plasma levels in the therapeutic range. Some patients can tolerate dosages being pushed well beyond this level so long as doses are increased at long enough intervals. Other patients seem mildly and chronically unwell with lower plasma phenobarbitone levels even though these are still within the therapeutic range for the population.

If desired, oral phenobarbitone loading doses may be used to obtain a more rapid effect. Probably double the daily maintenance dose could be given safely in the first 24 hours, but no plasma level data appear available to show how effective this is. It may produce unacceptable drowsiness in some subjects.

The therapeutic and toxic effects of penobarbitone do not appear to correlate as closely with phenobarbitone plasma levels as do phenytoin unwanted effects with plasma levels of that drug. Therefore there is perhaps a greater need to adjust phenobarbitone dosages in the light of the patient's clinical state than is the case with phenytoin. However plasma phenobarbitone concentration does provide a guide to the potential adequacy of therapy, and as to whether the patient is taking the drug.

At intervals during phenobarbitone therapy inquiry should be made of the patient and, if possible, of his relatives, as to whether there has been any personality change or deterioration in intellectual performance. These unwanted effects can develop insidiously, sometimes unnoticed by the patient, and may be troublesome enough to warrant replacement of the barbiturate anticonvulsant.

Methylphenobarbitone

It has been said that methylphenobarbitone doses need to be about twice phenobarbitone doses, on a weight basis, to produce comparable therapeutic effects in the same patient (Toman, 1970). The data of Figs. 8.3 and 8.11 suggest that the dosage ratio of the two drugs should be closer to $1 \cdot 6$ or $1 \cdot 7 : 1 \cdot 0$. Although methylphenobarbitone is an anticonvulsant in its own right its steady-state plasma levels usually are only $\frac{1}{7}$ to $\frac{1}{10}$ of the simultaneous plasma phenobarbitone levels. This does not necessarily mean that the brain levels of the two are in a similar ratio, since the higher apparent volume of distribution of methylphenobarbitone and its greater lipid solubility suggest that it may accumulate in certain tissues, including brain. However, some years' experience with methylphenobarbitone suggests that plasma phenobarbitone levels provide a sufficient guide to its therapeutic and unwanted effects. So far, measurement of simultaneous plasma methylphenobarbitone levels has not provided further assistance in interpreting the clinical situation. It should be pointed out that one enzyme immune-assay system for phenobarbitone measures methylphenobarbitone as phenobarbitone, as do gas chromatographic assays which involve the formation of methyl derivatives. Quantitatively, the error from this source is usually not great, since plasma methylphenobarbitone levels are often so much lower than simultaneous plasma phenobarbitone levels.

Methylphenobarbitone appears to exert most of its action by virtue of the phenobarbitone formed from it. Therefore the timing of drug doses, and the delay in achieving steady-state conditions when methylphenobarbitone is used, are approximately the same as when phenobarbitone is given. To achieve plasma phenobarbitone levels of 20 μg/ml, the average methylphenobarbitone dose required is just under 7 mg/kg/day for children and adolescents, 5·5 mg/kg/day for adults 15 to 40 years of age, and 3 mg/kg/day for older persons. As with phenobarbitone, it is preferable to use lower maintenance methylphenobarbitone doses initially to allow tolerance to develop and to reduce the unwanted sedative effects of the drug. Thus a 70 kg young adult might be given 60 mg of methylphenobarbitone twice daily at first, knowing he is likely to require a final dose of about 300–400 mg of the drug per day. If dose increments are made, plasma phenobarbitone levels should rise in direct proportion to methylphenobarbitone dose. This knowledge makes dose adjustment easier than when phenobarbitone itself is used.

Considerations for managing long term methylphenobarbitone therapy are similar to those which apply for continued phenobarbitone treatment.

Primidone

When used in long term therapy, primidone appears to have an anticonvulsant effect largely by virtue of the phenobarbitone formed from it. Clinical effects of primidone then seem to correlate adequately with plasma phenobarbitone levels. Phenobarbitone kinetics determine the time to achieve steady-state conditions when primidone is used. For most clinical purposes plasma phenobarbitone levels are a more useful adjunct to therapy than are plasma primidone levels. Virtually no work has been done on plasma phenylethylmalonamide levels in the steady-state, though this substance is probably an anticonvulsant.

The data of Fig. 8.19 suggest that for both children and adults a primidone dose of 10 mg/kg/day will yield a plasma phenobarbitone level of 20 μg/ml in the average patient. This primidone dose is virtually equivalent to the conventional 250 mg t.d.s. for a 70 kg adult. Thus one conventional primidone dosage unit, given three times a day, has a better chance of producing an adequate plasma phenobarbitone level than has one ordinary dosage unit of methylphenobarbitone (60 mg) given three times a day. This methylphenobarbitone dose will produce an average plasma phenobarbitone level of approximately 12 μg/ml in 70 kg adults. The typical 30 mg dosage unit of phenobarbitone itself, given three times a day, will produce an average plasma phenobarbitone level of approximately 11 μg/ml in a 70 kg adult. The reputation of primidone as a better anticonvulsant than phenobarbitone or methylphenobarbitone may be due largely to its more appropriately sized dosage unit, when the drugs are given in a traditional three times a day regime.

Many patients will not tolerate an initial primidone dose of 10 mg/kg/day.

Occasional patients may sleep for one or two days after their first 250 mg dose of primidone. Therefore it may be wise to begin primidone therapy with a single dose of 62·5 mg of the drug (a ¼ tablet). If severe drowsiness does not occur 125 mg b.d. might be given to an adult for a week, and then 250 mg b.d. till time for a steady-state to develop (3 weeks) has elapsed. The plasma phenobarbitone level could then be measured as a guide to any further dosage change. The relation of steady-state plasma phenobarbitone level to primidone dose increments in the individual is not known. Therefore primidone dose increments should be made cautiously and should not be made more often than at 3 weekly intervals to allow steady-state conditions for phenobarbitone to develop.

Primidone itself has a fairly short half-life and its steady-state plasma levels may show appreciable interdosage fluctuation depending on when the levels are measured in relation to the time of the last dose. This fluctuation decreases the usefulness of plasma primidone levels as a guide to therapy. From the viewpoint of the derived phenobarbitone it might seem that primidone would need to be given only once a day to keep plasma levels of the major anticonvulsant component within reasonable levels of fluctuation. However if this is done, there may be considerable variation in steady-state plasma primidone levels across the 24 hour dosage interval. There may be a problem with troublesome drowsiness at the time of the peak primidone level, unless the whole day's dose is taken at bedtime.

Long-term primidone therapy is conducted as is long-term phenobarbitone therapy, and plasma phenobarbitone level monitoring follows the guidelines indicated earlier.

If a barbiturate anticonvulsant, alone or in combination with other anticonvulsants, completely controls epilepsy without unduly severe side effects, the further management of the patient is as described for phenytoin in the same circumstances. Plasma drug concentrations and certain biochemical parameters (e.g. folate and calcium) should be monitored as suggested for phenytoin. However plasma drug levels should be measured 3 weeks after dosage changes, instead of after one week, to allow time for new steady-state conditions to apply for phenobarbitone.

Barbiturate anticonvulsants, like phenytoin, should be withdrawn slowly after a sufficient period of full control of the patient's epilepsy.

Carbamazepine

Carbamazepine induces its own elimination (Eichelbaum, Ekbom, Bertilsson, Ringberger and Rane, 1975). However the drug's half-life in the induced state is still about 15 to 20 hours. This suggests that twice daily carbamazepine administration should keep interdosage fluctuations in steady-state plasma drug level within acceptable limits. This is particularly so because the drug is slowly absorbed. Steady-state conditions should apply 4–5 days after dosage change. Perhaps there may be a longer delay (e.g. 10 days) when therapy is commenced, before increased elimination has had time to develop.

The data of Fig. 7.10 indicate that a wide range of drug doses will produce steady-state plasma carbamazepine levels in the provisional therapeutic range of 6–12 μg/ml in a majority of patients. The average dose required will be higher if the patient is taking phenytoin concurrently. For each 1 mg/kg/day of phenytoin taken, plasma carbamazepine will be lower by an average of 0·5 μg/ml. For adult patients who will be taking carbamazepine alone, an initial dose of 600 mg per day is likely to suffice. Half this dose might be used for the first week to allow the patient to develop tolerance to any drowsiness produced. Proportionately smaller doses may be used for children.

If patients are taking carbamazepine alone and it becomes necessary to increase the dose, steady-state plasma drug levels will probably be found to rise less than would be expected if plasma drug levels were directly proportional to dose in the individual (Fig. 7.15). However, if the patient is taking carbamazepine with phenytoin, carbamazepine dosage increase may produce a disporportionately great rise in plasma carbamazepine level, with risk of overdosage (Fig. 7.16). In order to control epilepsy it may be necessary to increase carbamazepine dosage to the patient's limit of tolerance of the drug. If plasma carbamazepine levels come to exceed 12 μg/ml one should suspect that the patient is unlikely to tolerate much more of the drug.

Clonazepam
At the present time clonazepam is unlikely to be used as sole therapy in the types of epilepsy here discussed unless the patient has experienced idiosyncratic reactions to phenytoin, carbamazepine, and to one of the barbiturate anticonvulsants, or else has refused to continue taking these drugs. Clonazepam use has been discussed earlier in relation to myoclonic epilepsy.

Anticonvulsant Combinations
If therapy with one of the major anticonvulsants discussed above fails to control epilepsy, and drug dosage has been taken to the patient's limit of tolerance, a second appropriate anticonvulsant from a different chemical family of drugs should be used. Dosage of the first drug is reduced to a level that leaves the patient free of unwanted effects. Generally it is not practicable to withdraw the first drug completely as soon as the second drug is begun. To do so may leave the patient unprotected against epilepsy while the optimal dosage of the second drug is being organised. If the patient's epilepsy comes under control, it is difficult to be sure that the first anticonvulsant is not having a useful effect. Therefore withdrawal of the first drug may still be to the patient's disadvantage, and most clinicians would therefore persist in using the combination.

When anticonvulsants are to be combined, dosage of the second drug should be adjusted as if it was the only drug used. Ordinary criteria for its therapeutic and toxic ranges of plasma levels seem to apply. However, when two drugs are given together to the one patient, pharmacokinetic interactions between the two are possible. Thus it is important to measure plasma levels of all the substances involved. Many of these interactions probably involve induction of the biotrans-formation of the first drug by increasing concentrations of the second drug. Such induction may not reach its maximum till a week or more after the second drug has achieved its steady-state conditions. By this time altered concentrations of the first drug may have occurred and may affect the pharmacokinetics of the second drug. Therefore, unless adverse effects occur earlier and necessitate a dosage change, it may be better to defer plasma level measurements till about 2 weeks after time for the expected appearance of the steady-state for the second drug. If doses of one drug are reduced it is possible that de-induction of the biotransformation of the other drug may occur. Little information is available regarding the time-course of this phenomenon. Again, it may be wise to defer measurement of plasma levels of the drugs involved for at least 2 weeks after the time of the expected steady state, calculated on the basis of the half-life of the more slowly eliminated drug. Should adverse effects occur in the interval, immediate plasma level measurement of the drugs involved would be desirable, as a guide to further dosage change.

The recorded interactions of the anticonvulsants have been set out in Section II of this book. They will not be considered in detail here. One may mainly indicate briefly that when phenytoin and phenobarbitone or methylphenobarbitone are combined there is likely to be little change in plasma levels of any of the substances concerned. If phenytoin is added to primidone therapy, plasma phenobarbitone levels may rise. If phenytoin is added to carbamazepine therapy, plasma carbamazepine levels are likely to fall significantly, necessitating revision of the the carbamazepine dose. Changes in plasma phenytoin levels are unpredictable when carbamazepine is added to phenytoin therapy. It may be unwise to assume that the above generalisations will apply to all individuals. It is always desirable to monitor plasma drug levels at appropriate times to help interpret the situation.

Valproate
At the present time the role of valproate as the sole anticonvulsant in patients is not established in the types of epilepsy here being considered (except perhaps for convulsive seizures of primary generalized epilepsy). Valproate would usually be given in conjunction with other anticonvulsants. Considerations as to valproate dosage are as dealt with earlier (page 298). When valproate is used it is important to monitor plasma levels of concurrently given anticonvulsants. These levels may show major changes (Chapter 12) making altered doses of the other anticonvulsants necessary.

Sulthiame
Sulthiame is often employed in combination with other anticonvulsants. The drug is commenced in a dose of 200 mg two or three times a day (with correspondingly lower doses, determined on a body weight basis, in children). Dosage adjustments are made on clinical grounds at weekly or fortnightly intervals thereafter. The common sulthiame side effects of hyperventilation and paraesthesiae sometimes necessitate a dosage reduction, and then a gradual subsequent dose increase. It should be remembered that sulthiame therapy may cause plasma phenytoin levels to rise. This may necessitate a revision in phenytoin dosages if that drug is taken with sulthiame.

If combinations of two anticonvulsants fail to control a patient's epilepsy a third, and even a fourth, appropriate anticonvulsant may have to be added. Considerations as to the further management are as when two drugs are combined.

EPILEPSY RESISTANT TO ALL DRUG TREATMENT

Anticonvulsant combinations given in doses that produce no side effects may fail to control epilepsy. It may then be necessary to increase the dose of one or more drugs to see if better control of the epilepsy can be obtained, even though some unwanted effects of treatment occur. This is an unsatisfactory situation, but it may be the best that can be offered some patients at the present time. These patients may have to accept life-long therapy, with the presence of some unwanted drug effects, yet only partial control of their epilepsy. However, they may still hope that some new, more effective drug, will be developed.

PROBLEMS OF COMPLIANCE

One of the great difficulties in long term anticonvulsant therapy is ensuring continued compliance with prescribed drug dosage. Several authors have commented on the extent of patient non-compliance with anticonvulsant regimes (Gibberd, Dunne, Handley and Hazelman, 1970; Lund, 1973; Wolf, Carr, Hanson, Dale, Davis, Goldenberg, Lulejian, Sharpe, Trietman and Weinstein, 1973; Wilson and Wilkinson, 1974; Eisler and Mattson, 1975; Dreissen and Höppner, 1977). All too often anticonvulsant dosages are found which completely control a patient's seizures. After some months or years attacks may recur and immediate measurement of plasma anticonvulsant levels show that these have fallen significantly. This suggests failure of compliance, whether or not the patient will admit this.

The ability to measure plasma anticonvulsant concentrations, and the realization that for most anticonvulsants the correct total dose need be taken only once or twice daily without the need for critical timing of doses, have helped considerably in reducing non-deliberate failures of compliance. The organization of a satisfactory dosage routine such as that described on page 306, which permits simple daily checking that each day's doses have been taken, further encourages compliance. However none of these measures is effective when the patient deliberately elects not to take his prescribed dosages. The only answer to this latter situation is education of the patient.

With increased availability of facilities for measuring plasma anticonvulsant concentrations, and the advent of new and better anticonvulsants, failure of compliance is becoming a major problem in contemporary anticonvulsant therapy. It is realistic to suggest that, whenever a patient's plasma anticonvulsant levels deviate too widely from what one has come to expect as the norm for his circumstances (i.e. age, body weight, dose, etc.), one should first suspect failure of compliance rather than some idiosyncracy of drug disposition (distribution and/or elimination).

SOME PARTICULAR THERAPEUTIC PROBLEMS

STATUS EPILEPTICUS

Status epilepticus consists of continuous epileptic seizures, or repeated generalized seizures which recur without intervening conscious periods.

CONVULSIVE STATUS
The immediate management of convulsive status epilepticus involves

1. protecting the patient from injury,
2. maintaining the airway and vital functions,
3. rapidly controlling the seizures with anticonvulsant drugs, and
4. trying to determine and treat the cause of the condition (e.g. omission of anticonvulsants, presence of a tumour or encephalitis).

Diazepam

Intravenous diazepam has been considered the treatment of choice for all varieties of status epilepticus (Gastaut, Naquet, Poire and Tassinari, 1965; Parsonage and Norris, 1967; Bell, 1969; Livingstone, 1972). This may at first seem surprising when oral diazepam is not a particularly effective anticonvulsant unless given in doses which produce drowsiness. However in dealing with status epilepticus one is prepared to make the patient quite drowsy for a time, in order to control the seizures. Such drowsiness could not be accepted in long term maintenance therapy. Diazepam is usually given intravenously in a dose of 1 mg per minute (in adults, and correspondingly less on a body weight basis in children). It is advisable to pause and assess the effect after the first 10 mg of diazepam in adults and after each subsequent 5 mg till the status epilepticus ceases or until respiratory or cardiovascular depression begins. It should be remembered that diazepam may potentiate the effects of other anticonvulsants given previously (Bell, 1969; Lalji, Hosking and Sutherland, 1967).

Clonazepam

Gastaut, Catier, Dravet and Roger (1970) found intravenous clonazepam to be even more effective than diazepam. The initial dose of clonazepam in adults is 1 mg, with additional 0·5 or 1 mg doses every 1–2 minutes till fitting ceases or respiratory or cardiovascular depression appears.

Amylobarbitone

If intravenous benzodiazepines fail, or are unavailable, intravenous sodium amylobarbitone may be used. The drug is given in a dose of 50 mg/minute in adults. Usually less than 500 mg is required. Amylobarbitone has the disadvantage that the solution (being unstable) must be made up just before use. There is a risk of producing respiratory depression if too much drug is given.

Phenytoin

Intravenous phenytoin does not have the disadvantage of depressing respiration unless given in great excess. However it can be inconvenient to use. A stable solution of phenytoin for parenteral use is available. It is often desirable to inject this solution into the tubing of an intravenous saline or glucose drip to dilute the drug and its solvent before they reach the circulation. However, if injected into a drip bottle the drug may precipitate out and not reach the patient. The average adult not already taking phenytoin is likely to require about 1000 mg of the drug to achieve a plasma phenytoin concentration in the therapeutic range (Wallis, Kutt and McDowell, 1968). Unless this amount of drug is given gradually over many minutes to several hours (which of course delays control of the status epilepticus) the amount of solvent that has to be injected with the phenytoin may cause cardiovascular collapse.

Chlormethiazole
Chlormethiazole (0·8 per cent solution in a 500 ml container) is given as a slow intravenous drip at a rate sufficient to stop the epilepsy without depressing vital functions. This can be an efficient method of controlling status epilepticus, but seizures may recur soon after the infusion is stopped.

Anaesthesia
Should the above measures fail, it may be necessary to anaesthetize the patient with intravenous thiopentone sodium. The patient should be maintained in this state until trial withdrawal of the anaesthetic shows that the seizures have ceased (Brown and Horton, 1967). Rarely in prolonged status epilepticus it may also be desirable to suppress the muscle jerking by curarisation, while employing artificial respiration (James and Whitty, 1961).

The intramuscular use of anticonvulsants (e.g. phenytoin, phenobarbitone or diazepam) appears a very uncertain way of treating status epilepticus. The drugs are often unpredictably and inefficiently absorbed. If a sufficient amount of these anticonvulsants is given by intramuscular injection to control status epilepticus fairly rapidly, so much may have been given that its subsequent absorption may leave the patient substantially overdosed for hours or days.

In the past, intramuscular injections of paraldehyde were used with some success in treating status epilepticus. This substance apparently absorbed rapidly enough to have a useful effect on epilepsy. However paraldehyde may produce local tissue damage at the injection site. Sharpless (1970) stated that the intravenous administration of paraldehyde is extremely hazardous.

The rectal administration of modern anticonvulsants has been relatively little explored, though Lennox-Buchthal (1973) suggested that rectal diazepam could absorb rapidly enough to be useful in treating epilepsy. Rectal administration of diazepam may be worth a trial in status epilepticus if intravenous administration is impracticable.

MINOR EPILEPTIC STATUS
In less severe forms of status epilepticus (e.g. serial unilateral motor seizures without respiratory impairment, *petit mal* absence status or myoclonic seizure status) therapy need not be so vigorous. However intravenous anticonvulsants are often required. Intravenous diazepam is likely to control *petit mal* absence status (Gastaut, Naquet, Poire and Tassinari, 1965). It should be noted that Tassinari, Dravet and Roger (1972) found that, in five children in a confused state associated with frequent slow spike and wave EEG discharges, intravenous diazepam or nitrazepam therapy precipitated tonic status epilepticus. All these patients previously had received benzodiazepine injections without adverse effect. Intravenous clonazepam has also been reported to have similar effects on occasions. If the patient can swallow, absence status could be possibly treated with large oral

ethosuximide doses, in view of the nature of the epilepsy and the rapid onset of action of this drug after oral administration (Wechselberg and Hubell, 1967).

Subsequent maintenance

Once status epilepticus has been controlled it is necessary to institute maintenance anticonvulsant therapy. One might, for example, continue to give diazepam or clonazepam by intravenous drip for one or two hours while preparing for maintenance therapy (e.g. with phenytoin or phenobarbitone). One may calculate the expected daily maintenance dose of either drug that should be given each 12 hours, give this by intravenous injection until the subject can swallow, and then commence oral dosage. Where possible, plasma anticonvulsant level monitoring should be used to guide the dosage adjustments. As experience with oral clonazepam grows it may prove to be the drug of choice in managing status epilepticus in previously untreated patients. Therapy could then continue long term with the same drug that was used initially. However patients who present in status epilepticus are often already taking several anticonvulsants. If these drugs appear appropriate for the patient's type of epilepsy the initial aim of maintenance therapy should be to achieve plasma levels of these drugs in their therapeutic ranges. If their plasma levels are already in their therapeutic ranges an additional appropriate anticonvulsant should be added.

'BENIGN' FEBRILE CONVULSIONS OF INFANCY

Such convulsions appear to be a form of generalized epilepsy, often based on an hereditary predisposition. They comprise bilateral tonic-clonic seizures which occur in infants as a complication of sudden fever. The infection causing this fever does not directly involve the nervous system. Febrile convulsions merit separate discussion because of their good prognosis and because there is argument over whether or not they need treatment.

The view is often expressed that 'benign' febrile convulsions of infancy do not need anticonvulsant treatment because the risk of subsequent non-febrile epilepsy is low (2·9 per cent, according to Livingstone, 1972). Further, no anticonvulsant treatment is reputed to be effective in preventing fevrile consulsions. If these assertions are examined more closely, it appears that Livingstone's (1972) figure was derived from 256 infants, each followed for at least 15 years from the time of the first febrile seizure. However these 256 in turn were part of a larger group of 622 children followed from the time of their first febrile seizure. This total group of 622 children was delineated only after children with known or probably intracranial lesions were excluded. The 256 infants with a very favourable prognosis all had initial brief generalized seizures only. None had clinical or laboratory evidence of neurological or acute general illness which might have affected the brain. All had an onset of the seizures within 24 hours of the onset of fever and all had a normal EEG one week after the seizures. Fifty-eight per cent of this group had a family history of febrile seizures. The above are more rigid criteria than those which clinicians often apply when diagnosing benign febrile convulsions. The other 366 of Livingstone's 622 children with febrile convulsions had prolonged or focal seizures. Of the children with prolonged seizures 97 per cent subsequently developed non-febrile epilepsy. This means that for the whole group of 622 children, 58·2 per cent subsequently developed epilepsy unrelated to fever. Other workers have not found so high an incidence of subsequent non-febrile epilepsy in children with febrile convulsions. Thus Wallace (1975) found a 17 per cent risk in such children over an 8 to 10 year follow-up period. Any individual child with brief febrile generalized seizures and all the other criteria of the good prognosis group may have a prolonged convulsion with a subsequent fever. If this happens the child's risk of later epilepsy is increased 3 or 4 times (Lennox-Buchthal, 1973). Nelson and Ellenberg's (1976) data suggest that the risk might be even higher in this circumstance. Ounsted, Lindsay and Norman (1966) emphasized that any individual child with previous 'benign' febrile seizures ran the hazard of later having a prolonged febrile convulsion. This might lead to hypoxic temporal lobe damage and subsequent non-febrile temporal lobe epilepsy. Ounsted (1967) found evidence that such events accounted for the aetiology of one-third of a series of 100 cases of temporal lobe epilepsy. This is an additional reason for attempting to prevent febrile convulsions. The need to prevent febrile seizures appears to be finding increasing acceptance (Wilson, 1972; Vaudour, Richardet, Ostre, Repesse, Bauvais, Costil, Debard and Brissaud, 1975).

Oral anticonvulsants are sometimes prescribed only at the onset of a fever in children who have previously had febrile convulsions (Ounsted, 1967). This is unlikely to be useful unless adequate loading doses are used, and this is almost never done. Even if a loading dose is given it is unlikely that an adequate plasma and tissue level of drug can be obtained before the febrile seizure occurs (unless so large a loading dose is given that overdosage effects appear later). Failure of anticonvulsants given only at the onset of fever is no evidence that they lack the potential for protecting against febrile convulsions. However it has been stated that continuous anticonvulsant therapy also fails to protect against febrile convulsions (Millichap, 1968). Melchior, Buchthal and Lennox-Buchthal (1971) showed that phenytoin, even when given in dosages sufficient to produce plasma phenytoin levels in the therapeutic range, did not prevent febrile convulsions of infancy. Phenobarbitone given in doses producing plasma levels over 15 μg/ml, however, did protect against febrile seizures (Faero, Kastrup, Lykkegaard Neilsen, Melchior and Thorn, 1972). Thorn (1975), Wallace (1975), Wolf (1977) and Wolf, Carr and Davis (1977) provided further evidence that phenobarbitone, given in a sufficient dose, had a prophylactic effect against febrile convulsions. Heckmatt, Houston, Clow, Stephenson, Dodd, Lealman and Logan (1976) could not confirm the occurrence of statistically-significant protection from the use of phenobarbitone in these circustances. Nonetheless their data suggested that the drug might have some prophylactic effect.

There seems to be a case for instigating continuous phenobarbitone therapy (or therapy with methylphenobarbitone or primidone) in doses which maintain plasma phenobarbitone levels above 15 μg/ml in all children who have even a single brief febrile convulsion. This therapy should continue until they are 3 or 4 years of age, even if no further epileptic manifestation occurs. If another anticonvulsant is shown to be effective, it may be preferable to phenobarbitone, which causes irritability and behaviour problems in many children (Livingstone, 1972). Cavazzuti (1975) has claimed that valproate is effective in preventing febrile convulsions.

It would largely avoid the undesirable sedative effects of phenobarbitone. However, while any suspicion exists that the use of valproate may possibly lead to testicular damage, one can hardly justify prescribing this drug in large numbers of children with benign febrile convulsions.

NEONATAL CONVULSIONS

In the neonatal period up to 1·4 per cent of infants suffer from tonic or clonic convulsions. These carry a grave prognosis. Death, or significant neurological or intellectual handicap in the survivors, occurs in 48–70 per cent (Brown, Cockburn and Forfar, 1972). Convulsions occurring in the first three days of life, or after the eighth day, are usually due to structural brain disease. Those occurring between the fifth and eighth days are likely to be due to metabolic disturbance. The exact nature of the metabolic disturbance in the individual cannot always be precisely defined. Some of the metabolic factors involved include hypocalcaemia, hypomagnesaemia, hypoglycaemia, hypo- or hypernatraemia and pyridoxine deficiency (Brown, Cockburn and Forfar, 1972). These factors may also contribute to the epileptic process in children with convulsions apparently due to organic brain disorder. The presence of such biochemical factors should be sought and treated in all instances of neonatal convulsions. Otherwise, apart from the treatment of underlying primary conditions (e.g. meningitis, hyperbilirubinaemia) the management of neonatal convulsions comprises the use of anticonvulsants. Studies of the pharmacokinetics of anticonvulsants in the human neonate are now beginning to appear but no completely adequate basis is yet available for rationalising therapy. Parenteral anticonvulsant therapy may be necessary at first. Anticonvulsants from the hydantoin, barbiturate or benzodiazepine groups may be used. Initial dosages are determined on a body-weight basis, where better data are not available to guide dosage selection. Thus Ouvrier and Goldsmith (1977) have shown that if neonates are given intramuscular phenobarbitone 10 mg/kg/day for 3 days, and then 6 mg/kg/day, the mean plasma phenobarbitone level after the first 24 hours is 7·5 μg/ml. After 3 days, mean plasma phenobarbitone levels become steady at 21 μg/ml. If the drug is given intravenously in the same dosages, reasonably similar plasma phenobarbitone levels occur, with a reasonably similar time course. Oral loading doses of anticonvulsants may be used if the drugs have not already been administered intravenously to control recurrent seizures, and if the neonate can swallow and is not vomiting. Obviously the ability to monitor drug comcentrations in body fluids may expedite the attaining of adequate tissue concentrations of anticonvulsant drugs in neonates. Changing drug elimination capacity in the first few days of life may necessitate dose adjustments during the first week or two of therapy. The further application of modern techniques of clinical pharmacology may greatly improve the management of neonates with convulsions.

EPILEPSY IN PREGNANCY

Pregnancy has been said to have unpredictable effects on epilepsy in the individual patient (Dimsdale, 1959). Knight and Rhind (1975) found that seizure frequency did not alter during pregnancy in 50 per cent of patients with the idiopathic disorder; seizures increased in frequency in 45·2 per cent and lessened in 4·8 per cent. However Loiseau, Legroux and Henry (1974) found that epilepsy did not increase during pregnancy. Monitoring plasma anticonvulsant levels during pregnancy (Mygind, Dam and Christiansen, 1975; Lander, Edwards, Eadie and Tyrer, 1977) has shown that anticonvulsant dosage requirements increase during pregnancy and fall again in the puerperium. Failure to recognize this phenomenon in the past may have been the explanation of the reports that epilepsy sometimes worsened during pregnancy.

A number of factors may contribute toward the increased anticonvulsant requirement during pregnancy (Eadie, Lander and Tyrer, 1977). These factors include an increased volume of maternal and fetal body in which the drug distributes, increased drug biotransformation due to possible induction of maternal liver enzymes by high levels of female sex hormones, possible drug metabolism in the placenta and fetal liver, and an effect of folic acid (which is often prescribed in pregnancy) in accelerating the elimination of phenobarbitone and phenytoin.

Recognition of the altered anticonvulsant dosage requirements as pregnancy advances makes monitoring of plasma anticonvulsant levels desirable at monthly intervals throughout pregnancy. Anticonvulsant doses should be adjusted when necessary to try to maintain plasma anticonvulsant levels at pre-pregnancy values throughout the whole course of pregnancy. After childbirth, plasma levels should be monitored weekly for the first month, and then every 2 or 3 weeks till rising plasma drug levels make resumption of the pre-pregnancy drug dosage advisable.

The question of anticonvulsant-associated dysmorphogenesis remains unsettled. Whether the association is causal, or coincidental, is not certain. If anticonvulsants are dysmorphogenic it is undesirable to have to increase their dosage during the period of fetal organ differentiation. However if drug doses are not increased there is a greater chance of the mother convulsing, and this could lead to hypoxic damage to the fetus. The wisest policy appears to be that the maternal epilepsy should be treated as effectively as possible. Certainly most authorities agree that anticonvulsants should not be withdrawn during pregnancy.

If the mother is correctly dosed with anticonvulsant drugs at term the neonate is not likely to experience any depression of consciousness from the drugs. Anticonvulsant levels in milk are not higher than anticonvulsant levels in maternal plasma, and are often a good deal lower. The breast fed child is unlikely to achieve plasma anticonvulsant levels as high as those to which it was exposed *in utero*. Unless the mother becomes badly overdosed, the child who has been exposed to anticonvulsants *in utero* should therefore not be adversely affected by the amounts of anticonvulsants provided by maternal milk. In fact breast feeding could be regarded as a convenient way of very gradually withdrawing anticonvulsants from the infant since, as the infant ages, maternal milk will comprise a decreasing component of the total dietary intake.

Because anticonvulsant intake in pregnancy may lead to coagulation factor deficiency and bleeding in the newborn, it is a sensible precaution to inject vitamin K into the mother early in labour.

REFERENCES

Bell, D. S. (1969) Dangers of treatment of status epilepticus with diazepam. *Brit. Med. J.*, i, 159–161.

Bower, B. D. & Jeavons, P. M. (1959) Infantile spasms and hypsarrhythmia. *Lancet*, i, 605–609.

Brown, A. S. & Horton, J. M. (1967) Status epilepticus treated by intravenous infusions of thiopentone sodium. *Brit. Med. J.*, i, 27–28.

Brown, J. K., Cockburn, F. & Forfar, J. O. (1972) Clinical and chemical correlates in convulsions of the neonate. *Lancet*, i, 135–139.

Buchanan, R. A., Fernandez, L. & Kinkel, A. W. (1969) Absorption and elimination of ethosuximide in children. *J. Clin. Pharmacol.*, 9, 393–398.

Buchanan, R. A., Kinkel, A. W., Goulet, J. R. & Smith, T. C. (1972) The metabolism of diphenylhydantoin (Dilantin) following once-daily administration. *Neurology* (Minneap.), 22, 126–130.

Buchanan, R. A. & Smith, T. C. (1971), cited by Chang, T., Dill, W. A. & Glazko, A. J. (1972) Ethosuximide. Absorption, distribution and excretion, in *Antiepileptic Drugs*, ed. Woodbury, D. M., Penry, J. K. & Schmidt, R. P. New York: Raven Press, 417–423.

Buchthal, F. & Lennox-Buchthal, M. A. (1972) Phenobarbital. Relation of serum concentration to control of seizures, in *Antiepileptic drugs*, ed. Woodbury, D. M., Penry, J. K. & Schmidt, R. P. New York. Raven Press, 335–343.

Butler, T. C., Makaffee, C. & Waddell, W. J. (1954) Phenobarbital: Studies of elimination, accumulation, tolerance and dosage schedules. *J. Pharmacol. exp. Therap.*, 111, 425–435.

Cavazzuti, G. B. (1975) Prevention of febrile convulsions with diprophylacetate (Depakine). *Epilepsia* (Amst.), 16, 647–648.

Coatsworth, J. J. (1971) Studies on the clinical efficacy of marketed antiepileptic drugs. *NINDS Monograph No. 12. Public Health Service, National Institute of Health*. Bethesda, Maryland.

De Negri, M., Lamedica, G. M. & Ravera, G. (1973) ACTH therapy in infantile epilepsy: its relationships with plasma cortisol levels. *Gaslini*, 5, 178–180.

Dimsdale, H. (1959) The epileptic in relation to pregnancy. *Brit. Med. J.*, xi, 1147–1150.

Driessen, O. & Höppner, R. (1977) Plasma levels of phenobarbital and phenytoin in epileptic outpatients. *Europ. Neruol.*, 15, 135–142.

Eadie, M. J., Lander, C. M. & Tyrer, J. H. (1977) Plasma drug level monitoring in pregnancy. *Clinical Pharmacokinetics*, 2, 427–436.

Eichelbaum, M., Ekbom, K., Bertilsson, L., Ringberger, V. A. & Rane, A. (1975) Plasma kinetics of carbamazepine and its epoxide metabolite in man after single and multiple doses. *Europ. J. Clin. Pharmacol.*, 8, 337–341.

Eisler, J. & Mattson, R. H. (1975) Compliance in anticonvulsant drug therapy. *Epilepsia* (Amst.), 16, 203.

Faero, O., Kastrup, K. W., Lykkegaard Neilsen, E., Melchior, J. C. & Thorn, I. (1972) Successful prophylaxis of febrile convulsions with phenobarbital. *Epilepsia* (Amst.), 13, 279–285.

Finne, P. H. (1963), *Nord. Med.*, 69, 197, cited by Jeavons & Bower (1964) *loc. cit.*

French, J. H., Grueter, B. B., Druckman, R. & O'Brien, D. (1965) Pyridoxine and infantile myoclonic seizures. *Neurology* (Minneap.), 15, 101–113.

Gastaut, H., Catier, J., Dravet, C. & Roger, J. (1970) Exception anticonvulsive properties of a new benzodiazepine. *Epilepsy Mod. Probl. Pharmacopsychiat.*, 4, 261–269.

Gastaut, H., Naquet, R., Poiré, R. & Tassinari, C. A. (1965) Treatment of status epilepticus with diazepam (Valium). *Epilepsia* (Amst.), 167–182.

Geller, M. D. & Christoff, N. (1971) Diazepam in the treatment of childhood epilepsy. *J. Amer. Med. Ass.*, 215, 2087–2090.

Gibberd, F. B., Dunne, J. F., Handley, A. J. & Hazleman, B. L. (1970) Supervision of epileptic patients taking phenytoin. *Brit. Med. J.*, i, 147–149.

Heathfield, K. W. G. & Jewesbury, E. C. O. (1964) Treatment of petit mal with ethosuximide: follow-up report. *Brit. Med. J.*, ii, 616.

Heckmatt, J. Z., Houston, A. B., Clow, D. J., Stephenson, J. B. P., Dodd, K. L., Lealman, G. T. & Logan, R. W. (1976) Failure of phenobarbitone to prevent febrile convulsions. *Brit. Med. J.*, i, 559–561.

Huttenlocher, P. R., Wilbourn, A. J. & Signore, J. M. (1971) Medium-chain triglycerides as a therapy for intractable childhood epilepsy. *Neurology* (Minneap.), 21, 1097–1103.

James, J. L. & Whitty, C. W. M. (1961) The electroencephalogram as a monitor of status epilepticus suppressed peripherally by curarisation. *Lancet*, ii, 230–241.

Jeavons, P. M. & Bower, B. D. (1964) Infantile spasms. *Clinics in Developmental Medicine No. 15*. London. William Heinemann Medical Books Ltd.

Kinkel, A. (1971), cite by Glazko, A. J. & Dill, W. A. (1972) in Woodbury, D. M., Penry, J. K. & Schmidt, R. P. *Antiepileptic drugs*. New York: Raven Press., 455–464.

Knight, A. H. & Rhind, E. G. (1975) Epilepsy and pregnancy: a study of 153 pregnancies in 59 patients. *Epilepsia* (Amst.), **16**, 99–110.

Kutt, H. & McDowell, F. (1968) Management of epilepsy with diphenylhydantoin sodium. *J. Amer. Med. Ass.*, **203**, 969–972.

Lalji, D., Hosking, C. S. & Sutherland, J. M. (1967) Diazepam (Valium) in the control of status epilepticus. *M. J. Australia*, **1**, 542–545.

Lance, J. W. (1968) Myoclonic jerks and falls: aetiology, classification and treatment. *M. J. Australia*, **1**, 113–120.

Lander, C. M., Edwards, V. E., Eadie, M. J. & Tyrer, J. H. (1977) Plasma anticonvulsant concentrations during pregnancy. *Neurology* (Minneap.), **27**, 128–131.

Lennox-Buchthal, M. A. (1973) Febrile convulsions. A reappraisal. *Electroenceph. Clin. Neurophysiol.* Suppl., **32**, 1–138.

Livingstone, S. (1972) *Comprehensive Management of Epilepsy in Infancy, Childhood and Adolescence*. Springfield. Charles C. Thomas.

Loeser, E. W. (1961) Studies on the metabolism of diphenylhydantoin (Dilantin). *Neurology* (Minneap.), **11**, 424–429.

Loiseau, P., Legroux, M. & Henry, P. (1974) Epilepsies et grossesses. *Bordeaux Med.*, **7**, 1157–1164.

Lorentz De Haas, A. M. & Kuilman, M. (1964) Ethosuximide (X-ethyl-X-methylsuccinimide) and grand mal. *Epilepsia* (Amst.), **5**, 90–96.

Ludden, T. M., Hawkins, D. W., Atlen, J. P. & Hoffman, S. F. (1976) Optimum phenytoin dosage regimens. *Lancet*, i, 307–308.

Lund, L. & Alvan, G. (1975) Phenytoin dosage nomogram. *Lancet*, ii, 1305.

Lund, M. (1973) Failure to observe dosage instruction in patients with epilepsy. The short term effect of a daily dispenser. *Acta Neurol. Scandinav.*, **49**, 295–306.

Lund, M., Jorgensen, R. S. & Kühl, V. (1964) Serum diphenylhydantoin (phenytoin) in ambulant patients with epilepsy. *Epilepsia* (Amst.), **5**, 51–58.

Melchior, J. C., Buchthal, F. & Lennox-Buchthal, M. A. (1971) The ineffectiveness of diphenylhydantoin in preventing febrile convulsions in the age of greatest risk, under three years. *Epilepsia* (Amst.), **12**, 55–62.

Millichap, J. G. (1968) *Febrile Convulsions*. New York: Macmillan Co.

Mullen, P. W. (1978) Optimal phenytoin therapy: A new technique for individualizing dosage. *Clin. Pharmacol. Therap.*, **23**, 228–232.

Mygind, K. I., Dam, M. & Christiansen J. (1976) Phenytoin and phenobarbitone plasma clearance during pregnancy. *Acta Neurol. Scandinav.*, **54**, 160–166.

Nelson, K. B. & Ellenberg, J. H. (1976) Predictors of epilepsy in children who have experienced febrile seizures. *New Engl. J. Med.*, **295**, 1029–1033.

Olesen, O. V. & Dam, M. (1967) The metabolic conversion of primidone (Mysoline) to phenobarbitone in patients under long-term treatment. *Acta neurol. Scandinav.*, **43**, 348–356.

Ounsted, C. (1967) Temporal lobe epilepsy: the problem of aetiology and prophylaxis. *J. roy. Coll. Phycns.*, **1**, 273–284.

Ounsted, C., Lindsay, J. & Norman, R. (1966) *Biological Factors in Temporal Lobe Epilepsy*. London: W. Heinemann Medical Books.

Ouvrier, R. A. & Goldsmith, R. (1977) Phenobarbitone dosage in the neonate. *Clin. Exptl. Neurol.*, **14**, 194–202.

Parsonage, M. J. & Norris, J. W. (1967) Use of diazepam in treatment of severe convulsive status epilepticus. *Brit. Med. J.*, iii, 85–88.

Penry, J. K., Porter, R. J. & Dreifuss, F. E. (1972) Ethosuximide. Relation of plasma levels to clinical control, in *Antiepileptic drugs*, ed. Woodbury, D. M., Penry, J. K. & Schmidt, R. P. New York: Raven Press. 431–441.

Porter, R. K., Penry, J. K. & Lacy, J. R. (1977) Diagnostic and therapeutic reevaluation of patients with intractable epilepsy. *Neurology* (Minneap.), **27**, 1006–1011.

Richens, A. (1975) A study of the pharmacokinetics of phenytoin (diphenylhydantoin) in epileptic patients, and the development of a nomogram for making dose increments. *Epilepsia* (Amst.), **16**, 627–646.

Richens, A. & Dunlop, A. (1975) Serum-phenytoin levels in management of epilepsy. *Lancet*, ii, 247–248, and *Lancet*, ii, 1305–1306.

Rieder, J. (1973) Plasma levels and derived pharmacokinetic parameters of unchanged nitrazepam in man. *Arzneim.-Forsch.*, **23**, 212–218.

Rodin, E. A. (1968) *The Prognosis of Patients with Epilepsy*. Springfield: Charles C. Thomas.

Schmidt, R. P. & Wilder, B. J. (1968) *Epilepsy*. Philadelphia. F. A. Davis Co.

Scott, D. F. & Swash, M. (1972) Febrile convulsions in early childhood. *Brit. Med. J.*, iii, 415–416.

Seitelberger, F. (1968) Myoclonus body disease, in *Pathology of the nervous system*, ed. Minckler, J. Vol. 1. New York: McGraw-Hill Book Co. 1121–1134.

Sharpless, S. K. (1970) Hypnotics and Sedatives, in *The pharmacological basis of therapeutics*, ed. Goodman, L. S. & Gilman, A. 4th edition. London: Macmillan., 121–134.

Sherwin, A. L. & Robb, J. P. (1972) Ethosuximide: Relation of plasma level to clinical control in *Antiepileptic drugs*, ed. Woodbury, D. M., Penry, J. K. & Schmidt, R. P. New York: Raven Press. 443–448.

Sherwin, A. L. & Robb, J. P. (1972) Ethosuximide: Relation of plasma level to clinical control, in ethosuximide. *Arch. Neurol.* (Chic.), 28, 178–181.

Sugita, E. T. & Neibergall, P. J. (1973) Prednisone, in *The Biovailability of drug products*. Washington. American Pharmaceutical Association., 36–38.

Sutherland, J. M. & Bowman, D. A. (1963) Sulthiame (Ospolot) in the treatment of temporal lobe epilepsy. *Med. J. Aust.*, 2, 532–533.

Tassinari, C. A., Dravet, C. & Roger, J. (1972) Tonic status epilepticus precipitated by intravenous benzodiazepine in five patients with Lennox Gastaut syndrome. *Epilepsia* (Amst.), 13, 421–435.

Terrence, C. & Alberts, M. (1978) Phenytoin dosage in ambulant epileptic patients. *J. Neurol. Neurosurg. Psychiat.*, 41, 463–465.

Thorn, I. (1975) A controlled study of prophylactic long-term treatment of febrile convulsions with phenobarbital. *Acta Neurol. Scandinav.* Suppl., 60, 67–73.

Toman, J. E. P. (1970) Drugs effective in convulsive disorders, in *The pharmacological basis of therapeutics*, ed. Goodman, L. S. & Gilman, A. 4th edition. London and Toronto: MacMillan Co., 204–225.

Tudor, I., Milea, S. & Stoica, I. (1974) ACTH therapy in some non-hypsarrhythmic forms of epilepsy. *Rev. Roum. Neurol. Psychiat.*, 11, 147–156.

Vajda, F. J. E., Merory, J. & Bladin. P. F. (1975) Fluctuation of plasma phenytoin levels on single dose and twice daily dosage regimes. *Proc. Aust. Assoc. Neurol.*, 12, 61–64.

Vadour, G., Richardet, J.–M., Ostre, C., Repesse, G., Beauvais, P., Costil, J., Debard, A. & Brissaud, H.-E. (1975) Traitement préventif des récidives des convulsions fébriles du nourrisson et de l'enfant par le phénobarbital. *Ann. Pédiat.*, 22, 915–923.

Wallace, S. J. (1975) Continuous prophylactic anticonvulsants in selected children with febrile convulsions. *Acta Neurol. Scandinav.*, 52, Suppl., 60, 62–66.

Wallis, W., Kutt, H. & McDowell, F. (1968) Intravenous diphenylhydantoin in treatment of acute repetitive seizures. *Neurology* (Minneap.), 18, 513–525.

Wechselberg, K. & Hübel, G. (1967) Zur Resorption und Verteilung von Methyl-Älthyl-Succinimid (MAS) im Serum und Liquor bei Kindern. *Z. Kinderheilkd.*, 100, 10–19.

Wilson, J. (1969) Drug treatment of epilepsy in childhood. *Brit. Med. J.*, iv, 475–477.

Wilson, J. T. & Wilkinson, G. R. (1974) Delivery of anticonvulsant drug therapy in epileptic patients assessed by plasma level analyses. *Neurology* (Minneap.), 24, 614–623.

Wolf, S. M. (1977) Effectiveness of daily phenobarbital in the prevention of febrile seizure recurrences in simple febrile convulsions and epilepsy triggered by fever, *Epilepsia* (Amst.), 18, 95–99.

Wolf, S. M., Carr, A. & Davis, D. C. (1977) The value of phenobarbital in the child who has had a single seizure: a controlled prospective study. *Pediatrics*, 59, 378–385.

Wolf, S. M., Carr, A. C., Hanson, R. A., Dale, E. P., Davis, D. C., Goldenberg, E. D., Lulejain, G. A., Sharpe, K. S., Trietman, P. & Weinstein, A. W. (1973) Parental compliance in the continuous administration of phenobarbital for the prevention of febrile seizures. *J. Pediat.*, 83, 1085–1086.

Wulff, K., Flachs, H., Würtz-Jorgensen, A. & Gram, L. (1977) Clinical pharmacological aspects of valproate sodium. *Epilepsia* (Amst.), 18, 149–157.

17

Conclusions

Until recently clinicians were accustomed to treat epilepsy on purely clinical grounds, adjusting anticonvulsant dosages on the basis of frequency and severity of seizures and on the presence of unwanted effects of therapy. Often such a therapeutic practice was reasonably adequate, particularly when the epileptic seizures were minor and occurred frequently enough to permit ready clinical assessment of the effectiveness or otherwise of seizure control. At times hesitancy in deviating from standard pharmacopoeal dosages made the policy less adequate.

In the past few years the monitoring of plasma anticonvulsant levels has become widely used in many Western countries. The measurement of plasma anticonvulsant levels has led to significant changes in the practice of anticonvulsant therapy, particularly in relation to types of epilepsy in which seizures may recur at long intervals. The range of inter-individual variation in plasma drug levels produced by standard doses of anticonvulsants has now been recognized. More appropriate anticonvulsant doses can be prescribed for individual patients and the potential adequacy of doses can be determined more rapidly. Atypical adverse effects due to drug overdosage can be detected, even though the drug dose may not be excessive in terms of pharmacopoeal recommendations. Failures of patients to comply with prescribed doses may be easily detected. Pharmacokinetic interactions involving anticonvulsants need no longer perplex the clinician diagnostically. Monitoring of plasma anticonvulsant levels should make the treatment of epilepsy safer and more effective. Studies such as that of Lund (1974) show that skilled manipulation of anticonvulsant doses, guided by plasma anticonvulsant levels, can substantially improve control of epilepsy in a series of patients. At least in newly diagnosed adults with epilepsy, the need for polypharmacy may be reduced (Shorvon, Chadwick, Galbraith and Reynolds, 1978).

Unfortunately, the benefits that could accrue from measuring plasma anticonvulsant levels have not always been realized. There has sometimes been a tendency to regard the achieving of particular plasma anticonvulsant levels as the chief aim of therapy. Thus one has seen doses of an anticonvulsant reduced when a patient's epilepsy finally was fully controlled and he was experiencing no adverse effects whatsoever, simply because the plasma drug level exceeded what was regarded as the therapeutic range for that drug. Lack of pharmacokinetic knowledge has led to a rather substantial occurrence of drug overdosage when doses have been altered without realizing that the relation between plasma level and drug dose in the individual may not be linear, or when doses were altered on the basis of plasma drug levels which were measured before a steady state obtained.

Thus the availability of facilities for monitoring plasma anticonvulsant levels has not always yielded the dividends of which it is capable. More information about the pharmacokinetics of some of the anticonvulsants is still required, and more rigorous statistical definition of their therapeutic ranges. Those who treat epilepsy need an increased appreciation of pharmacokinetic principles and increased skill in applying these principles in clinical situations. The attempt at a scientific approach to anticonvulsant therapy should remain subordinate to clinical common sense. Plasma anticonvulsant levels are a most helpful guide to therapy, but they are not the final criterion of the success of therapy.

As anticonvulsant therapy, guided by plasma drug level measurements, becomes more efficient, a new problem is assuming increasing importance in the control of epilepsy. This is failure of compliance. No matter how adequately anticonvulsant dosage can be prescribed, failure to take the prescribed dosage will almost inevitably deny the patient the optimal available benefits. The time has come when an attempt to improve patient compliance with prescribed anticonvulsant dosage may yield very useful dividends.

The optimal treatment of epilepsy is still being evolved. As knowledge and experience accumulate and are analysed, therapeutic practice changes. A book such as the present one can only collate and try to interpret the data available at the time of its writing. It may thus serve a purpose, and may also indicate gaps in knowledge and deficiencies in practice which should be remedied in the future. One therefore hopes that the book may provide a point of departure on the road towards the total control and cure of epilepsy.

REFERENCES

Lund, L. (1974) Anticonvulsant effect of diphenylhydantoin relative to plasma levels. A prospective three-year study in ambulant patients with generalized epileptic seizures. *Arch. Neurol.* (Chic.), **31**, 289–294.

Shorvon, S. D., Chadwick, D., Galbraith, A. W. & Reynolds, E. H. (1978) One drug for epilepsy. *Brit. Med. J.*, **i**, 474–476.

Index

Pharmacokinetic parameters of the more commonly used anticonvulsants
The figures shown are approximate, and are based on best available values for adults

Drug (and metabolites)	Nature		Absorption		T_{max} (hours)	V_d (L.kg^{-1})	% protein bound	$T\frac{1}{2}$ (hours)	Clearance (L.kg^{-1}hr^{-1})	% excreted unchanged
	Acid/base	pk$_a$	$T\frac{1}{2}$ (hours)	Bioavailability (%)						
Carbamazepine	Neutral	—	2–7	60–85	6–30	0·8	72–76	25–50	0·010–0·022	2
Clonazepam	Base	1·5;10·5	-	100	1–2	~2·0	47;80	24–36	0·09	1
Ethosuximide	Acid	9·3	—	—	1–3	0·7	0	30–70	0·010–0·015	17–38
Methylphenobarbitone	Acid	7·6	—	See Phenobarbitone	<8	~2·0	—	30–60	0·025	2
phenobarbitone				See Phenobarbitone						
Phenobarbitone	Acid	7·2	1·4	—	6–12	0·5–1·0	60	70–100	0·006	25
Phenytoin	Acid	8·3 or 8·6	1·6	95	4–12	0·5–0·7	90–93	15–20*	0·02	5
Primidone	Neutral	—		92		0·6	0	6–12		15–66
phenobarbitone				See Phenobarbitone						
phenylethylmalonamide	—									
Sulthiame	Acid	—	—	>90	—	—	—	20–30	—	—
Troxidone	Neutral	—	—	—	—	—	—	—	—	60–70
dimethadione	Acid	6·13	—	—	0·5	—	—	16	—	—
Valproate	Acid	4·95	0·4	68–100	1–4	0·15	85–95	8–10	0·010–0·015	3–7

*follows Michaelis-Menten Kinetics